Therapeutic Exercise for Parkinson's Disease and Related Disorders

César Alonso Aguilar Mejía

Therapeutic Exercise for Parkinson's Disease and Related Disorders

A Comprehensive Clinical Strategy for Preventing and Reversing Neurodegeneration

Springer

César Alonso Aguilar Mejía
Bogotá, Colombia

ISBN 978-3-031-62118-5 ISBN 978-3-031-62119-2 (eBook)
https://doi.org/10.1007/978-3-031-62119-2

This Springer imprint is published by the registered company Springer Nature Switzerland AG
The registered company address is: Gewerbestrasse 11, 6330 Cham, Switzerland

Comprehensive health manifests itself through physical, mental, social, and SPIRITUAL well-being, while limited and selfish health is mediocre and partial.

César Alonso

Preface

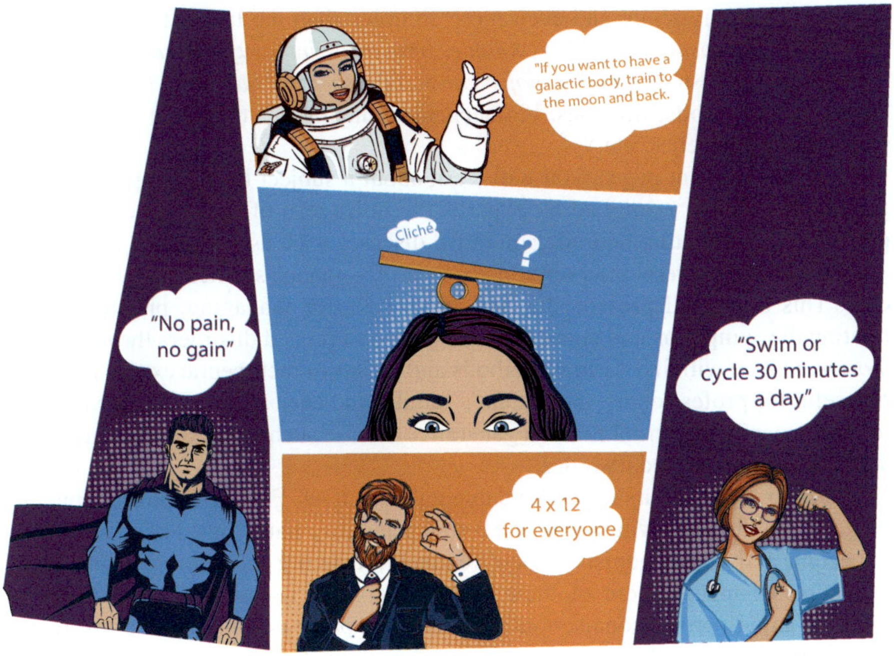
"If you want to have a galactic body, train to the moon and back.
Cliché
?
"No pain, no gain"
"Swim or cycle 30 minutes a day"
4 x 12 for everyone

Do exercise! The cliché phrase on everyone's voice.

Do exercise! is a cliché phrase recommended by doctors, physical therapists, trainers, physical educators, influencers, actors, accountants, shoemakers, butchers, parents, children, grandparents, neighbors, friends, and even the milkman. Such a phrase has become a meaningless assertion, as we all aim to be experts in prescribing exercise, without asking ourselves:

- Is exercise focused on health the same as exercise for aesthetic or performance purposes?

- What is the minimum or maximum dosage of exercise required for it to fulfill its objective?
- Should your training be continuous and mild or intermittent and intense?
- What is the individual capacity to perform certain exercises?
- Which loading dynamics are most recommended?
- Is a medical endorsement sufficient to determine if we are fit for a particular type of training?
- Do you perform or prescribe exercises correctly based on the pathology?
- Can any type of exercise be practiced by patients with neurodegenerative pathologies?

The dosing of physical exercise and/or training is based on observation, evidence, and reasoning within an inexact science, given that its particularity is essential for its success. Therapeutic exercise doesn't have fixed parameters, but it is true that its precise and quantifiable aspect is as effective as the pharmacological dosage provided by a physician, and even more complex than the latter. This complexity arises from its *dosing variables (volume, frequency, intensity, and density)*, which are continually tested in every *biopsychosocial aspect of human beings* (age, culture, customs, habits, illnesses, biomechanics, mental health, social environment, surroundings, genetics, etc.).

In the subsequent pages, you will learn about a subject that is frequently disregarded and seldom examined by experts: the utilization of therapeutic exercise in preventing and treating neurodegenerative diseases such as Parkinson, a condition that necessitates several interventions from professionals, sciences, treatments, and care. This book will provide the building blocks for managing, preventing, and treating the symptoms and signs of the disease and related disorders through *dosed movement*. You will find various methods and means of therapeutic exercise that can be useful for professionals, the patient's family, and even more so if you've started to notice manifestations of neurodegenerative disease such as Parkinson's or already suffering from a related disorder.

Together, we will pursue two fundamental objectives. Firstly, to motivate patients diagnosed with or showing signs of neurodegenerative pathologies like Parkinson's to become active protagonists in their treatment, fostering autonomy, independence, and personal management of their health. Secondly, to sow the seed of critical thinking among professionals, non-professionals, patients, and within myself, aiming to unveil thoroughly the significance and impact of the most recommended phrase to "do exercise" in approaching and treating the disease.

Bogotá, Colombia César Alonso Aguilar Mejía

Ethics Approval and Rights

Thank you for reading this book and purchasing the original. This book is the result of the hard work of professionals, professors, and researchers. Copying this book is disregarding and violating intellectual property rights.

The editors have made every effort to locate the owners of the copyrighted source material used. If they have inadvertently omitted any, the editors will make the necessary arrangements at the earliest opportunity.

The concepts, guidance, proposals, methods, and therapies presented in this book are not intended to substitute or replace a consultation, recommendation, or medical care from a qualified professional. Anything related to your health necessitates medical supervision. The author and publisher are not liable for any loss, damage, adverse reaction, injury, syndrome, symptom, sign, or medical condition arising from the information or recommendations presented in this book. The information contained in this book is solely for informational purposes with the objective of improving physical and mental health. Any recommendation or suggestion regarding exercise or any other treatment should be followed only after consulting a physician to ensure that the treatment is appropriate. This book and its contents do not assure specific outcomes in the health of patients.

The content referenced in this book does not represent an endorsement, assumption, or support for the seriousness and suitability of third-party sources, treatments, entities, studies, research, guides, or other sources used for creating this book, by the author or the editor. The author have verified the reliability of the sources of information used in this work. However, due to the constant changes and advances in the field of health, and the possibility of human error, neither the author nor the editors certify the accuracy and completeness of the information provided. Furthermore, they are not responsible for any errors or omissions, or for any results achieved using this information. To ensure accuracy, it is recommended that readers verify the information presented in this book by consulting other sources.

This book refers to various studies conducted by different authors. It is asserted that all studies mentioned in this book were conducted in accordance with the ethical guidelines of the Declaration of Helsinki or other comparable ethical standards. The integrity and ethics of research are fundamental aspects in the collection and presentation of information in this work, and emphasis is placed on the importance of respecting ethical principles at all stages of research involving human participants.

It is the reader's responsibility to check the original sources for detailed information on the ethical approval of each study mentioned. It is strongly recommended that readers directly consult the reports and original documents of the studies to gain a full understanding of the ethical considerations involved in each of the studies cited.

Acknowledgments

It is necessary to acknowledge our God in an essential and fundamental manner for the glory and grace shown in the writing of this work. Without His support, our scientific knowledge would be lacking.

We also address ourselves to all the readers, who are already part of this work. Their reading and application are essential so that these words will not be ephemeral and will come to life.

We express our gratitude to the researchers referenced in this book, whose dedication and efforts have yielded results.

Additionally, special thanks are due to:

- Cristian Yáñez, for consistently developing an interest in research.
- Catalina Gutiérrez, for providing valuable insights into an extract of the book.
- Elkin Londoño, for shedding light on the actualities of sports in Colombia.
- Cesar Lovera, for cultivating enthusiasm and professionalism in us throughout the process.
- Carlos Cruz, for enabling us to understand the significance of teaching.
- Rozo Omayra, for instilling a passion for movement as a therapeutic pillar.
- Camilo Morales, for sharing his academic and moral values with us.
- Cesar Villa, for placing a small step on my path to professionalism.
- The editors of Springer Nature, especially Érica de Cássia Ferraz. Their collaboration and support were essential to the quality of this book.
- Sahara Ocampo, for always being willing to listen and for her decisive suggestions in the writing of the book.
- Eliana Mejía, for her contribution to developing the tool that made this work possible.

I appreciate your interest and commitment. Thank you very much.

About This Book

This work presents a comprehensive training program and clinical strategy aimed at helping readers understand how therapeutic exercise can effectively reverse and mitigate both motor and non-motor symptoms of neurodegenerative diseases such as Parkinson's. The work is organized into eight logically structured chapters that facilitate the acquisition of specialized knowledge on the subject.

The first chapter provides an overview of the pathophysiological mechanisms of Parkinson's disease. The aim is to familiarize the reader with the biopsychosocial aspects and characteristics, including biological, psychological, and social factors, which should be considered before planning and administering therapeutic exercise.

Chapter 2 presents tools and protocols for diagnosing, monitoring, and controlling the symptoms and signs of the disease, which helps determine the patient's stage and select an effective method of therapeutic physical training.

Chapter 3 discusses the physiological benefits obtained through controlled and appropriately dosed therapeutic exercises. This section examines how practicing these exercises can have a positive impact on the body, addressing both motor and non-motor symptoms associated with neurodegenerative diseases such as Parkinson's. It is closely linked to the second chapter, as detailed diagnosis, monitoring, and control are not only tools to understand the progression and origin of the disease but also serve as crucial indicators of improvement. These indicators effectively evaluate whether therapeutic exercise benefits meet specific needs identified during the evaluation and control phase.

Chapters 4 and 5 focus on planning physical training safely, effectively, and efficiently to prevent risks and accidents during the execution of the therapeutic exercise plan.

Chapters 6 and 7 provide evidence-based therapeutic exercises to reduce, prevent, and reverse motor and non-motor symptoms of neurodegenerative diseases, such as Parkinson's. The proposed methods are structured to include an explanation of the method, examples, effects, and dosing, making practical implementation easier. Chapter 7 concludes with a summary table of all proposed therapeutic exercise methods to aid in creating a therapeutic training plan model, which is further explained in Chap. 8.

Chapter 8 represents the ultimate goal of the training acquired in the previous chapters. It explains the science behind creating a training plan under the proposed model. The objective is to plan a therapeutic training that is evidence-based and applicable, translating theory into practice. This chapter includes an Excel format that facilitates planning a 3-month training under the ATR (Accumulation, Transformation, and Realization) model. It guides the construction of therapeutic proposals and/or treatments through exercise in a step-by-step manner.

Contents

About the Author

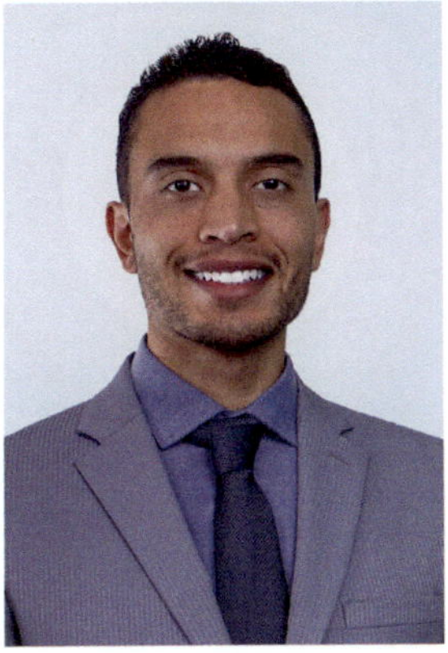

César Alonso Aguilar Mejía César Alonso is a distinguished professional in the fields of physiotherapy, therapeutic exercise, and clinical as well as sports training. He is recognized as an expert in preventing and treating patients with neurodegenerative and neurodevelopmental pathologies. His extensive training in primary care physiotherapy as a Master, a specialist in nutrition, pain management, geriatric physiotherapy, and a professional in movement and exercise sciences has enabled him to make valuable contributions in this field. As an author of innovative scientific research, he has left a significant mark with his study titled *Plyometric and Proprioception Training in Cognitive Disabilities, Down Syndrome and Autism*, which has been widely recognized in the scientific community. His dedication and excellence are also reflected in his role as a therapist and functional evaluator in different foundations, where he has excelled in prescribing exercises, correcting postures, and improving the quality of life for people with cognitive disabilities, Parkinson's disease, Down syndrome, and autism.

Aside from his exceptional professional accomplishments, César Alonso is an enthusiastic practitioner of Jiu-Jitsu, a discipline of combat sport. His fervor for the sport motivated him to initiate research and make contributions to the field of high-performance sports. One of his remarkable studies, *Determination of the physical profile in elite athletes for the detection and selection of talents in Jiu-Jitsu* has been fundamental in promoting the professionalism of the *Colombian* sports.

Abbreviations

%AT	Percentage of anaerobic threshold
%HRR	Percentage of heart rate reserve
%MAV	Percentage of maximum aerobic velocity
%MHR	Percentage of maximum heart rate
$\%VO_2^{max}$	Percentage of maximum oxygen consumption
[Lact-] $mmol{\cdot}L^{-1}$	Lactate concentration in millimoles per liter
µs	Microsecond
AR	Augmented reality
ATP	Adenosine triphosphate
ATR	Accumulation, transformation, and realization
BDNF	Brain-derived neurotrophic factor
bpm	Beats per minute
CAREN	Computer-assisted rehabilitation environment
cm	Centimeters
CNS	Central nervous system
COMT inhibitors	Catechol-O-methyltransferase inhibitors
COPD	Chronic obstructive pulmonary disease
EMST	Expiratory muscle strength training
FDA	Food and Drug Administration
FOG	Freezing of gait
GABA	Gamma-aminobutyric acid
HIIT	High-intensity interval training
HR	Heart rate
Hz	Hertz
LED	Light-emitting diode
LSVT	Lee Silverman voice treatment
m	Meters
mA	Milliamperes
MAOIs	Monoamine oxidase inhibitors
MHR	Maximum heart rate
ME	Muscle electrostimulation

MIBG	Metaiodobenzylguanidine
min.	Minutes
MOCA	Montreal cognitive assessment
MPTP	1-Methyl-4-phenyl-1,2,3,6-tetrahydropyridine
MSA	Multiple system atrophies
mTOR	Mammalian target of rapamycin
N/A	Not applicable
N°	Number
NGF	Nerve growth factor
NICE	National Institute for Health and Care Excellence
NSAIDs	Non-Steroidal Anti-Inflammatory Drugs
PA	Physical activity
Perflex	Perceived effort of flexibility
PKG	Personal KinetiGraph
PNF	Proprioceptive neuromuscular facilitation
PNS	Peripheral nervous system
PSP	Progressive supranuclear palsy
REHACOP	Rehabilitation cognitive program for psychosis
REM	Rapid eye movement
Reps.	Repetitions
RM	Repetition maximum
ROM	Range of motion
ROT	Reality orientation therapy
SSRIs	Selective serotonin reuptake inhibitors
SUA	Serum uric acid
T′	Time
tDCS	Transcranial direct current stimulation
TMS	Transcranial magnetic stimulation
UPDRS	Unified Parkinson's disease rating scale
VAST	Video-assisted swallowing therapy
VR	Virtual reality
WHO	World Health Organization

List of Figures

List of Tables

Chapter 1
Exploring and Diving Deeper into Parkinson's Disease Mechanisms

Initial Questions

- How does Parkinson's disease affect the body and what are the most common signs?
- What factors influence predisposition to and protection against neurodegenerative diseases, particularly Parkinson's disease?
- How can a deep understanding of the pathological mechanisms of Parkinson's disease improve the diagnosis, monitoring, control, and treatment of its effects on patients?

Neurodegenerative Diseases

Neurodegenerative diseases are characterized by progressively affecting the physiological deterioration of the central and peripheral nervous system [1, 2]. As an analogy, the neurological decline caused by neurodegenerative pathologies is compared to the programmed obsolescence of a cell phone, where fortunately human lives do not end after 2 years of use but are in continuous morphological and physiological wear and tear.

Continuing with the similarities, the central nervous system is like a computer's motherboard (which processes information and regulates memory), and the peripheral nervous system bears resemblance to video, sound, and network cards. When a virus or malicious program enters a computer, the device's functionality becomes slower, data processing becomes erroneous, and applications fail to start properly. The same process occurs when the central and peripheral nervous systems are infected with a virus, gradually leading the patient to manifest signs and symptoms of a neurodegenerative pathology, progressively impairing cognitive executive functions (such as problem-solving, the ability to structure, create, plan, and evaluate information), the quality of neuronal synapses, basic motor skills, physical

C. A. A. Mejía, *Therapeutic Exercise for Parkinson's Disease and Related Disorders*, https://doi.org/10.1007/978-3-031-62119-2_1

conditioning, and coordination capabilities. These aspects determine the useful range of joint movement, static and dynamic balance, strength, power, speed, proprioception, phonation and praxis, respiratory capacity, cardiovascular functionality, and metabolic dysfunction, in short, the quality of life [3, 4].

Personal electronic devices (cell phones, computers, tablets, or televisions) become useless due to two underlying factors. The first factor is planned obsolescence, which is analogous to the hereditary and genetic etiology of a neurodegenerative disease. Genes contain information that predisposes and contributes to the development of a neurodegenerative disease, leading to the emergence of comorbidities and mortality. In contrast, personal electronic devices have a replaceable nature, whereas our neurons and circuits are currently irreplaceable.

Fortunately, or unfortunately, there exists a second etiological factor of a neurodegenerative pathology that is under the control of the device owner and determined by good usage and care habits (such as cleaning the cache, history, temporary files, malware, device cleaning, avoiding impact, and proper care of charging connectors). This factor is comparable to the preventive measures and causative factors of a neurodegenerative disease, such as dietary habits, physical activity, smoking, alcohol consumption, prevention or early detection of malignant tumors, environmental factors like continuous exposure to pesticides, insecticides, heavy metals, industrial chemicals (polychlorinated biphenyls), air pollution, and associated comorbidities or etiological factors of a stroke [1, 2].

Several neurodegenerative diseases share similar molecular, pathophysiological, and clinical characteristics, which increase the level of morbidity, mortality, and physical disability. The treatment of these diseases is not singular or isolated since the causal factors involved in their etiology are multifactorial and include genetic, environmental, social, and psychological factors.

Although there is no scientifically validated cure for these pathologies, there are numerous treatments and preventive methods available. Among these methods, properly prescribed therapeutic physical exercise is included [5]. In the following pages, the prescription of exercise for Parkinson's disease (PD) as a neurodegenerative pathology will be illustrated. It is essential to note that the prescription of therapeutic physical exercise for Parkinson's disease aims to alleviate, reduce, and treat symptoms and associated comorbidities while preventing neurological decline.

Parkinson's Disease

Parkinson's disease in everyday life is like a poorly maintained bicycle. Over time, the bike shows signs of wear on its components, and its operation becomes less efficient. The brakes may become stiff and unresponsive, making control and stability difficult when stopping. Pedals may stick or move slowly, affecting the ability to accelerate smoothly. Similarly, the patient with Parkinson's disease or "paralysis agitans" (PA), named after the key symptoms of the pathology, is affected by this neurodegenerative disease that alters the central nervous system, causing muscle rigidity, postural instability, bradykinesia (slowness of movement due to altered muscle tone, usually leading to "paralysis"), and sporadic and irregular tremors ("agitation"). The name Parkinson's disease is commonly attributed to the physician James Parkinson, who studied the disease for many years and described it in 1817 [6].

Parkinson's disease (PD) is a chronic, progressive disease that typically affects patients over the age of 40, with a higher prevalence in people over the age of 60. Approximately 2–3% of the world's population over the age of 60 has PD. It is also important to note that Parkinson's disease is the second most common neurodegenerative disease worldwide, with Alzheimer's disease being the first. The prevalence of Parkinson's disease is expected to increase in the coming decades as the population ages. As life expectancy increases, so does the number of people over the age of 60, which may lead to an increase in the incidence and burden of the disease in the future. The prevalence of this pathology was 1.5 cases per 1000 inhabitants in 2021, and it is estimated that it will affect 12 million people worldwide by 2040 [1, 2, 6–8].

On the other hand, Parkinson's disease has a significant socioeconomic impact due to the medical costs associated with the treatment and management of the disease, the loss of work productivity of patients, the financial and emotional burden on informal caregivers, the social and emotional costs associated with the quality of life of patients and their families, and the additional burden on health-care systems due to the increasing prevalence in an aging population. It is essential to address these challenges through a comprehensive approach that includes access to appropriate medical care, support for caregivers and patients, public awareness, and continued investment in research [1].

Physiopathology

Parkinson's disease is like a complex medical puzzle with several pieces that are not yet fully understood. This multifactorial disease (the origin of which is unknown in 90% of patients) has two key pieces: a loss of dopaminergic neuronal activity (dopamine is a neurotransmitter responsible for controlling various cognitive and sensorimotor functions) and an increase in cholinergic activity (choline is a precursor of acetylcholine, a neurotransmitter responsible for cognitive functions such as memory and muscle control). Typically, Parkinson's patients have reduced levels of dopamine, ranging from 70% to 80% lower than healthy individuals [6, 9].

Another piece of the puzzle is the formation of Lewy bodies, which are abnormal aggregations and deposits of alpha-synuclein proteins within nerve cells.

Parkinson's disease develops in stages, with symptoms ranging from mild to severe. Mild stages typically develop within about 5 years of the onset of the disease, while more advanced stages with characteristic symptoms may appear after the first 5 years. According to Hammer and McPhee [7], the most severe symptoms may manifest from 5 years or more after the onset of the disease. On the other hand,

Galimberti and Scarpini [1] report that the average age of Parkinson's disease onset is between 60 and 65 years, and the more chronic or severe effects of the disease usually appear between the ages of 70 and 79.

In addition to the stages of the disease and the age of onset, it is important to note that the progression of Parkinson's disease can vary greatly from patient to patient. Some people may experience a slower progression of symptoms, while others may experience more rapid progression.

The severity of symptoms can also vary widely, meaning that some patients may experience a greater impact on their quality of life and daily functioning than others. This is partly due to the heterogeneity of the disease and how it affects different systems of the body, including both motor and non-motor systems.

Protective and Risk Factors

According to Galimberti and Scarpini [1], there are several *risk factors* that increase the predisposition to Parkinson's disease. Some of these factors include:

Exposure to Toxins Such as Carbon Disulfide, Carbon Monoxide, and 1-Methyl-4-Phenyl-1,2,3- and 6-Tetrahydropyridine

- Carbon disulfide: An industrial chemical used as a solvent and raw material in the manufacture of chemicals and fibers. It can be found in industrial environments.
- Carbon monoxide: An odorless, colorless gas produced by the incomplete combustion of fossil fuels. It is dangerous in confined or poorly ventilated environments, such as homes with faulty appliances or garages with running vehicles.
- 1-methyl-4-phenyl-1,2,3,6-tetrahydropyridine (MPTP): A neurotoxin that affects dopamine-producing nerve cells. It is used in research to model Parkinson's disease in animals but is not safe for human use. It is a synthetic neurotoxin that does not occur naturally in the environment or in common foods.
- 6-tetrahydropyridine: A toxic by-product of MPTP, also a neurotoxin that damages dopamine-producing nerve cells.

The Long-Term Use of Drugs Like Reserpine, Phenothiazines, Tetrabenazine, Butyrophenones, and Metoclopramide

The long-term use of those drugs may aggravate or cause symptoms of Parkinson's disease by interfering with the dopaminergic neurotransmission system in the brain. Dopamine is a crucial neurotransmitter responsible for controlling movement and various cognitive functions.

- Reserpine: It blocks the storage of dopamine in nerve cells, reducing its release in synapses and leading to symptoms similar to Parkinson's disease, such as slow movements and muscular rigidity.
- Phenothiazines: These are antipsychotic medications that block dopamine receptors in the brain, leading to extrapyramidal symptoms resembling those of Parkinson's disease.
- Tetrabenazine is a medication used to treat Huntington's chorea. It works by reducing dopamine levels in the brain, which can result in symptoms similar to Parkinson's disease. Tetrabenazine, which is used to treat Huntington's chorea, reduces dopamine levels in the brain.
- Butyrophenones are another class of antipsychotic drugs that block dopamine receptors. This interference with dopaminergic function can lead to symptoms similar to Parkinson's disease.
- Metoclopramide is a medication used to treat nausea and gastrointestinal issues. Metoclopramide can affect dopamine receptors in the brain, causing extrapyramidal symptoms such as involuntary movements and muscular rigidity.

Traumatic Brain Injuries

Head injuries that involve the brain, like concussions or severe blows to the head, can damage nerve cells and circuits in the brain. Some severe brain traumas, especially repetitive ones that can occur in high-impact sports or dangerous work activities, have been observed to increase the risk of developing Parkinson's disease years after the event. However, the exact relationship remains not fully understood.

Cerebrovascular Accidents

Blood flow interruptions to the brain can impact areas related to motor function and dopamine production, potentially leading to Parkinson's symptoms. However, the relationship between cerebrovascular accidents and Parkinson's is complex and multifactorial.

Wilson's Disease

Wilson's disease is a genetic disorder responsible for disruptions in copper metabolism resulting in toxic metal concentration in different organs. Symptoms of this disease can affect the nervous, hepatic, or ocular systems, leading to Parkinson's-like symptoms, such as muscle stiffness and slow movements, due to the involvement of dopaminergic pathways.

Huntington's Disease

Huntington's disease is a genetic disorder that causes neurodegeneration and impairs certain brain areas controlling movement, resulting in symptoms similar to Parkinson's. Despite the different mechanisms underlying Huntington's disease and Parkinson's, both disorders affect some shared brain areas, resulting in similar motor symptoms. Some common symptoms of both diseases are involuntary movements, muscle rigidity, and difficulties in coordination and balance.

Multiple System Atrophies (MSA)

MSA are a group of rare neurodegenerative disorders that progressively degenerate multiple brain and nervous systems. In some cases, MSA subtypes may exhibit motor symptoms that resemble those seen in Parkinson's disease. This can cause confusion or misdiagnosis.

Suffering from Progressive Supranuclear Palsy (PSP)

PSP is a neurological disorder that damages neurons, leading to the loss of motor skills, balance, and cognitive executive functions. The degeneration mainly affects the brain region known as the subthalamic nucleus as well as other areas that are involved in controlling movement. This impairment in the subthalamic nucleus may result in issues in coordinating eye movements, which can cause characteristic ocular symptoms of PSP, such as a fixed gaze or difficulty in moving the eyes vertically.

Alterations in Certain Genes

Alterations in certain genes such as PARK2, PARK6, PARK7, PARK19, PARK4, PARK8, PARK17, PARK18, PINK1, LRRK2, PARK-CHCHD2, PARK-RAB39B, and SNCA have been linked to the hereditary forms of Parkinson's disease and play a crucial role in regulating various cellular functions. These genes can impair the normal functioning of nerve cells, especially those that produce dopamine in the brain, leading to worsening of symptoms of Parkinson's disease over time. Although the hereditary forms of Parkinson's disease are rare compared to sporadic cases. The study of these genes has improved our understanding of the disease and holds significant implications for future treatment options.

Having an Infection Caused by the Hepatitis C Virus

There is evidence-based among researchers that hepatitis C virus can damage nerve cells in the brain. The virus is also capable of triggering an inflammatory reaction in the brain, which is thought to contribute to the development of Parkinson's disease.

Studies have found that individuals with hepatitis C are at a higher risk of developing Parkinson's disease compared to those without the infection. The risk is higher in individuals who have been infected with hepatitis C for an extended period.

Intestinal Microbiota Dysbiosis

Intestinal microbiota dysbiosis refers to an imbalance in the composition and function of bacteria within the gut. This imbalance might have a connection with the pathogenesis of Parkinson's disease. Factors that increase the risk of intestinal dysbiosis include a poor diet, for example, low intake of soluble and insoluble fiber and high consumption of simple sugars and saturated fats, which are typical characteristics of a Western American diet. Alterations in the gut microbiota can be detected many years prior to the onset of Parkinson's disease, presenting with symptoms such as constipation. The chronic inflammation associated with intestinal constipation can cause damage to the intestinal mucosa as well as the brain's immune system. This, in turn, can lead to death or loss of dopaminergic neurons responsible for regulating movement [10].

Age

Age is one of the most significant risk factors for Parkinson's disease. The risk of developing this neurodegenerative disease increases as a person ages. Although Parkinson's disease can affect people of all ages, the incidence of its occurrence notably increases in individuals over 60 years old. The gradual deterioration of nerve cells in the brain over time is believed to contribute to the development of Parkinson's disease.

Gender

Gender is another risk factor to consider; studies have shown that men have a higher risk of developing Parkinson's disease than women. Nevertheless, the cause of this gender difference is still not fully comprehended. According to some researchers, sex hormones and other biological differences may contribute to this inequality.

Exposure to Pesticides

Exposure to pesticides, in particular for farmers, has been linked to an increased risk of developing Parkinson's disease due to chronic and frequent exposure to certain chemicals used in agriculture. Individuals working in the agricultural industry, especially farmers, face a greater risk due to prolonged exposure to these toxic substances. It is believed that pesticides could damage nerve cells and contribute to the development of the disease.

Residing in Rural Areas

Residing in rural areas is usually linked to air and water pollution, as well as lifestyle and dietary factors.

Daily Consumption of Dairy Products

Daily consumption of dairy products may increase the risk of Parkinson's, based on several research studies. Nevertheless, the evidence to establish a definitive relationship between the two is still inconclusive and further studies are necessary to understand it more fully.

Individuals with a Family or Personal History of Melanoma

Individuals with a family or personal history of melanoma, a type of skin cancer, may have an increased risk of developing Parkinson's disease. Despite not fully understanding the reason behind this association, there could be genetic or environmental factors shared that contribute to this relationship.

On the other hand, Galimberti and Scarpini [1], Ko [11], and Zhou et al. [12] present certain *protective factors* against Parkinson's disease, such as:

The Effects of Coffee Consumption

Caffeine has been researched for its ability to delay the onset of Parkinson's disease by possessing neuroprotective properties. This is attributed to its ability to inhibit adenosine receptors, reducing inflammation and cellular damage in the brain. Although some positive effects of caffeine have been observed in patients with pre-existing Parkinson's disease, its benefit is not as significant compared to the effects if it had been consumed prior to the onset of the disease. Different mechanisms of caffeine could explain this, where it acts as an anti-inflammatory agent to protect dopaminergic neurons, which are typically severely affected at the onset of the disease, and also inhibits GABA signaling.

A study conducted on patients with advanced Parkinson's disease using the A2aR antagonist Istradefylline showed a reduction in "off" time dyskinesia. However, it did not significantly affect the severity of symptoms when they were present. As caffeine primarily acts through the same mechanism, it may have comparable effects on the progression of the disease. Another study found no significant changes in the score of Unified Parkinson's Disease Rating Scale (UPDRS) with caffeine consumption, although a nearly significant improvement was observed in activities of daily living associated with the disease score.

However, it is important to exercise caution while consuming high doses of caffeine because it may lead to an increased risk of developing cardiovascular diseases. Although caffeine may have beneficial effects on patients with preexisting Parkinson's disease, it has limited ability to halt the progression of the disease. The association between caffeine and Parkinson's disease is still under active investigation, and more research is required to fully comprehend its effects.

Blood Urea Level

A meta-analysis by Zhou et al. [12] examined the association between serum uric acid (SUA) levels and the risk of dementia and its different forms. Twenty-three studies with a total of 5575 participants were reviewed. The results showed that people with dementia had lower levels of SUA than people without dementia. In addition, a significant association was found between low SUA levels (<292 μmol/L or 4.91 mg/dL) and Alzheimer's disease and Parkinson's disease with dementia, but not vascular dementia. Lower SUA levels were negatively associated with the presence of dementia and its neurodegenerative subtypes, whereas higher SUA levels were positively associated with dementia. These findings suggest that SUA levels may play an important role in the risk of developing certain types of dementia. However, more research is needed to confirm these findings and to better understand the mechanisms involved.

Daily Exercise

Daily exercise prevents and protects against Parkinson's disease through several physiological mechanisms that are activated during regular physical activity:

- *Brain stimulation*:
  Regular physical activity leads to brain activation that promotes the release of important neurotransmitters such as dopamine, serotonin, and endorphins. These neurotransmitters play a critical role in mood regulation, cognitive function, and motor control. In Parkinson's disease, which is characterized by the loss of dopaminergic neurons in the substantia nigra, exercise may partially counteract this loss by promoting the production and release of dopamine, thereby improving both motor and non-motor symptoms of the disease.

- *Protection from oxidative stress*:
  Exercise stimulates the body's production of antioxidants, which play an important role in neutralizing free radicals and reducing oxidative stress. Oxidative stress has been linked to the progression of Parkinson's disease and cellular damage caused by the accumulation of free radicals. Regular exercise can counteract this phenomenon and help maintain cellular integrity.

- *Increase brain plasticity*:
  Regular physical activity promotes brain plasticity, or the brain's ability to adapt and reorganize itself. This plasticity is critical for compensating the areas affected by Parkinson's disease and making new neural connections that can improve motor and cognitive function.

- *Reduce inflammation*:
  Studies have shown that exercise has an anti-inflammatory effect on the body, which may be beneficial for people with Parkinson's disease, as chronic inflammation has been linked to the progression of the disease. By reducing inflammatory markers, exercise may help reduce cellular damage and lessen the effects of the disease.

- *Improve balance and coordination*:
  Exercise, especially exercise that involves balance and coordination training, strengthens muscles and improves motor skills. This is particularly important for people with Parkinson's disease, who often have difficulty with balance and experience stiffness or slowness of movement. Appropriate physical activity can help improve these problem areas.

The Consumption of a Mediterranean Diet

Consumption of a Mediterranean diet has been associated with prevention and protection against Parkinson's disease due to several physiological factors:

- *Antioxidants*:
  The Mediterranean diet is rich in antioxidant foods such as fruits, vegetables, nuts, and olive oil. Antioxidants help neutralize free radicals, unstable molecules that can damage brain cells and contribute to the development of neurodegenerative diseases such as Parkinson's.

- *Anti-inflammatory*:
  This diet is characterized by its content of omega-3 fatty acids, found in fatty fish such as salmon and sardines, and in foods rich in healthy fats such as olive oil. These components have anti-inflammatory properties that may protect the brain from chronic inflammation, which has been linked to neuronal damage in Parkinson's disease.

- *Cardiovascular protection*:
  The Mediterranean diet has been shown to benefit cardiovascular health by helping to lower cholesterol and blood pressure. A healthy heart also contributes to better blood flow to the brain and a lower likelihood of developing vascular disease, which can increase the risk of Parkinson's disease.

- *Blood sugar regulation*:
  This diet is based on foods with a low glycemic index, such as whole grains, legumes, and fresh fruits. This helps maintain stable blood sugar levels, which may be beneficial for brain health, as there has been a possible link between insulin resistance and Parkinson's risk.

- *Beneficial gut bacteria*:
  The Mediterranean diet includes foods rich in fiber, such as fruits, vegetables, and legumes, which can promote the growth of beneficial gut bacteria. The health of the gut microbiome has been shown to significantly influence brain function and reducing the risk of neurodegenerative diseases, including Parkinson's.

The Use of Nonsteroidal Anti-inflammatory Drugs (NSAIDs)

The role of nonsteroidal anti-inflammatory drugs (NSAIDs) in preventing and protecting against Parkinson's disease has been the subject of different researches because of their potential to modulate inflammatory processes in the brain. NSAIDs are pharmacological agents that inhibit the activity of cyclooxygenase enzymes, which are responsible for the synthesis of pro-inflammatory prostaglandins. By reducing the activity of these enzymes and decreasing the production of prostaglandins, NSAIDs can exert anti-inflammatory effects in the brain and other tissues. In addition to their anti-inflammatory effects, some NSAIDs have demonstrated antioxidant properties and the ability to modulate mitochondrial function, which may contribute to their potential protective effect against Parkinson's disease.

It is important to note that although the results from preclinical studies and animal models are promising, clinical trials in humans have yielded mixed and sometimes contradictory results regarding the effect of NSAIDs in preventing and protecting against Parkinson's disease. Therefore, the relationship between the use of NSAIDs and their effect on Parkinson's disease is still not fully understood and requires further in-depth and exhaustive research.

Signs and Symptoms

According to Ehrman et al. [9], patients with Parkinson's disease present with characteristic motor and non-motor symptoms, which are outlined below.

Motor Symptoms and Signs

- *Muscle and joint stiffness*:
  Muscle and joint stiffness in Parkinson's disease occurs due to increased muscle tone, known as hypertonia. This abnormal muscle tone causes resistance to movement, resulting in a feeling of stiffness and tension in the muscles. This stiffness can affect various joints in the body, with the knees, elbows, wrists, ankles, and neck being particularly common sites.

  Muscle stiffness in Parkinson's disease can be detected through a clinical evaluation by a health-care professional. During the physical examination, the doctor may perform passive movements in the patient's joints to assess resistance to movement and the presence of stiffness. In addition, the patient may report a sensation of stiffness and lack of flexibility in the joints.

- *Resting muscle tremor*:
  One of the classic motor symptoms of Parkinson's disease is resting muscle tremor. These tremors are rhythmic and involuntary movements that occur when the patient is at rest, that is, when they are not performing any activity with their limbs. Parkinson's disease tremor typically occurs at a frequency of 4–6 Hz per second and tends to be more noticeable in the extremities, such as the hands and fingers.

  Detection of resting muscle tremor is by direct observation of the patient. The physician may notice these tremors while the patient is sitting or lying in a resting position. In addition, the patient may report the presence of tremor and how it affects their daily quality of life. It is important to differentiate Parkinson's disease tremor from other types of tremors that may have different causes. To do this, the following clinical assessments and specialized tests are performed:

  - *Accelerometry test*: Uses accelerometers to measure and record the patient's movements and tremors.
  - *Electromyography*: Measures the electrical activity of muscles to distinguish Parkinson's tremor from other muscular conditions.
  - *Magnetic resonance imaging and computed tomography*: Imaging tests used to rule out structural causes of tremor, such as brain tumors.
  - *Transcranial Doppler*: Uses ultrasound to measure cerebral blood flow and evaluate blood flow to specific areas of the brain.
  - *Video electroencephalography*: Combines video recording and electroencephalography to assess electrical activity in the brain.
  - *DaTSCAN scan*: Imaging technique that uses a radioactive substance to differentiate Parkinson's tremor from other types of tremors related to dopamine deficiency.

- *Tremor that starts suddenly and unilaterally*:
  Tremors are one of the most characteristic motor symptoms of Parkinson's disease and manifest as rhythmic and oscillating movements of a body part that usually begin suddenly and initially affect only one side of the body. Detecting

tremor in a person with suspected Parkinson's disease can be done by direct observation of uncontrolled and rhythmic movements of a limb, such as the hands, legs, or jaw. Tremors tend to worsen at rest and improve with voluntary movement.

In addition, it is important to note that in the early stages of the disease, there are unilateral changes in the body (tremor, muscle rigidity, and bradykinesia), whereas in the later stages of the disease, there are bilateral changes in the body (tremor, muscle rigidity, and bradykinesia).

The treatment of tremor associated with Parkinson's disease usually involves the use of medication, with levodopa being one of the most prescribed drugs. However, it is important to note that prolonged use of levodopa can lead to the development of continuous involuntary movements known as dyskinesia. Dyskinesia is an unwanted side effect of levodopa treatment and can make it difficult to control movements, negatively impacting a patient's quality of life [13].

- *Bradykinesia*:
  Bradykinesia is a characteristic motor symptom of Parkinson's disease that manifests as a voluntary slowing of the patient's movements. A decrease in the range of optimal movement (ROM) and the speed of motor activities is observed. Bradykinesia is caused by sensorimotor dysfunction in Parkinson's disease patients and commonly occurs unilaterally in 1% of the population over the age of 55 [13].

  To detect bradykinesia in a patient, tests of movement and coordination can be performed. The patient's performance of voluntary movements, such as opening and closing their hands, walking, or getting up from a chair, is observed. Slowness and reduced ROM in movements may be observed during these tests. It is important to note whether bradykinesia is unilateral or bilateral, as it is more common in the early stages of Parkinson's disease.

  It is crucial to remember that bradykinesia in Parkinson's disease can affect basic activities of daily living and others complex tasks that lead to a significant impact on a patient's quality of life. Health-care professionals should be alert to the presence of this symptom in individuals over the age of 55, as it may serve as an early indicator of Parkinson's disease.

- *Postural alteration*:
  Postural alteration in patients with Parkinson's disease is a clinical manifestation characterized by difficulties in maintaining an upright and balanced posture. Unlike postural alterations that may be caused by proprioceptive, visual, or vestibular deficits, in Parkinson's, the underlying cause lies in a disorder of muscular tone, specifically due to the involvement of dopaminergic neural pathways. Altered muscular tone, along with other motor deficits such as muscular rigidity and bradykinesia, contributes to the development of a stooped posture and progressive postural instability. This difficulty in maintaining proper body alignment can lead to a tendency to lean forward and walk with a flexed posture, known as "flexion posture."

The detection of postural alteration in Parkinson's is accomplished through careful clinical observation during the patient's physical examination. The patient's ability to maintain an upright and balanced posture while standing or walking should be evaluated. It is also relevant to perform specific tests to assess the patient's balance and gait, such as the Tinetti Test or the 10-Meter Walk Test. Furthermore, it is important to consider the patient's medical history, including any previous incidents of frequent falls or musculoskeletal injuries related to postural alteration. Information provided by the patient and their caregivers can be of great assistance in obtaining a complete picture of the manifestation of this symptom.

Early identification of postural alteration in Parkinson's is crucial, as this condition can lead to an increased risk of falls and musculoskeletal injuries. An integrated approach that includes specific treatment strategies to improve posture and balance, along with appropriate pharmacological therapy to address Parkinson's motor symptoms, is essential for enhancing the patient's quality of life and reducing the negative impact of this symptom on their functionality.

- *Altered gait pattern*:
  Parkinsonism significantly affects a person's ability to walk smoothly and in a coordinated manner. The altered gait pattern in Parkinson's disease is characterized by a series of changes in the way the patient walks due to a combination of motor and muscular factors that affect locomotion.

  - *Reduced stride length*: Parkinson's disease patients tend to take shorter and faster steps, known as "stepping." This can be seen in the distance they travel with each step and their walking speed.
  - *Decreased hip abduction*: Parkinson's disease may limit this movement, resulting in a narrower and stiffer gait.
  - *Inadequate foot pressure and positioning during stride*: Patients may have difficulty placing their feet properly on the ground while walking, resulting in increased pressure on certain areas of the foot and an increased risk of tripping and falling.
  - *Lack of arm swing*: The patient's arms may remain still or have little movement while walking, contributing to stiffness and lack of fluidity in movement.
  - *Reduced muscle strength in the lower limbs*: Parkinson's disease can affect muscle strength, especially in the legs, making it difficult to support body weight and provide propulsion for forward movement while walking.
  - *Lack of lower limb coordination during gait*: Coordination of the leg muscles is critical to maintaining a stable and safe gait. In Parkinson's disease, lack of coordination can lead to irregular steps and imbalance.
    It is important to note that these changes in gait pattern can vary in intensity depending on the degree of disease progression and can significantly impact a patient's mobility and quality of life. Early recognition of these signs and symptoms is essential for proper disease management and implementation of therapeutic interventions to improve walking ability and reduce the risk of falls [14].

- *Micrography*:
  The significantly reduced size of handwriting, known as micrography, is a characteristic and early motor symptom of Parkinson's disease. It refers to an impairment in the ability to write with legible and appropriately sized letters, resulting in small and closely spaced handwriting.
  Micrography can be identified by a visual assessment of the patient's handwriting. The health-care professional can ask the patient to write a sentence or paragraph on paper. It is important to observe the size and legibility of the writing. In people with Parkinson's disease, handwriting may be noticeably smaller than usual, and letters may be closer together, making the writing appear cramped. In addition to visual observation, standardized rating scales, such as the Columbia Micrography Scale, can be used to quantify and objectively measure the degree of micrography in the patient.

- *Hypomimia*:
  Reduced or absent facial expression, known as "hypomimia" or "poker face," is a characteristic motor symptom of Parkinson's disease. It refers to the difficulty or inability to display a full range of facial expressions, resulting in a rigid facial appearance with a lack of natural facial movements.
  To identify hypomimia in a patient, one should carefully observe the patient's face while performing various emotional expressions, such as smiling, frowning, or raising the eyebrows. Limited or unchanging facial expressions, especially during emotional interactions, may indicate the presence of hypomimia and could suggest possible Parkinson's disease.

- *Dorsal hyperkyphosis*:
  Dorsal hyperkyphosis, also known as "stoop" or "hunchback," is a motor symptom often seen in people with advanced Parkinson's disease. It refers to an exaggerated curvature of the spine, especially in the dorsal region of the back, resulting in a stooped and forward leaning posture.
  To detect dorsal hyperkyphosis in a patient, one should observe their posture while standing or walking. Excessive curvature in the upper part of the back, leading to a forward-leaning posture, can be an indication of dorsal hyperkyphosis associated with Parkinson's. Additionally, a detailed physical evaluation can be performed to measure the magnitude of the curvature and determine the severity of the symptom.

- *Hypotonia and weakness of the orofacial, esophageal, gastric, and facial muscles*:
  Parkinson's patients may experience a decrease in muscle tone and strength in the muscles that control the mouth, throat, esophagus, stomach, and face. This condition, called hypotonia, can manifest as a deeper voice, constant drooling, and difficulty swallowing (dysphagia). Health-care professionals can detect orofacial hypotonia and muscle weakness through clinical observation and specific tests that assess the strength and function of facial muscles.

- *Erectile dysfunction*:
  Erectile dysfunction is a serious complication that significantly affects the quality of life of people with Parkinson's disease. This condition, characterized by the inability to achieve or maintain an erection sufficient for satisfying sexual activity, can have a profound emotional and psychological impact on affected individuals.

  Erectile dysfunction in Parkinson's disease can be multifactorial, with several interrelated causes. One of the most important factors is the impairment of the autonomic nervous system, which regulates sexual function, among other bodily functions. The degeneration of dopaminergic neurons in Parkinson's disease affects the nerve pathways that control the sexual response, leading to difficulties with arousal, erection, and ejaculation. In addition, the presence of tremors and muscular rigidity characteristic of Parkinson's disease can cause anxiety and stress in the patient, which in turn can affect sexual performance and worsen erectile dysfunction. In addition, some medications used to treat Parkinson's disease may have side effects that affect sexual function, further contributing to erectile dysfunction.

  It is important to emphasize that erectile dysfunction in Parkinson's disease affects not only the patient but also the partner, which can create tension in the relationship and affect intimacy and communication between partners. Treatment of erectile dysfunction in Parkinson's disease patients requires a comprehensive assessment and multidisciplinary approach. Health-care professionals should approach the issue openly and sensitively, providing a trusting environment in which patients can express their concerns and needs. In addition, specific pharmacological therapy for erectile dysfunction may be considered in some cases, although interactions with other Parkinson's disease medications should be considered. Physical therapy and exercise can play an important role in the management of erectile dysfunction, especially when it is associated with neuromuscular conditions such as Parkinson's disease. Although erectile dysfunction can have a variety of causes, physiotherapy and exercise can be beneficial in the context of Parkinson's disease in several ways:

  - Improving blood circulation in the genital region, which promotes a firmer erection.
  - Strengthening the pelvic floor muscles, which enhances erectile function and control.
  - Reducing stress and anxiety, psychological factors that can contribute to erectile dysfunction.
  - Enhancing neuromuscular function, especially relevant in neurological diseases like Parkinson's.
  - Promoting self-confidence, which can be beneficial in overcoming psychological barriers that affect sexual function.

Non-motor Symptoms and Signs

- *Anosmia*:
  Loss of the sense of smell, also known as anosmia, is a non-motor symptom often associated with Parkinson's disease. It refers to a decrease or inability to properly perceive odors. This olfactory alteration results from the progressive degeneration of neuronal structures in the olfactory system, affecting the transmission and processing of sensory signals related to smell. Loss of the sense of smell can be detected by specific olfactory assessment tests, such as the use of standardized odor panels or odor identification tests. Patients may undergo a comprehensive olfactory evaluation by a neurologist or otolaryngologist to identify any changes in olfactory function.

- *Hyposmia*:
  Hyposmia refers to a decreased sense of smell and is one of the most common non-motor symptoms of Parkinson's disease. As the disease progresses, many people with Parkinson's disease may experience a gradual loss of smell, affecting their ability to recognize familiar odors. Hyposmia can be assessed through standardized olfactory tests in which different odors are presented and the patient must correctly identify them. These tests quantify the decline in the sense of smell and provide valuable information for diagnosing and monitoring Parkinson's disease.

- *Sleep and mood disorders*:
  Patients may experience sleep disturbances such as insomnia, excessive daytime sleepiness, periodic leg movements during sleep, and REM sleep behavior disorder. These sleep disturbances may result from changes in the brain circuits that regulate sleep and wakefulness. On the other hand, mood changes are also common in Parkinson's disease. Patients may experience depressive symptoms, anxiety, irritability, and changes in emotional regulation. These changes may be due to dysfunction in dopaminergic pathways and other neurotransmitters that regulate mood and emotional responses.

  Identifying sleep and mood disorders in people with Parkinson's disease involves a detailed assessment of sleep patterns, sleep quality, and affective symptoms. Patients may be interviewed about their sleep quality, sleep duration, and possible depressive or anxiety symptoms. In addition, the use of standardized mood and sleep scales can provide a more objective and quantitative assessment of these symptoms. It is important for Parkinson's patients to be evaluated regularly to identify and properly address these changes, as they can have a significant impact on a patient's quality of life and overall well-being.

- *Frequent shoulder pain*:
  Shoulder pain is a common symptom in Parkinson's patients and may be related to the muscle stiffness.

Shoulder pain can be identified by asking patients about the presence of discomfort or pain in this area of the body. It may also be evident during the physical examination, where the doctor can palpate and assess the mobility of the shoulders for signs of stiffness and pain.

- *Gastrointestinal dysfunction*:
  Parkinson's disease can affect the gastrointestinal system, causing a variety of symptoms. These symptoms may include:
  - *Dysphagia,* which is difficulty swallowing, resulting in the sensation that food is stuck in the throat or esophagus.
  - *Reduced ability to properly empty the contents of the stomach,* known as delayed gastric emptying. This can cause bloating, nausea, and vomiting.
  - *Excessive salivation, also known as sialorrhea.* This symptom presents as an overproduction of saliva, which causes discomfort and negatively affects the patient's quality of life.
  - *Difficulty with bowel movements*, which may manifest as constipation or steatorrhea (fatty stools).
    These symptoms may result from decreased motor activity in the gastrointestinal tract due to degeneration of dopaminergic neurons in the central nervous system.

    Early detection of these digestive symptoms is essential for proper management of Parkinson's disease and for improving the patient's quality of life. It is critical for health-care professionals to be vigilant for these symptoms and to perform a detailed evaluation of gastrointestinal function during the diagnosis and follow-up of Parkinson's patients. To detect dysphagia, specific swallowing tests such as video fluoroscopy or endoscopy can be performed to assess the coordination and safe passage of food through the esophagus. Delayed gastric emptying can be evaluated by gastric emptying studies, which measure the time it takes for the stomach to empty its contents. Sialorrhea, or excessive salivation, can be determined by clinical observation and assessment of salivation at rest and with food intake. About bowel problems, it is important for patients to inform their physicians of any changes in bowel habits, and health-care professionals can assess this through history and physical examination. In addition, complementary tests such as stool analysis may be used to determine the presence of steatorrhea.

- *Arterial hypotension*:
  Arterial hypotension, also known as low blood pressure, is another non-motor symptom observed in some patients with Parkinson's disease. It is characterized by a decrease in both systolic and diastolic blood pressure below what is considered normal. To detect arterial hypotension in Parkinson's patients, blood pressure is measured in the resting, standing, and lying positions. Significant drops in blood pressure while standing may indicate the presence of orthostatic hypotension, which is particularly common in people with this condition.

- *Chronic fatigue*:
  Chronic fatigue is a common non-motor symptom of Parkinson's disease. It is characterized by a persistent feeling of physical and mental exhaustion that does not improve with adequate rest. Often, Parkinson's patients experience debilitating fatigue that negatively affects their quality of life and ability to perform daily activities.

  To identify chronic fatigue in Parkinson's disease patients, health-care professionals must conduct a thorough assessment of the patient's reported symptoms. It is important to inquire about perceived energy levels, the degree of fatigue during the day, and the impact of fatigue on daily activities. Fatigue assessment scales can also be used to provide a more objective measure of fatigue severity.

- *Neuropsychiatric disorders*:
  Neuropsychiatric disorders are common in Parkinson's disease patients and can include symptoms such as depression, anxiety, apathy, and psychosis. These problems can have a significant impact on a patient's emotional well-being and quality of life, as well as their relationship with caregivers and loved ones.

  - *Depression*: Depression is one of the most common symptoms of Parkinson's disease. Patients may experience persistent sadness, loss of interest in activities they once enjoyed, changes in appetite and sleep, and feelings of hopelessness and helplessness.
  - *Anxiety*: Anxiety is another common neuropsychiatric manifestation of Parkinson's disease. Patients may experience excessive worry, restlessness, irritability, and physical symptoms such as heart palpitations or sweating.
  - *Apathy*: Apathy is characterized by a lack of motivation and interest in participating in activities. Patients may appear discouraged and show a general decrease in energy and engagement in social activities.
  - *Psychosis*: Psychosis can manifest in patients with advanced Parkinson's disease in the form of hallucinations and delusions. These symptoms can be frightening and confusing to the patient and those around them.
    The identification of neuropsychiatric disorders in patients with Parkinson's disease requires a comprehensive evaluation by trained health-care professionals. Thorough clinical interviews should be conducted, and specific questionnaires and rating scales should be used for each symptom, such as the Hamilton Depression Scale to measure depression and the Hamilton Anxiety Scale to assess anxiety. In addition, it is important to assess cognitive function to detect behavioral changes and possible signs of psychosis. Early detection and appropriate treatment of these disorders are essential to improve patients' quality of life and optimize their medical care.

- *Impulse control behaviors caused by disease or medication use*:
  Some people with Parkinson's disease may experience behavioral changes that manifest as impulsivity, obsessions, and repetitive behaviors. These behaviors may be a direct result of the disease itself or may be related to medications used

to treat motor symptoms. In particular, some dopaminergic medications commonly prescribed to control Parkinson's motor symptoms may have side effects that affect judgment and decision making, leading to impulsive and inappropriate behaviors. It is important for health-care professionals, caregivers, and patients to be vigilant about these behaviors and to adjust treatment as needed to minimize adverse effects on the patient's quality of life and social environment.

Behavioral changes should be carefully evaluated during follow-up visits with the Parkinson's disease patient. Health-care professionals should conduct a thorough review of the patient's medical history and medications to identify potential side effects related to impulsivity and compulsivity. It is also important to involve family members and caregivers in the assessment process, as they can provide valuable information about changes in the patient's behavior. If problematic impulsive behaviors are identified, adjustments in pharmacologic treatment and other therapeutic options should be considered to minimize these adverse effects.

- *Nephrotic disorders*:
  Nephrotic disorders, characterized by the presence of proteinuria (excess protein in the urine), hypoalbuminemia (low levels of albumin in the blood), edema, and elevated blood lipids, are a group of kidney diseases that may be associated with Parkinson's disease. Although the exact relationship between Parkinson's disease and nephrotic disorders is not fully understood, some clinical and epidemiologic studies have observed associations between the two.

  Detection of nephrotic disorders in patients with Parkinson's disease can be achieved through laboratory testing, including urine analysis to detect proteinuria and blood tests to assess albumin and lipid levels. It is important for health-care professionals caring for patients with Parkinson's disease to be aware of this possible association and to evaluate renal function on a regular basis, especially if the patient presents with symptoms or risk factors suggestive of nephrotic disorders. If evidence of kidney damage is detected, a more thorough evaluation should be performed and, if necessary, the patient should be referred to a nephrologist for appropriate and timely management.

- *Urinary dysfunction due to altered response of continence reflexes*:
  Urinary dysfunction associated with an altered response of the continence reflex is a commonly observed and clinically relevant symptom in patients with Parkinson's disease. These dysfunctions may result from the central and peripheral nervous system involvement that characterizes this neurodegenerative disease. Dysfunction of continence reflexes in Parkinson's disease is primarily manifested by hypotonia of the urogenital muscles and disruption of detrusor muscle synapses, which are responsible for bladder contraction and emptying. This muscular hypotonia leads to weakened bladder control, resulting in urinary continence problems.

  Early detection of this urinary dysfunction is critical to effective treatment and improved quality of life for Parkinson's patients. Some key indicators for detecting this problem are:

- *Uncontrolled nighttime urination*: Patients may experience episodes of urinary incontinence during the night, resulting in involuntary urination during sleep.
- *Constant urinary frequency*: The constant need to urinate is a characteristic sign of urinary dysfunction in Parkinson's disease.

  Once these symptoms are identified, it is important to perform a comprehensive evaluation of the Parkinson's patient, including a detailed review of the patient's medical history and a complete physical examination. In addition, urodynamic studies are essential to obtain objective information about the functioning of the urinary system and to confirm the diagnosis. The clinical management of these urinary dysfunctions in Parkinson's disease patients requires a multidisciplinary approach involving neurologists, urologists, and specialized therapists. Therapeutic options include the use of medications to improve detrusor function, pelvic floor rehabilitation and, in more severe cases, the use of incontinence devices.

- *Decreased pelvic floor muscle tone, urinary and fecal incontinence, and increased risk of prolapse*:

  Parkinson's disease can affect pelvic floor muscle tone, leading to a decrease in sphincter control and resulting in urinary and fecal incontinence. In addition, weakening of the pelvic floor increases the risk of prolapse, which is the displacement of pelvic organs due to lack of muscular support.

  Urinary and fecal incontinence are diagnosed by a detailed review of the patient's symptoms and medical history. Physicians may also perform physical examinations and specialized tests to assess pelvic floor function and detect prolapse. Early detection and appropriate treatment can improve the quality of life for Parkinson's patients facing these complications.

- *Lack of cognitive executive function*:

  Executive function is a term that encompasses a set of higher mental processes that allow us to perform complex activities and control our behavior to achieve goals. In Parkinson's disease, the reduction of dopamine, a key neurotransmitter for neuronal communication, can negatively affect these executive functions. This results in difficulty organizing tasks, planning activities, making decisions, and solving problems efficiently.

  Symptoms of executive function deficits may include problems with daily organization, difficulty prioritizing tasks, delays in making decisions, and difficulty maintaining focus on complex activities. Changes in work or academic performance and difficulty adapting to new situations can also be signs of changes in executive functioning. Professionals and specialists can assess these abilities through specific neuropsychological tests that evaluate working memory, mental flexibility, and planning ability [4].

- *Dementia*:
  As Parkinson's disease progresses, some individuals may develop dementia, which is a broader and more significant cognitive impairment beyond the characteristic motor deficits of the disease. Dementia in Parkinson's disease may be related to the accumulation of abnormal proteins in the brain and may affect various cognitive functions.

  While not all Parkinson's patients develop dementia, those who do experience progressive cognitive decline that affects memory, language, attention, and other mental functions. The exact cause of dementia in Parkinson's disease is not fully understood, but it is believed to be related to the accumulation of abnormal proteins, such as alpha-synuclein, in the brain.

  Early detection of dementia in Parkinson's disease is essential to provide the best care and treatment for patients. Signs of dementia may include significant memory loss, difficulty performing everyday tasks, changes in personality and behavior, problems with language and communication, and difficulties with time and spatial orientation. Neurology and neuropsychology specialists can perform detailed assessments to identify cognitive changes and determine if dementia is present and at what stage.

Competing Interests The author have no conflicts of interest to declare that are relevant to the content of this chapter.

References

1. Galimberti D, Scarpini E. Neurodegenerative diseases. 2nd ed. Springer; 2018.
2. Singh S, Joshi N. Pathology, prevention and therapeutics of neurodegenerative disease. Singapore: Springer; 2018.
3. Josefina A, Alonso P. Epilepsias y discapacidades neurológicas en el niño. Cuba: Ciencia mé; 2007.
4. Vladisauskas M, Goldin AP. 20 Años De Entrenamiento Cognitivo: Una Perspectiva Amplia. J Neuroeduc. 2020;1:130–5. https://doi.org/10.1344/joned.v1i1.31628.
5. Heemels M-T. Neurodegenerative diseases. Nature. 2016;539:7628.
6. Rojas JE, Goméz SR. Las 100 enfermedades más frecuentes, First. Bogotá: Penguin Random House Grupo Editorial S.A.S; 2017.
7. Hammer GD, McPhee SJ. Pathophysiology of disease. 8th ed. McGraw-Hill Education; 2019.
8. Organización mundial de la salud (2022) Enfermedad de Parkinson, datos y cifras. https://www.who.int/es/news-room/fact-sheets/detail/parkinson-disease.
9. Ehrman JK, Gordon PM, Visich PS, Keteyian SJ. Clinical exercise physiology. 4th ed. Human Kinetics; 2019.
10. Albani G, Albani S, Keshavarzian A. Editorial: role of diet, physical activity and immune system in Parkinson's disease. Front Neurol. 2020;11:1–3. https://doi.org/10.3389/fneur.2020.611349.
11. Ko TK. Does drinking coffee reduce the incidence of Parkinson's disease? Cureus. 2023; https://doi.org/10.7759/cureus.34296.
12. Zhou Z, Zhong S, Liang Y, et al. Serum uric acid and the risk of dementia: a systematic review and meta-analysis. Front Aging Neurosci. 2021;13:625690.

13. Cusso ME, Donald KJ, Khoo TK. The impact of physical activity on non-motor symptoms in Parkinson's disease: a systematic review. Front Med (Lausanne). 2016;3:1–9. https://doi.org/10.3389/fmed.2016.00035.
14. Rigby BR, Davis RW, Avalos MA, et al. Acute cardiometabolic responses to three modes of treadmill exercise in older adults with Parkinson's disease. Adapted Phys Activity Quart. 2018;35:424–36. https://doi.org/10.1123/apaq.2017-0200.

Chapter 2
Diagnosis, Monitoring, and Control

Initial Questions

- How does the multidisciplinary approach to Parkinson's disease diagnosis influence the creation of personalized therapeutic exercise programs for patients?
- How do Parkinson's diagnostic, monitoring, and control devices and tools contribute to therapeutic exercise decision making?
- How can the clinical course of Parkinson's disease be applied to the planning, implementation, and adaptation of therapeutic exercise programs?

The diagnosis of Parkinson's disease is a complex process that requires a multidisciplinary approach due to its multifactorial nature. Unlike other diseases with clearer and more specific causes, Parkinson's disease does not have a single biomarker that can definitively confirm its etiology. Instead of relying on a single indicator, healthcare professionals must carefully consider and evaluate multiple clinical and physiological aspects to arrive at a more accurate and certain diagnosis (see Fig. 2.1).

The initial diagnosis of Parkinson's disease is a clinical challenge, as an error range of approximately 24% has been observed in many specialized centers [5]. For this reason, the International Parkinson and Movement Disorder Society emphasizes the importance of not being limited to an early diagnosis, but to thoroughly evaluate both motor and non-motor symptoms that manifest over time and gradually, considering the clinical progression.

The diagnostic process for Parkinson's disease must not only analyze the characteristic symptoms of the disease, such as motor problems and tremor, but also pay attention to non-motor symptoms that can occur in early and advanced stages. These symptoms include cognitive impairment, emotional changes, sleep disturbances, and gastrointestinal problems, among others.

To achieve a more accurate and differential diagnosis in the clinical progression of Parkinson's disease, it is essential to understand and consider the different pathological stages (see Fig. 2.2). This is crucial for the prescription of exercise, the

C. A. A. Mejía, *Therapeutic Exercise for Parkinson's Disease and Related Disorders*, https://doi.org/10.1007/978-3-031-62119-2_2

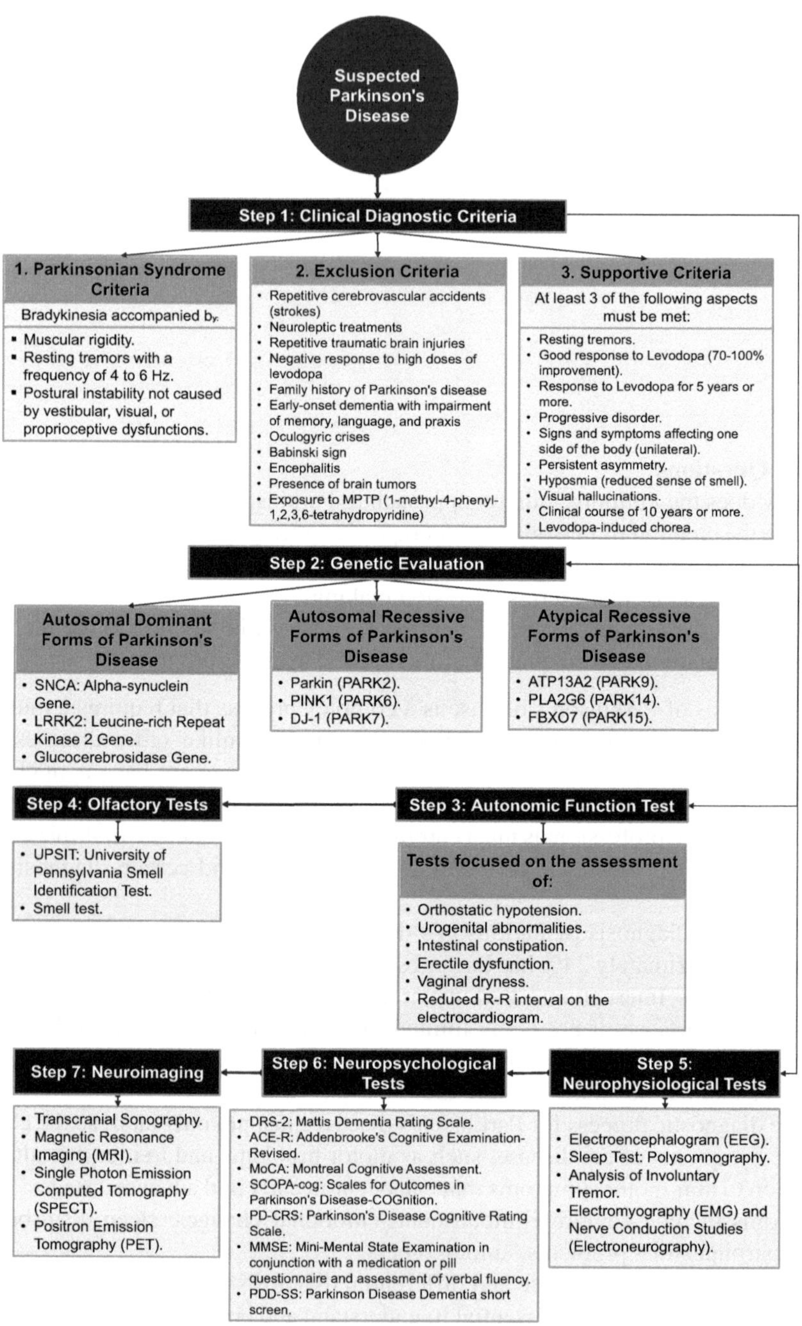

Fig. 2.1 Algorithm for the diagnosis of Parkinson's disease, inspired from Berardelli et al. [1], Hammer and McPhee [2], Perera Pintado et al. [3], and Singh and Joshi [4]

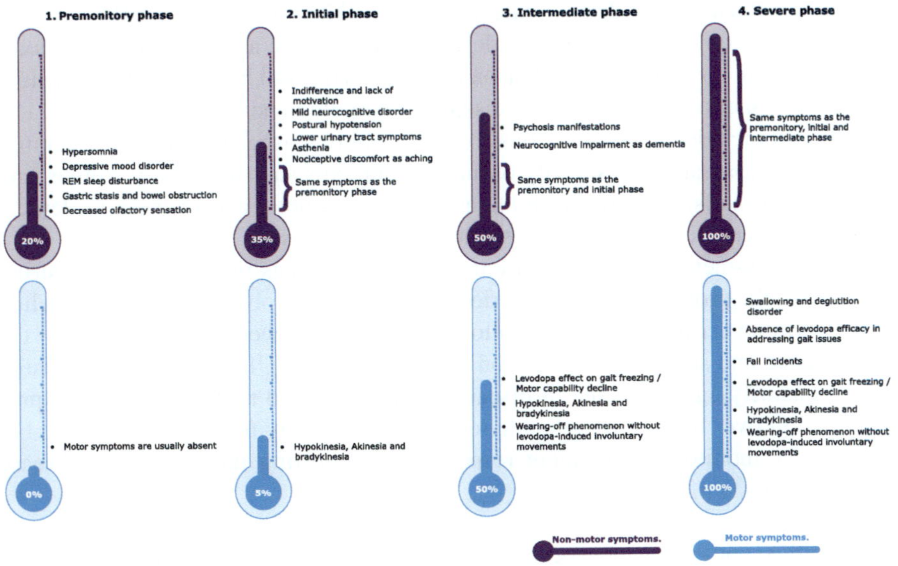

Fig. 2.2 Clinical progression of Parkinson's disease, showing both motor and non-motor symptoms according to stages of pathology. Note that quality of life deteriorates dramatically as the disease progresses. (Adapted from Galimberti and Scarpini [5])

accurate determination of the load dosage, the necessary care, the contraindications, and the therapeutic goals. This consideration is important in the early stages of the disease, when symptoms can be subtle and easily confused with other conditions [1].

In addition to the tests listed in the algorithm in Fig. 2.1, the following tests may be performed:

- **Meta-iodobenzylguanidine (MIBG) myocardial scintigraphy:** Myocardial scintigraphy with meta-iodobenzylguanidine (MIBG) is an advanced diagnostic imaging technique used to evaluate the sympathetic functions of the heart, which tend to be altered in people with Parkinson's disease. The procedure is based on the administration of a special radiopharmaceutical called MIBG, which is injected into the patient's vein. Once inside the body, MIBG selectively concentrates in the sympathetic nerve endings of the heart, providing information about the activity of these nerve cells. In patients with Parkinson's disease, a decrease in MIBG uptake has been observed due to the degeneration of sympathetic neurons, a characteristic phenomenon of this neurodegenerative disease.

  MIBG myocardial scintigraphy is performed in specialized nuclear medicine centers. After injection of the radiopharmaceutical, images of the heart are taken with a gamma camera, allowing visualization of the distribution of MIBG and evaluation of the sympathetic function of the heart. These images provide valuable information about the state of the sympathetic neurons and can therefore confirm the diagnosis of Parkinson's disease and rule out other diseases with similar symptoms [6, 7].

- **Unified Parkinson's disease rating scale (UPDRS) test:** The UPDRS is a comprehensive rating scale that is widely used to measure and quantify both motor and non-motor aspects of Parkinson's disease. This tool has become an essential standard measure for evaluating disease progression and treatment efficacy. The UPDRS includes several sections covering different aspects of the disease, ranging from assessing the severity of motor symptoms such as rigidity, tremor, and bradykinesia (slow movements) to assessing non-motor aspects such as depression, anxiety, cognitive problems, and sleep problems.
  This assessment is performed by trained professionals or neurologists. During the test, the professional asks a series of questions and observes the patient while performing certain motor tasks, allowing for a comprehensive assessment of the presence and severity of Parkinson's symptoms. The UPDRS score is essential for quantifying the degree of disease involvement and monitoring disease progression over time. This valuable tool is used not only for initial diagnosis, but also for monitoring treatment response and adjusting therapy as the disease progresses.

Significant advances have been made in the use of technology and artificial intelligence to monitor the signs and symptoms of Parkinson's disease, complementing traditional diagnostic and monitoring methods. While these devices are still in the research phase, they show great potential for improving early detection and patient monitoring. An experimental 12-month study by Adams et al. [8] evaluated the efficacy of a smartwatch and smartphone application in 82 untreated early-stage Parkinson's patients and 50 age-matched controls. The devices recorded data on movement and motor skills, as well as language and cognitive tests. The results showed significant differences between Parkinson's patients and controls in involuntary arm movements, tremor duration, and finger dexterity, suggesting that these digital measures could provide objective and continuous assessments to complement early Parkinson's diagnosis. However, longitudinal analyses and patient participation are needed to identify the most relevant digital measures for evaluating therapies in this growing population.

In addition, the National Institute for Health and Care Excellence (NICE) in the United Kingdom has published an article suggesting the use of evidence-based technological devices based on experimental studies to monitor the signs and symptoms of Parkinson's disease. Among these devices, those based on motion sensors stand out, allowing the detection of dyskinesia (involuntary movements), bradykinesia (slowing of complex voluntary movements), involuntary tremor, gait freezing, sleep disturbances, speech, and communication difficulties, among others [9].

These wearable devices offer a valuable tool to improve early detection, monitoring, and assessment of disease progression, contributing to more personalized and effective treatment for Parkinson's patients. The focus on using motion sensing technology opens new possibilities in medical care and promises to improve the quality of life for people affected by this neurodegenerative disease.

Among the devices recommended by NICE and supported by scientific evidence are:

- **STAT-ON (Sense4care):** STAT-ON® is an autonomous and noninvasive Holter-type device worn on the patient's waist to continuously record motor symptoms, particularly the "on-off" and "wearing-off" phenomena experienced by patients taking levodopa as part of their Parkinson's disease treatment. It also records other motor symptoms such as bradykinesia, dyskinesia, gait parameters (speed, cadence, stride length, etc.), number of falls, energy expenditure, and gait freezing.
  Using advanced algorithms and signal processing methods, STAT-ON accurately monitors and records the patient's motor symptoms. This device is particularly useful for detailed monitoring of disease progression and evaluation of treatment response in each patient. It also provides valuable information for the appropriate prescription of therapeutic exercises and allows the monitoring of benefits related to "on-off" phenomena, "wearing-off," gait changes, fall risk, and dyskinesia.
  In Parkinson's disease, "on-off" phenomena are characterized by fluctuations in motor activity in which the patient alternates between moments of normal mobility and periods of motor difficulty, sometimes even freezing and being unable to initiate movements. These fluctuations are related to changes in levodopa levels in the blood, making the effects of the medication unpredictable throughout the day.
  On the other hand, the "wearing-off" phenomenon refers to a gradual decrease in the effectiveness of levodopa toward the end of the dose. As the disease progresses, the intervals between doses become more pronounced and the patient may experience fluctuations in treatment efficacy.

- **The Personal KinetiGraph (Global Kinetics Corporation):** The Personal KinetiGraph® (PKG) is an FDA-cleared device in the United States and is widely used in Australia and Europe. It uses algorithms to monitor and quantify symptoms of movement disorders, sleep, and other symptoms in Parkinson's patients. It is a system that records movement over several days and generates data-driven reports to make more personalized treatment and management decisions.
  The PKG resembles a smartwatch that is worn on the wrist most affected by Parkinson's symptoms and is equipped with a three-axis accelerometer to measure acceleration. The device generates scores for bradykinesia, dyskinesia, and tremor, and presents the data graphically and numerically in an intuitive) way for clinical staff. Bradykinesia and dyskinesia scores are generated every 2 min and presented in a final report over a 6-day period. This report shows average bradykinesia and dyskinesia scores throughout the day, as well as scheduled medication times, allowing for detailed tracking of patient progress. In addition, the PKG is useful for classifying Parkinson's patients as controlled or uncontrolled based on their motor scores.

- **Kinesia 360 (Great Lakes Neurotechnologies):** The Kinesia 360® system is a tool that provides continuous and remote measurement of patient symptoms. It uses wrist and ankle sensors, along with a mobile application, to continuously collect data and assess tremor, slowness of movement, dyskinesia, and mobility.

This data is sent to the Kinesia app, where algorithms detect symptoms and calculate severity scores every 2 min, providing a detailed assessment of the patient's motor signs and symptoms. This device can monitor changes in symptoms, making it a useful tool for monitoring and early detection of other characteristic Parkinson's symptoms.

- **PDMonitor (PD Neurotechnology):** The PDMonitor® is a portable device and software that provides continuous, noninvasive monitoring of patients with Parkinson's disease and other movement disorders. The device uses five lightweight monitoring sensors placed on different parts of the body to collect three-dimensional motion data. This data, combined with information about the patient's lifestyle and treatment compliance, is analyzed to provide physicians with a comprehensive view of each patient's disease progression. The PDMonitor® monitors various symptoms such as bradykinesia, dyskinesia, involuntary tremor, gait freezing, gait changes, loss of postural balance, on-off phenomena, and others. This tool is valuable for clinical decision making and personalized treatment design.

Competing Interests The author have no conflicts of interest to declare that are relevant to the content of this chapter.

References

1. Berardelli A, Wenning GK, Antonini A, et al. EFNS/MDS-ES recommendations for the diagnosis of Parkinson's disease. Eur J Neurol. 2013;20:16–34. https://doi.org/10.1111/ene.12022.
2. Hammer GD, McPhee SJ. Pathophysiology of disease. 8th ed. McGraw-Hill Education; 2019.
3. Perera Pintado A, Torres Aroche L, Vergara Gil A, et al. SPECT/CT: principales aplicaciones en la medicina nuclear. Nucleus (La Habana). 2017:2–9.
4. Singh S, Joshi N. Pathology, prevention and therapeutics of neurodegenerative disease. Singapore: Springer; 2018.
5. Galimberti D, Scarpini E. Neurodegenerative diseases. 2nd ed. Springer; 2018.
6. AlMahadin G, Lotfi A, Zysk E, et al. Parkinson's disease: current assessment methods and wearable devices for evaluation of movement disorder motor symptoms—a patient and healthcare professional perspective. BMC Neurol. 2020;20:1–13. https://doi.org/10.1186/s12883-020-01996-7.
7. Khalil H, Alomari MA, Khabour O, et al. The association between physical activity with cognitive function and brain derived neurotrophic factor in people with Parkinson's disease, a pilot study. J Aging Phys Act. 2017;0:1–24. https://doi.org/10.1123/japa.2016-0121.
8. Adams JL, Kangarloo T, Tracey B, et al. Using a smartwatch and smartphone to assess early Parkinson's disease in the WATCH-PD study. NPJ Parkinsons Dis. 2023;9:64. https://doi.org/10.1038/s41531-023-00497-x.
9. National Institute for Health and Care Excellence. NICE recommends NHS collects real-world evidence on devices that monitor people with Parkinson's disease. In: Article. 2022

Chapter 3
The Influence of Therapeutic Exercise

Initial Questions

- What are the specific physiological effects of exercise that can benefit patients with neurodegenerative diseases such as Parkinson's?
- How can exercise influence both motor and non-motor aspects of Parkinson's, and to what extent does it translate into concrete improvements in the quality of life for patients?
- How can an understanding of the therapeutic effects of exercise provide insight into the treatment and management of patients with Parkinson's?

Traditional treatment for Parkinson's disease has been based on pharmacotherapy (dopaminergic and non-dopaminergic medications, catechol-*O*-methyltransferase inhibitors, and levodopa) and surgery to implant neurostimulators in the brain, such as deep brain stimulation, to control involuntary movements, emotions, and pain through electrical signals. However, with scientific and technological advances in areas such as exercise prescription, physical therapy, occupational therapy, speech therapy, kinesiotherapy, and others non-pharmacological and minimally invasive treatments have experienced a remarkable resurgence. Among these, therapeutic exercise stands out as a valuable tool for the prevention, treatment, and improvement of motor and non-motor symptoms of diseases such as Parkinson's disease [1].

Therapeutic exercise presents itself as a highly beneficial option for controlling the motor signs and symptoms of Parkinson's disease. This approach includes a wide variety of tools as functional electrical stimulation, sensorimotor exercises, movement-based neurorehabilitation, hydrotherapy, manual therapy, balance and coordination exercises, muscle strengthening therapies, resistance training, flexibility and stretching exercises, relaxation and mindfulness techniques, proprioception exercises, cognitive stimulation therapies, and cardiovascular rehabilitation exercises, among others. These diverse therapeutic tools can be customized for each patient, allowing for the development of personalized and effective treatment plans to improve the quality of life for people with Parkinson's disease. In this context,

C. A. A. Mejía, *Therapeutic Exercise for Parkinson's Disease and Related Disorders*, https://doi.org/10.1007/978-3-031-62119-2_3

therapeutic exercise becomes an important ally in the comprehensive management of the disease, helping to improve the functionality and well-being of affected patients [1].

Several beneficial effects of therapeutic exercise can be identified, such as:

Increased Range of Motion (ROM)

- *Explanation:* ROM refers to the distance and direction a joint can move between its most extended and most flexed positions. Parkinson's disease can cause muscle stiffness and progressive loss of ROM due to neuronal degeneration and neurotransmitter imbalances. This rigidity and loss of movement limits the individual's functionality and independence.
- *Useful tools:* Stretching and joint mobility exercises can be used to increase and improve ROM. These exercises focus on stretching and relaxing muscles, which helps to reduce stiffness and increase ROM in the affected joints. Some methods to help improve ROM include:
  - Static stretches: Exercises that involve stretching a muscle to its maximum point and holding the position for a period of time, which helps improve flexibility and increase joint range of motion.
  - Dynamic stretches: Active and controlled movements that move the joint through its full range of motion, helping to reduce muscle stiffness and improve joint range of motion.
  - Joint mobilization: Techniques performed by a trained therapist to apply passive and controlled movements to the joints to improve mobility and flexibility.
  - Proprioceptive neuromuscular facilitation (PNF) techniques: Methods that combine isometric contractions and passive movements to improve coordination and ROM in affected joints.
  - Controlled range of motion (ROM) exercises: Controlled movements in which the joint is moved to the limit of its ROM and held for a few seconds before returning to the starting position to gradually increase flexibility.
- *Benefits:* By improving ROM, people with Parkinson's disease can regain or maintain mobility in their joints, allowing greater freedom of movement and facilitating daily tasks and activities. In addition, improved ROM may reduce the risk of injury associated with muscle stiffness and limited range of motion.

Improve Passive and Active Joint Mobility

- *Explanation:* Passive joint mobility refers to the movement of a joint when it is moved by an external force, such as a therapist or a mobilization device. Active joint mobility, on the other hand, is the movement a joint can achieve on its own through voluntary muscle contraction. Parkinson's disease can affect both forms of mobility because of loss of motor control and muscle stiffness.

- *Useful tools:* Specific exercises that promote joint mobility, such as flexion, extension, rotation, and gliding movements, can be used to improve both passive and active joint mobility. Some tools for improving the quality of joint mobility include:
  - Manual therapy: Techniques used by healthcare professionals, such as physical and occupational therapists, to manipulate and mobilize joints and soft tissues to improve movement quality and reduce stiffness.
  - Postural self-correction exercises: Activities that allow patients to become aware of their posture and make adjustments to improve alignment and movement quality.
  - Pulley and elastic band therapy: These devices are used to provide controlled resistance and assistance to joint movements, facilitating mobility improvement and muscle strength development.
  - Assisted active mobilization exercises: Movements performed by the patient with the assistance of a therapist or device to improve coordination and quality of movement.
  - Mirror therapy: A method that uses the visual illusion of a mirror to improve perception and control of movement in affected limbs, potentially leading to improved mobility.
- *Benefits:* Improving the quality of joint mobility promotes greater coordination and precision in movement, resulting in increased functional independence. In addition, improved passive joint mobility can make it easier for therapists to work with patients, resulting in more effective therapy.

Proprioceptive and Balance and Stability Improvement

- *Explanation:* Proprioception is the sense that allows us to perceive the position, movement, and orientation of our body in space. In Parkinson's disease, decreased proprioception can lead to problems with balance and stability. Therapeutic exercise, especially exercises that involve sensorimotor activities, has the potential to improve proprioception by stimulating sensory receptors in muscles, joints, and tendons.
- *Useful tools:* Therapeutic exercise may include specific exercises that challenge proprioception, such as working on unstable surfaces, single-leg balance exercises, or movements that require more precise coordination. Some tools that can help improve proprioception, balance, and stability include:
  - Unstable platform: Using an unstable platform, such as a cushion or balance board, to perform balance exercises while standing or sitting.
  - Bosu or balance hemisphere: Exercises on an inflatable hemisphere known as a bosu, which provides an additional challenge for stability and control of movement.

- Single-leg exercises: Perform balance and strengthening exercises on one leg to improve proprioception and strength.
- Sensory training: Incorporating exercises that stimulate the senses, such as closing your eyes while performing a balance exercise, to increase body awareness.
- Coordination exercises: Performing coordinated movements and specific sequences that require good proprioceptive control.
- Virtual reality (VR) and augmented reality (AR): Using virtual reality or augmented reality devices to perform balance and coordination exercises in virtual environments, providing an immersive and stimulating experience to improve proprioception.
- Interactive balance platforms: Interactive platforms that connect to a mobile device or computer to perform balance and proprioceptive control exercises while receiving real-time performance data.
- Exercise video games: Exercise video games that require precise movement and balance to stimulate proprioception while having fun.
- Motion sensors: Use motion sensors placed on different parts of the body to monitor and improve posture, balance, and alignment during exercise.

• *Benefits:* By improving proprioception and sensory control, people with Parkinson's can experience significant improvements in balance and stability in both static and dynamic situations. This can reduce the risk of falls and help patients perform daily activities with greater confidence and safety.

Increased Walking Speed and Stride Length; Reduced Freezing of Gait Episodes

• *Explanation:* In Parkinson's disease, there is a change in the function of the basal ganglia, which affects the initiation and coordination of movement. This can result in a slow gait, short steps, and in some cases, freezing of gait episodes (moments when the patient feels that the feet are stuck to the ground and has difficulty moving forward).
• *Useful tools:* Therapeutic exercise may include gait training programs specifically designed to improve walking speed and stride length. In addition, incorporating endurance and flexibility exercises can promote smoothness and coordination of movement while walking. Some tools that can help improve walking speed and stride length include:

- Walking to the rhythm of music: Walking to the beat of music can help improve gait cadence and fluidity.
- Cone or step markers: Placing cones or step markers on the floor at a set distance for the patient to walk past encourages wider strides and increased speed.
- Zigzag walking: Creating a zigzag path that requires changes in direction, which can help improve agility as the ability to turn while walking.

- Assisted treadmill walking: Using a treadmill with a support and assistance system to train for faster and longer strides.
- Hip and ankle mobility exercises: Incorporates specific exercises to improve hip and ankle mobility, allowing for a greater range of motion while walking.
- Gait vibrating belt: A wearable device placed around the waist that provides rhythmic vibrations to help maintain gait rhythm and speed.
- Walking exoskeletons: Lightweight and wearable exoskeletons that conform to the body and assist with hip and leg movements during walking.
- Noninvasive brain stimulation: The use of noninvasive brain stimulation, such as transcranial direct current stimulation (tDCS) or transcranial magnetic stimulation (TMS), to improve brain plasticity and motor function in people with Parkinson's disease.
- Mixed reality walking games: Applications that combine virtual reality with physical reality, where patients interact with virtual objects while walking, promoting a more active and fluid gait.

• *Benefits:* By increasing walking speed and stride length, Parkinson's patients can experience a smoother and safer gait. This can significantly reduce the frequency and severity of gait freezes, improving overall independence and quality of life.

Increased Reaction Speed

• *Explanation:* Physiologically, the increased reaction speed observed with exercise in Parkinson's patients is due to several factors. During exercise, there is greater neuronal activation in brain areas responsible for coordination and motor response, such as the cerebellum and motor cortex. In addition, exercise promotes the release of neurotransmitters such as dopamine, which plays a critical role in modulating movement speed and precision.

• *Useful tools:* To improve reaction time, specific exercises that promote coordination and agility can be used. Examples of useful tools include:

  - Arm and leg coordination exercises: Activities that involve coordinating arm and leg movements simultaneously can improve agility and reaction time. For example, performing cross-pattern movements with arms and legs, such as touching the right foot with the left hand and vice versa.
  - Obstacle course walking: Placing low obstacles in the way while walking can stimulate quick decision-making and movement adaptation. Walking safely around or over the obstacles improves agility and speed of movement.
  - Agility exercises: Using cones, tape, or hoops to mark a course with rapid changes in direction can be very effective in improving agility and reaction time.
  - Reaction games: Games that require quick and accurate responses, such as throwing and catching a ball, making quick movements in response to visual or auditory cues, or simulation games with changing stimuli can be excellent tools for training reaction speed.

- Explosive strength training: Incorporating explosive strength exercises, such as vertical jumps, lateral jumps, or plyometric exercises, can improve rapid reaction and force generation in fast movements.
- Gait speed training: Conducting specific sessions to improve gait speed can be beneficial. Visual or auditory feedback can be used to adjust pace and gradually increase speed.
- Interactive games and mobile applications: Many mobile applications and video games are specifically designed to improve agility and reaction time. These games can be tailored to the individual needs of the patient and provide an entertaining way to perform therapeutic exercises.
- Motion sensors and wearable devices: Using wearable devices with motion sensors, such as smartwatches or activity wristbands, to monitor and measure reaction speed during exercise. These devices can provide real-time feedback and allow for accurate progress tracking.
- Biofeedback training: The use of biofeedback devices that help patients visualize and better understand their performance during exercise. For example, sensors that detect movement and provide real-time information on reaction speed and movement accuracy.
- Exergaming: The combination of physical exercise and interactive video games. Specialized platforms and devices allow patients to participate in games that require quick and coordinated movements while engaging in physical activity.
- Interactive training systems: Using interactive projections on walls or screens to create challenges that require quick decision-making and motor responses in real time.

• *Benefits:* Increased reaction time facilitates the performance of daily tasks, reduces the risk of falls, and improves functional independence in people with Parkinson's disease. In addition, the stimulation of neural pathways associated with fast responses helps maintain brain plasticity and counteract cognitive decline associated with the disease.

Better Activation of Mitochondrial Oxidative Pathways During Endurance Exercise, Which Reduces Autophagy and Activates MTOR (Mammalian Target of Rapamycin) Pathways

• *Explanation:* Physiologically, endurance training induces beneficial changes in mitochondrial function in Parkinson's patients. Mitochondria are cellular organelles responsible to produce energy in form of adenosine triphosphate (ATP) through the oxidation of nutrients. With aging and certain health conditions, such as Parkinson's disease, mitochondrial function can be compromised, leading to

increased autophagy, a process by which cells break down and recycle damaged or dysfunctional cellular components.
Long-term endurance exercise increases energy demand and stimulates the activity of mitochondrial oxidative pathways. This leads to an improvement in mitochondrial function and a reduction in cellular autophagy. In addition, resistance training also activates MTOR pathways, which are critical for cell growth and protein synthesis, promoting maintenance and repair of muscle and neural tissue [2].

- *Useful tools:* To promote the activation of mitochondrial oxidative pathways and MTOR pathways, progressive resistance training can be used. It is important that the training program is progressive and personalized, considering the level of physical fitness and the specific needs of each patient. Some useful examples are:
  - Brisk walking or Nordic walking: Brisk walking or using Nordic walking poles can be an excellent option for activation of mitochondrial oxidative pathways. These exercises are low-impact and allow you to maintain a steady pace for an extended period, activating mitochondrial oxidative pathways and improving cardiovascular function.
  - Stationary cycling: Using a stationary bike is an effective way to exercise large muscles in the body, such as the legs and glutes, while maintaining sustained activity. This type of exercise helps stimulate mitochondrial function and improve cardiovascular endurance.
  - Swimming: Swimming is a low-impact, full-body option that can significantly improve cardiovascular endurance.
  - Treadmill or elliptical: These machines allow for a gradual increase in effort and can be adjusted to maintain a steady pace.
- *Benefits:* Improving mitochondrial function and reducing autophagy help maintain cellular health and protect neurons from oxidative stress associated with Parkinson's disease. In addition, resistance training strengthens muscles and improves functional capacity, resulting in greater independence and quality of life for patients affected by this neurodegenerative disease.

Enhanced Dopaminergic Function, Which Increases Dopamine Activity in the Brain

- *Explanation:* Physiologically, dopamine is a key neurotransmitter that plays a critical role in the coordination of movement, motor control, and cognitive functions. In Parkinson's disease, there is a decrease in dopaminergic neurons in certain regions of the brain, particularly in a structure known as the substantia nigra. This decrease leads to a reduction in the amount of dopamine available to transmit signals between neurons. Therapeutic exercise has been shown to be a beneficial stimulus for dopaminergic function because it promotes greater release of dopamine in the brain. When we exercise, we activate neural pathways associated with movement and coordination, leading to an increase in dopamine production and release.

- *Useful tools:* In this regard, exercises that activate mitochondrial oxidative pathways are prescribed at moderate to high intensity. It has also been observed that exercises involving wide and coordinated movements, such as dance, Tai Chi, and yoga, are beneficial for stimulating dopaminergic function.

Low Scores on the Unified Parkinson's Disease Rating Scale (UPDRS)

One of the highlighted benefits of exercise for people with Parkinson's disease is a reduction in scores on the Unified Parkinson's Disease Rating Scale (UPDRS), particularly on Parts 2 and 3 of the questionnaires. These findings suggest a reduction in disability experienced by patients with this neurodegenerative disease [3].

Preventing and Reducing the Risk of Falls

Parkinson's disease is associated with several motor impairments that significantly increase the risk of falls. These impairments, such as bradykinesia (slow movements), muscle rigidity, and balance problems, can compromise a patient's stability and make it difficult to perform daily activities safely. However, therapeutic exercise can address these physiological challenges and prevent falls. Regular exercise, especially balance, coordination, and strength training, has a positive effect on the neuromuscular system. Balance exercises stimulate and strengthen the neural connections between the brain and muscles responsible for balance and posture. Similarly, strength training promotes muscle strengthening and improves the ability of muscles to respond to challenging situations.

Reduced Dependency and Increased Patient Functionality

- *Explanation:* Another important benefit of therapeutic exercise is its ability to reduce dependence on daily activities and improve overall patient functionality. As disease progresses, patients may experience a decline in their ability to perform simple tasks, affecting their quality of life and autonomy. Exercise, by improving cardiovascular endurance and muscle strength, provides patients with the physical capacity to meet daily demands. In addition, exercise helps release neurotransmitters and endorphins in the brain, contributing to a sense of well-being and reducing symptoms of depression and anxiety that are common in Parkinson's patients.

- *Useful tools:*
  - Active therapies: Involve the use of movements and functional exercises that resemble activities of daily living, allowing the patient to improve their ability to perform these tasks.
  - Resistance therapies: Involve long-duration exercises such as walking, swimming, or cycling that improve cardiovascular endurance and lung capacity.

Improving Transfers

Parkinson's disease is closely associated with a decrease in the patient's ability to move, both actively and passively. This is manifested by several motor and non-motor symptoms characteristic of the disease. One of the primary goals for people with Parkinson's disease is to regain independence in their daily activities. This not only reduces the burden on their families, but also has a significant impact on their quality of life.

To better understand the importance of this independence in daily activities, we can refer to the term "transfers," which the International Classification of Functioning, Disability, and Health defines as the ability to move a person's body actively (with autonomy and independence), passively (where someone else performs the movement all the time), or mixed (where the patient receives partial assistance from another person). These transfers include position changes, such as moving from sitting to lying in bed, moving from one chair to another, moving from a wheelchair to a bed or another seat, and moving to the toilet or within a vehicle, among other essential activities of daily living [4].

The ability to perform these transfers effectively, especially active transfers, is critical to the independence and quality of life of people with Parkinson's disease. However, the degree of success in achieving this ability is influenced by the severity of the disease and the stage the patient is in, as well as the effectiveness of training the necessary skills to perform safe and efficient transfers that preserve the physical and mental integrity of the individual [5].

At this point, therapeutic exercises play a fundamental role in the recovery, restoration or substitution of motor functions and abilities that may have been affected by the disease. Training conditional physical abilities (strength, speed, flexibility, and endurance) and coordination abilities (coupling, differentiation, orientation, reaction, adaptation, rhythm, and balance) through dual-task methods (where mobility training is combined with cognition, such as walking while holding a conversation) significantly facilitates the ability to perform active transfers and ultimately improves the quality of life and independence of people with Parkinson's disease [6].

Improve Cognitive Abilities

- *Explanation:* Physical exercise stimulates several changes in the brain that promote cognitive enhancement. During exercise, blood flow to the brain increases, which improves oxygenation and the availability of nutrients essential for neuronal function. In addition, neurotrophins such as Brain-Derived Neurotrophic Factor (BDNF) are released, promoting the growth and connection of new neurons, especially in brain regions associated with learning and memory.
- *Useful tools*: To improve cognition in people with Parkinson's disease, exercises that combine mental stimulation with physical activity can be implemented. Useful tools include cognitive training programs during exercise, activities that require coordination and concentration, such as dancing or Tai Chi, and performing dual tasks that involve physical and cognitive actions simultaneously.
- *Benefits*: By improving cognitive abilities, people with Parkinson's disease may experience increased mental clarity, problem-solving skills, sustained attention, and information retention. These benefits not only impact patients' daily lives but can also contribute to greater autonomy and emotional well-being.

Increase in Neural Activity and Brain Volume

- *Explanation:* Regular physical activity promotes neuroplasticity, which refers to the brain's ability to adapt and reorganize itself structurally in response to experience and external stimuli. During exercise, different areas of the brain are activated, leading to the production and release of neurotransmitters and growth factors. This repeated and specific neuronal activity over time can result in increased brain volume and greater connectivity between different brain regions.
- *Useful tools*: To take advantage of these benefits, it is recommended that the exercise program include a variety of activities that stimulate different parts of the brain. Resistance training, along with balance and coordination exercises, are particularly useful for promoting neural activity in different brain areas.
- *Benefits*: Increasing neuronal activity and brain volume may have a positive effect on overall brain function in people with Parkinson's disease. Those who exercise regularly have been observed to show improvements in executive function, motor control, and memory, as well as increased resistance to the neurodegenerative effects associated with the disease. This brain plasticity may also contribute to the adaptation and compensation of areas affected by the pathology, helping to maintain functionality and independence in daily life.

Regulation of Neurotrophic Factors Responsible for Neuronal Proliferation and Survival

- *Explanation:* One of the notable benefits is the regulation of neurotrophic factors, which are intimately involved in neuronal proliferation and survival. Physiologically, neurotrophic factors are key proteins that play a critical role in the maintenance and function of nerve cells in the brain. Among the most prominent are BDNF and nerve growth factor (NGF). These proteins are responsible for stimulating the growth, survival, and maintenance of neurons, which is essential for the proper functioning of the nervous system.
  Therapeutic exercise triggers several beneficial physiological responses by activating and physically stimulating the body. During exercise, there is an increase in the metabolic and energetic demands of neuronal tissue, leading to an increased release of neurotrophic factors such as BDNF. This increased release of BDNF has been directly linked to promoting neuronal growth and survival, facilitating the formation of new synaptic connections, and protecting existing neurons.
- *Useful tools:* Doing moderate to high-intensity exercise that activate mitochondrial oxidative pathways (aerobic), such as walking, jogging, cycling, and swimming, has been shown to be particularly effective in stimulating the release of BDNF and other neurotrophic factors in the brain. In addition, resistance and strength training can also contribute to this neuronal stimulation by increasing the physical and energetic demands on the nervous system.
- *Benefit:* The ultimate benefit of regulating neurotrophic factors through exercise is to improve brain plasticity and protect neurons vulnerable to damage and degeneration, which are common features of Parkinson's disease. By promoting nerve cell survival and growth, therapeutic exercise helps preserve cognitive and motor function, slowing disease progression and improving quality of life for patients.

Competing Interests The author have no conflicts of interest to declare that are relevant to the content of this chapter.

References

1. Fox SH, Katzenschlager R, Lim SY, et al. The movement disorder society evidence-based medicine review update: treatments for the motor symptoms of Parkinson's disease. Mov Disord. 2011;26:2–41. https://doi.org/10.1002/mds.23829.
2. Oddo S. The role of mTOR signaling in Alzheimer disease. Front Biosci Schol. 2012;4(S):941–52. https://doi.org/10.2741/s310.
3. Fahn S, Elton RL. Unified Parkinson's disease rating scale (UPDRS). Encyclop Clin Neuropsychol. 2017;2:1–3.

4. World Health Organization. Clasificación internacional del funcionamiento de la discapacidad y de la salud: CIF: versión abreviada, Versión abreviada. 1st ed. Organización Mundial de la Salud; 2001. https://iris.who.int/handle/10665/43360
5. Echemendía del Valle A, Sentmanat Belisón A, Yumila Noa Pelier B, Gómez Pérez R. Programa de ejercicios para las transferencias y la marcha en los pacientes lesionados medulares. Rev PODIUM Rev Cienc Tecnol Cult Física. 2022;17:876–91.
6. Fritz NE, Cheek FM, Nichols-Larsen DS. Motor-cognitive dual-task training in persons with neurologic disorders: a systematic review. J Neurol Phys Ther. 2015;39:142–53.

Chapter 4
Guidelines for Safe Training

Initial Questions

- What is the impact of pharmacological interactions on the effectiveness and safety of treatments focused on therapeutic exercise for patients with neurodegenerative diseases, such as Parkinson's?
- Additionally, what is the relationship between deficits in dynamic and static stability and the quality of life of individuals affected by neurodegenerative diseases?
- Could therapeutic exercise help reduce the side effects of pharmacotherapy and improve static and dynamic stability in Parkinson's patients? Please provide your reasoning.

Consider the Pharmacological Interaction

It is important to consider the positive and negative pharmacologic interactions in Parkinson's patients when prescribing exercise. For example, there is evidence that therapeutic exercise combined with levodopa pharmacotherapy controls and reduces the motor signs and symptoms of Parkinson's disease. On the other hand, in certain situations, pharmacological treatment may be a factor that limits and/or delays the effectiveness of therapeutic exercise and some physical therapy procedures [1].

The most used drug for the treatment of Parkinson's disease is levodopa. It is crucial to consider the precise control of the pharmacological dosage, comparing what the patient is currently consuming with the medical dose prescribed by the specialist. Too much or too little, depending on the stage of the disease, could limit the beneficial effects of therapeutic exercise. When levodopa is taken appropriately in the early stages of the disease and combined with therapeutic exercise, it has been shown to significantly improve quality of life and safely reduce future motor disability [1].

C. A. A. Mejía, *Therapeutic Exercise for Parkinson's Disease and Related Disorders*, https://doi.org/10.1007/978-3-031-62119-2_4

Detailed knowledge of how long a person has lived with Parkinson's disease and the specific dosage of levodopa they have received are fundamental and critical factors in the prescription process for therapeutic exercise. In the early stages, proper administration of levodopa can help improve quality of life, relieve symptoms, and slow the progression of motor problems. In more advanced stages, however, controlling the dosage of levodopa becomes a challenge, as the body may develop tolerance to the medication and therapeutic effects may diminish over time.

The specific dosage of levodopa prescribed to the patient is a critical factor in determining functional capacity and the amount of energy available to participate in therapeutic exercise. An inadequate supply of levodopa may limit the patient's ability to perform certain physical activities or reduce the patient's motivation to participate in exercise programs. Conversely, too much levodopa can cause undesirable side effects, such as involuntary movements or dyskinesias, which can make it difficult to perform certain types of exercise or even be detrimental to the patient's overall health [2].

Therefore, when designing a therapeutic exercise program for a person with Parkinson's disease, the physician or health-care professional must carefully assess the time since diagnosis and the current dose of levodopa. This will allow for an accurate and safe adjustment of the exercise plan, considering the patient's individual needs and abilities, with the goal of improving overall well-being, mobility, and quality of life. It is important to emphasize that any change in levodopa dosage or exercise program should be made under appropriate medical supervision and guidance.

Below Figs. 4.1, 4.2, 4.3, 4.4, and 4.5 are the side effects and mechanisms of action of the most used medications for the treatment of Parkinson's disease. This important information must be considered when prescribing any type of active therapy, exercise, and/or training [3].

- **Key considerations when prescribing therapeutic exercise alongside dopamine agonists:**
  - *Synergistic benefits:*

    Exercise has also been associated with an increase in brain dopamine levels, which may complement the effects of dopamine agonists and enhance therapeutic benefits.

    Both dopamine agonists and exercise can improve motor function in people with Parkinson's disease. Dopamine agonists reduce muscle stiffness and bradykinesia, while regular exercise helps improve muscle strength, coordination, and balance, improving mobility and the ability to perform activities of daily living.

    Dopamine agonists may reduce neuronal degeneration and, when combined with exercise, which also promotes the release of neurotrophic factors, may improve nerve cell survival and function.

Therapeutic exercise may help improve Parkinson's symptoms, which may allow a reduction in the dosage of dopamine agonists or other medications used in the treatment.

Physical activity promotes the release of endorphins, which can improve emotional well-being, while medications help control both motor and non-motor symptoms associated with Parkinson's disease, contributing to overall well-being.

– *Detrimental effects:*

Intense exercise may interfere with the absorption or metabolism of dopamine agonists, which could alter their effectiveness or increase the risk of side effects. Therefore, it is important for the physician to adjust the medication dosage based on individual needs and changes in physical activity levels.

Some dopamine agonists can cause orthostatic hypotension (a drop in blood pressure when you stand up), and exercise can also affect blood pressure, especially in people who are sensitive to sudden changes. The combination of both interventions may require special attention to prevent falls or dizziness, especially in patients with preexisting cardiovascular problems.

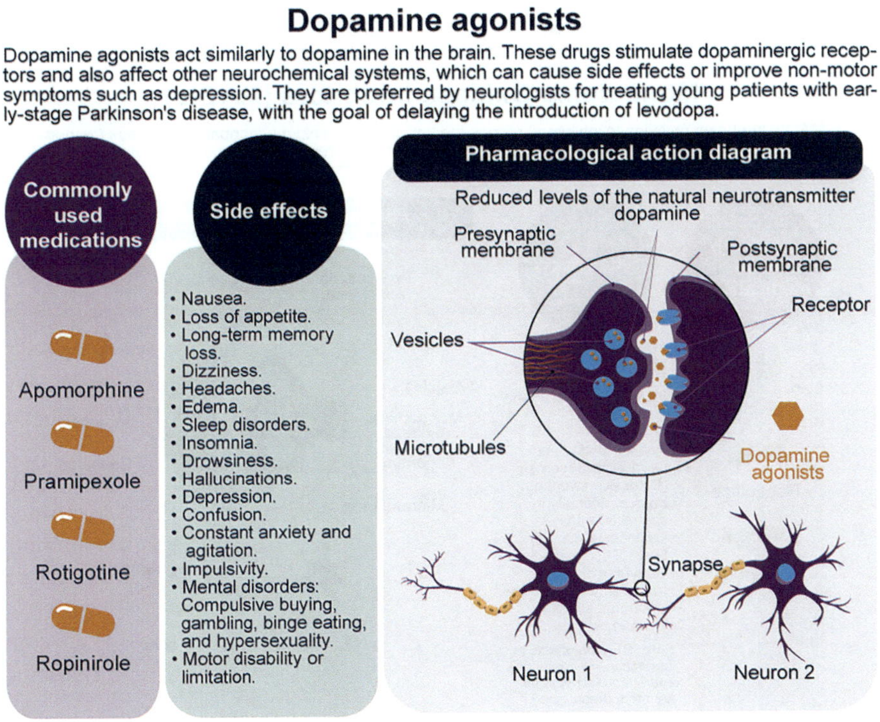

Fig. 4.1 Dopamine agonists (most used drugs, side effects, and pharmacological action diagram)

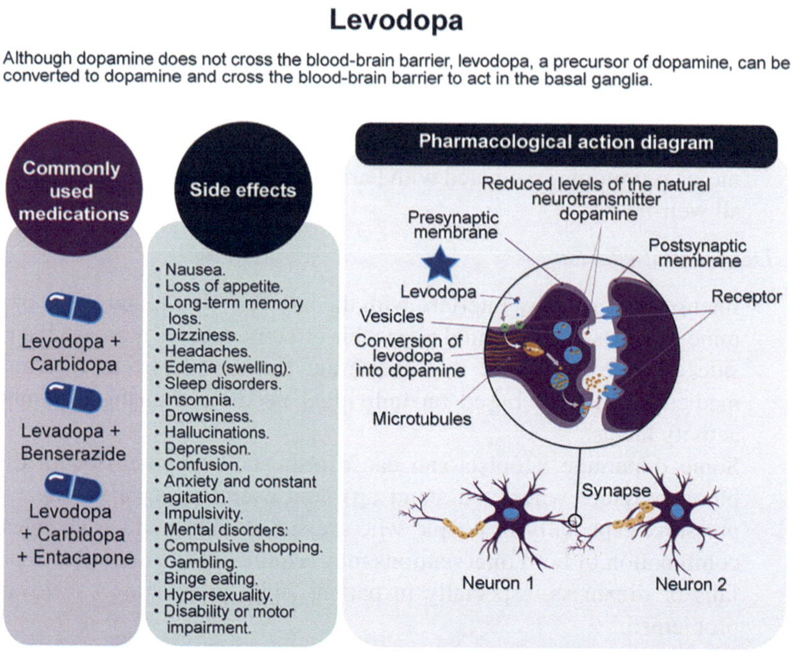

Fig. 4.2 Levodopa (most used drugs, side effects, and pharmacological action diagram)

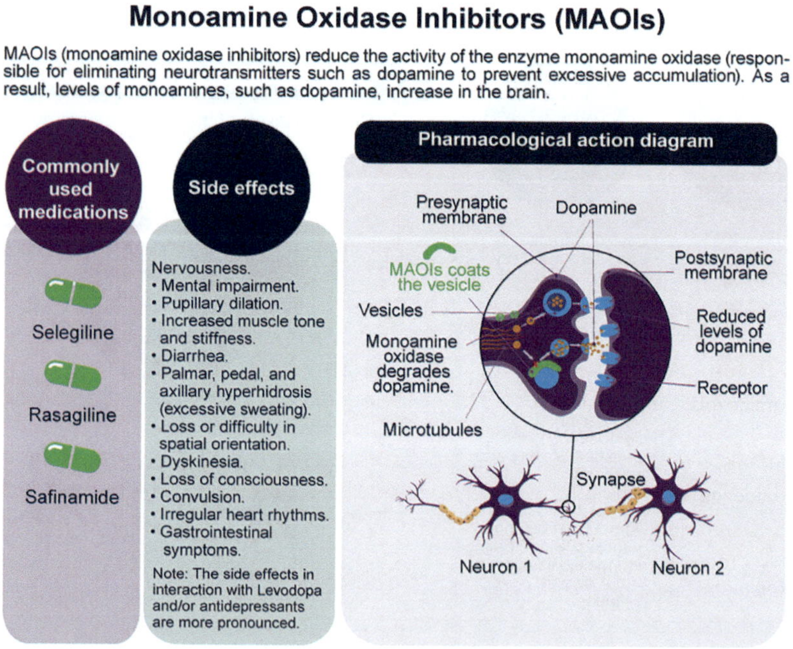

Fig. 4.3 Monoamine oxidase inhibitors—MAOIs (most commonly used drugs, side effects, and pharmacological action diagram)

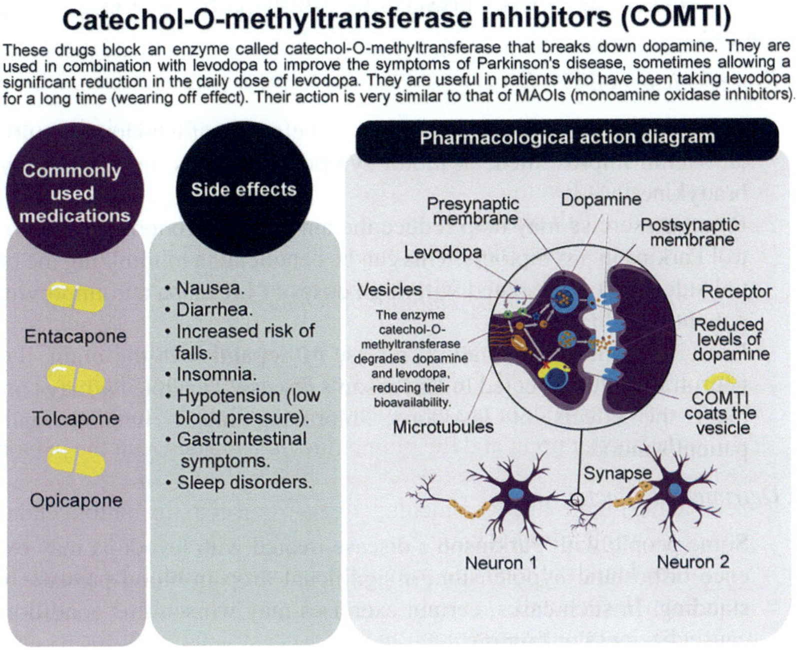

Fig. 4.4 Catechol-*O*-methyltransferase inhibitors (most commonly used drugs, side effects, and pharmacologic action diagram)

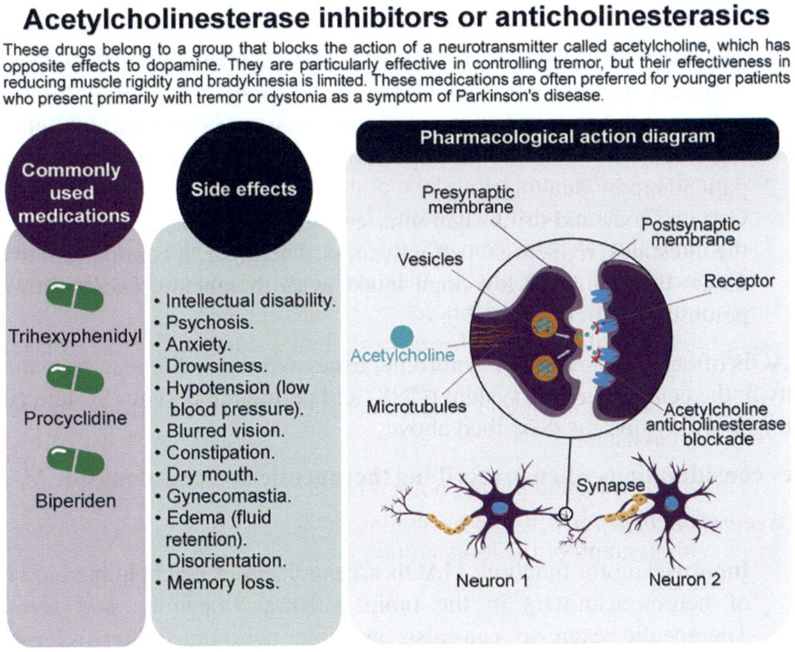

Fig. 4.5 Acetylcholinesterase inhibitors or anticholinesterasics (most commonly used drugs, side effects, and pharmacologic action diagram)

- **Key considerations when prescribing therapeutic exercise alongside levodopa:**
  - *Synergistic benefits:*

    Exercise can increase the absorption and efficacy of levodopa, resulting in an overall improvement in motor symptoms such as muscle rigidity and bradykinesia.

    Regular exercise may help reduce the amount of levodopa needed to control Parkinson's symptoms. This can be beneficial in minimizing the potential side effects associated with high doses of levodopa and improving the patient's quality of life.

    Exercise promotes the natural release of dopamine in the brain, the key neurotransmitter affected in Parkinson's disease. This release may complement the effects of levodopa, improving motor function and the patient's mood.

  - *Detrimental effects:*

    Some people with Parkinson's disease treated with levodopa may experience orthostatic hypotension, a significant drop in blood pressure when standing. In such cases, certain exercises may worsen this condition and cause dizziness or fainting.

    Fatigue is a common symptom of Parkinson's disease, and some patients may find that therapeutic exercise worsens their fatigue, especially when taking levodopa. In these cases, it is important to adjust the exercise routine to avoid excessive fatigue and to find the right balance between activity and rest.

    In advanced stages of Parkinson's disease, when mobility is severely impaired, the pharmacological dose of levodopa is increased. As a result, certain exercises may become difficult or unsafe to perform. In such cases, it is important to work with a specialized therapist to tailor exercises to the patient's individual needs.

    Certain foods and drinks can interfere with the absorption of levodopa in the intestines, reducing its effectiveness. Therefore, it is important to coordinate the timing of levodopa intake with therapeutic exercise to avoid potential conflicts.

MAOIs often cause serotonin syndrome; excessive serotonin neurotransmission activity in the central nervous system (CNS) and peripheral nervous system (PNS), resulting in the symptoms described above.

- **Key considerations when prescribing therapeutic exercise alongside MAOIs:**
  - *Synergistic benefits:*

    Improved motor function: MAOIs are medications that help increase levels of neurotransmitters in the brain, such as dopamine and serotonin. Therapeutic exercise can also promote neurotransmitter release and improve motor function in people with Parkinson's disease.

Reduced muscle stiffness: MAOIs may help reduce muscle stiffness by increasing dopamine levels in the brain, while therapeutic exercise may help maintain flexibility and reduce muscle stiffness through stretching and exercise.
Mood improvement: Both MAOIs and therapeutic exercise may have a positive effect on the mood of people with Parkinson's disease. MAOIs increase serotonin levels, which can improve emotional well-being, and exercise releases endorphins, which have a positive effect on mood.
Neuroplastic stimulation: Therapeutic exercise stimulates brain plasticity, by promoting the formation of new neural connections, which may complement the effects of MAOIs.

– *Detrimental effects:*

  Interactions with certain foods: MAOIs may interact with foods rich in tyramine, such as aged cheeses, cured meats, and red wine, which may trigger a hypertensive crisis. It is important for patients or caregivers to inform prescribers about this.
  Risk of hypertension: MAOIs may increase blood pressure, and therapeutic exercise may temporarily increase blood pressure during activity.
  Drug interaction: MAOIs may interact dangerously with other medications, including some antidepressants and medications for other conditions. Patients should tell their doctor about all medications they are taking before starting treatment with MAOIs or a therapeutic exercise program.
  MAOI side effects: MAOIs may cause side effects such as nausea, dizziness, insomnia, and confusion. It is important to assess the patient's tolerance to these medications and adjust the dosage as necessary to avoid adverse effects during exercise, physical activity, or training.

- **Key considerations when prescribing therapeutic exercise alongside catechol-o-methyltransferase inhibitors:**

  – *Synergistic benefits:*

    Improved motor control: Catechol-O-methyltransferase inhibitors (COMT inhibitors) are drugs that increase dopamine availability in the brain, which may complement the beneficial effects of exercise in improving motor control in Parkinson's disease patients.
    Potentiation of treatment effects: Combining COMT inhibitors with therapeutic exercise can enhance the effects of pharmacological treatment, resulting in greater reductions in motor symptoms such as tremor and rigidity.
    Cognitive benefits: Regular physical activity has been shown to improve cognitive function in Parkinson's patients. Combining this activity with COMT inhibitors, which may also have beneficial effects on brain function, may provide a synergistic effect in cognitive improvement.

- *Detrimental effects:*

  Pharmacologic interactions: COMT inhibitors) may interact with other medications the patient is taking for Parkinson's disease or other medical conditions. Caution should be exercised and doses should be adjusted appropriately to avoid adverse effects during therapeutic exercise.
  Risk of orthostatic hypotension: Both exercise and COMT inhibitors can lower blood pressure. When combined, there is an increased risk of orthostatic hypotension (low blood pressure while standing), which may increase the risk of falls and injury in patients.
  Side effects: COMT inhibitors may cause side effects such as nausea, vomiting, and diarrhea. Exercise, especially vigorous exercise, may exacerbate these side effects and affect tolerability and adherence.

• **Key considerations when prescribing therapeutic exercise alongside anticholinesterasics:**

- *Synergistic benefits:*

  Potentiation of neuroprotection: Acetylcholinesterase inhibitors have demonstrated neuroprotective effects in preclinical models of Parkinson's disease by reducing the death of dopaminergic neurons. Therapeutic exercise has also been shown to be neuroprotective and may complement these effects, resulting in enhanced neuronal protection in Parkinson's patients.
  Control of motor and non-motor symptoms: The combination of acetylcholinesterase inhibitors and exercise may lead to a general improvement in motor symptoms, such as rigidity and bradykinesia, and non-motor symptoms, such as depression and anxiety. This synergy may contribute to an improved quality of life for patients.

- *Detrimental effects:*

  Cardiovascular problems: Some Parkinson's patients receiving acetylcholinesterase inhibitors may experience hypotension. In such cases, it is important to perform therapeutic exercise under appropriate supervision and to avoid intense exertion that may increase cardiovascular risk.
  Fragility and risk of falls: Parkinson's patients may be more prone to falls due to motor symptoms and postural instability. When acetylcholinesterase inhibitors are combined with physical exercise, especially exercises that require balance and coordination, the potential risk of falls should be considered and the exercise program should be adjusted based on the individual patient's abilities.
  Drug interactions: Acetylcholinesterase inhibitors may interact with other medications the patient is taking for Parkinson's disease or coexisting medical conditions. Close monitoring and dose adjustment may be necessary to avoid adverse interactions.

Other Pharmacotherapeutic Agents Used

1. **Amantadine:** Amantadine is a drug with antiviral properties that was originally developed to combat certain types of viruses, specifically influenza type A. However, during its clinical use, it was found to have a moderate but beneficial effect in the treatment of Parkinson's disease. In addition, it has been observed to have a notable effect in reducing dyskinesias, which are involuntary and troublesome movements associated with prolonged levodopa therapy in Parkinson's patients.

   (a) *Pharmacokinetics:* The pharmacokinetics of amantadine include its absorption, distribution, metabolism, and excretion in the body. Quantitative data on these aspects are presented below:

   - Absorption: Amantadine is rapidly absorbed after oral administration. It reaches peak plasma concentration approximately 2–4 h after ingestion. The oral bioavailability of amantadine is close to 90%, meaning that most of the administered drug reaches the bloodstream and is available to exert its therapeutic effects.
   - Distribution: Amantadine has a large volume of distribution, suggesting widespread distribution in the tissues of the body. Approximately 50% of the drug binds to plasma proteins, while the remaining 50% is in a free and active form to exert its pharmacological action.
   - Metabolism: Amantadine is metabolized primarily in the liver, where it undergoes hydroxylation to form inactive metabolites. The primary metabolite formed is 1-adamantylamine, which is considered less active than the original amantadine. This metabolite is excreted in the urine along with unchanged amantadine.
   - Elimination: Amantadine and its metabolites are primarily eliminated by the kidneys. Approximately 90% of the administered drug is excreted in the urine in unchanged form or as inactive metabolites within the first 24–48 h after administration. The elimination half-life of amantadine varies on average from 10 to 14 h in individuals with normal renal function.

It is important to note that patients with renal impairment may have prolonged elimination of amantadine, which may require dose adjustments to avoid accumulation and potential adverse effects. Understanding these pharmacokinetic parameters is critical to understanding the dynamics of the drug in the body and determining the appropriate dosage in the treatment of Parkinson's disease and other conditions in which amantadine is used. This detailed knowledge allows health-care professionals to design an optimal and safe therapeutic regimen for patients, ensuring better efficacy and minimizing the risk of side effects [2, 3].

   (b) *Mechanism of action:* The exact mechanism of action of amantadine in the treatment of Parkinson's disease is not fully understood. However, it has been proposed that its therapeutic effect may be related to its ability to increase dopamine release in certain areas of the central nervous system and to block dopamine reuptake. This may improve dopaminergic function and help alleviate the characteristic symptoms of Parkinson's disease and reduce the dyskinesias caused by prolonged levodopa use.

(c) *Contraindications:* The prescription of amantadine is contraindicated in patients with a known allergy to the drug or those who have experienced severe adverse reactions to its use in the past. In addition, caution should be exercised in patients with severe or moderate renal insufficiency, as amantadine is mainly eliminated through the kidneys and its accumulation could increase the risk of side effects.

(d) *Side effects:* As with any drug, amantadine may cause side effects in some patients. The most common side effects include dizziness, drowsiness, insomnia, dry mouth, and gastrointestinal disturbances such as nausea and constipation. In some cases, psychiatric effects such as agitation, hallucinations, and confusion have been reported.

(e) *Key considerations when prescribing therapeutic exercise:*

- Interaction with exercise: Amantadine has a relatively short half-life and its elimination is primarily through the kidneys. Exercise may affect blood circulation and renal function, which could affect the rate of elimination of the drug. If the patient engages in intense and prolonged exercise, it may accelerate the elimination of amantadine, thereby affecting its concentration in the body. Therefore, it is important to consider how physical activity may alter the pharmacokinetics of amantadine and, if necessary, adjust the dosage or timing of drug administration.
- Potential for side effects: Amantadine may cause side effects such as dizziness or drowsiness. If therapeutic exercise involves activities that require a high degree of alertness or coordination, it is important to be aware of the potential sedative effects of amantadine. If a patient experiences excessive drowsiness, it may be dangerous to perform certain physical activities during this time.
- Optimize therapeutic response: Understanding the pharmacokinetics of amantadine helps to maximize its therapeutic effect. By knowing its half-life and duration of action, health-care professionals can suggest the best time to administer the medication in relation to exercise sessions. This ensures that the patient receives the maximum benefit from both treatments: amantadine to control Parkinson's symptoms and therapeutic exercise to improve motor function and quality of life.
- Assessment of patient tolerability: By knowing the pharmacokinetic parameters, health-care professionals can be alert to any unexpected changes in the patient's response to amantadine and therapeutic exercise. If unusual side effects or lack of improvement in symptoms are observed, a review of the dosing regimen or exercise intensity may be considered.

2. **Continuous pharmacological infusion:** Continuous pharmacological infusion has emerged as a highly effective strategy for the treatment of advanced Parkinson's disease, particularly in patients with complex motor fluctuations and severe dyskinesias. This therapy utilizes drug delivery systems through infusion pumps that allow for continuous dopaminergic stimulation, significantly improving motor fluctuations and dyskinesias [2, 3].

   (a) Benefits demonstrated in clinical trials: Clinical trials have demonstrated the efficacy of this therapy by significantly reducing the time that symptoms are present, allowing for the reduction or even elimination of other antiparkinsonian medications that may cause unwanted side effects.
   (b) Available systems: Currently, two continuous pharmacological infusion systems are available for the treatment of Parkinson's disease:

      - Subcutaneous apomorphine infusion: This system continuously delivers apomorphine, a dopaminergic agonist, through a programmable syringe pump and subcutaneous needle. Despite its benefits, it is important to note that it has side effects similar to those of dopaminergic agonists. In addition, regular erythrocyte monitoring is required and adequate patient education is necessary to avoid subcutaneous nodules at the puncture site. However, it is important to mention that apomorphine infusion is contraindicated in patients with dementia or severe psychiatric disorders.
      - Intraduodenal levodopa infusion: This system continuously delivers levodopa directly into the duodenum through a gastrostomy tube and a programmable syringe pump. Side effects are similar to oral levodopa, and this treatment is not appropriate for patients with severe dementia.

   (c) *Key considerations when prescribing therapeutic exercise:*

      - Improved quality of life: Continuous pharmacological infusion therapy can significantly reduce motor symptoms and fluctuations, allowing patients to participate in exercise more effectively and comfortably, thereby improving their quality of life.
      - Less interference with daily activities: By reducing motor symptoms, infusion therapy can facilitate the patient's participation in physical activities and exercises without the limitations and obstacles that may have been present with previous treatments.
      - Reduced medication burden: The efficacy of continuous infusion therapy may lead to the reduction or elimination of other antiparkinsonian medications, thereby reducing the possibility of drug interactions with prescribed exercise.
      - Improved mobility: Infusion therapy can improve motor function, making it easier for the patient to perform exercises that may have previously been difficult due to stiffness and other Parkinson's symptoms.
      - Coordination and balance: By reducing motor fluctuations, infusion therapy can improve a patient's coordination and balance, increasing the safety and effectiveness of prescribed exercises.

(d) *Potential side effects:*

- Drowsiness and dizziness: Both infusion therapy and some antiparkinsonian medications can cause drowsiness and dizziness. It is important to consider these effects when prescribing exercises that require alertness and coordination.
- Fatigue: Some patients may experience fatigue as a side effect of continuous infusion therapy. Health-care professionals should consider this when designing exercise programs that do not overload the patient.
- Nausea and gastrointestinal disturbances: Intraduodenal levodopa infusion may cause gastrointestinal effects similar to oral levodopa. It is important to consider these potential effects when prescribing plyometric and/or high-intensity exercise to avoid discomfort or additional complications.

3. **Pharmacologic treatment of non-motor symptoms**: Non-motor symptoms of Parkinson's disease can have a significant impact on patients' long-term quality of life. These symptoms include a variety of disorders, including sleep disturbances, autonomic dysfunction, mood and behavioral changes, cognitive impairment, and other symptoms such as pain, fatigue, and drooling. Treatment of these symptoms is individualized for each patient and may involve the use of different medications based on specific needs [2, 3].

(a) *Sleep disturbances:* Benzodiazepines such as clonazepam, which have been shown to be effective in improving sleep quality and relieving insomnia, may be used to treat sleep disturbances in people with Parkinson's disease. Clonazepam works by increasing the activity of gamma-aminobutyric acid (GABA) in the brain, producing a calming and relaxing effect that helps improve sleep. Common side effects of clonazepam include daytime drowsiness, dizziness, memory and coordination problems, and in rare cases, dependence when used for long periods of time.

- *Important considerations when prescribing therapeutic exercise:* Exercise planning should consider times of day when the patient is more alert and less likely to experience drowsiness to ensure safe and effective participation in exercise sessions.

(b) *Depression and anxiety:* Treatment of depression and anxiety in Parkinson's disease often involves the use of antidepressants such as selective serotonin reuptake inhibitors (SSRIs), which have been shown to be effective in relieving depressive symptoms and reducing anxiety. SSRIs increase serotonin levels in the brain, which helps to improve mood and reduce anxiety. SSRIs can cause side effects such as nausea, insomnia, agitation, and in some cases, decreased libido.

- *Important considerations when prescribing therapeutic exercise:* Regular exercise has been associated with improved mood and reduced anxiety overall, but potential additional effects should be monitored in each patient, as the combination of exercise and medication could potentiate or alter the therapeutic response.

(c) *Psychotic symptoms:* In cases where psychotic symptoms are present, antipsychotics such as quetiapine may be used to control the psychosis. However, it is important to note that some antipsychotics can cause parkinsonism as a side effect, so the risk-benefit ratio should be carefully assessed before administration. For example, quetiapine is an antipsychotic that works by blocking dopamine and serotonin receptors in the brain, helping to control psychotic symptoms, but it can cause drowsiness, dizziness, weight gain, and in some cases may increase the risk of type 2 diabetes.

- *Important considerations when prescribing therapeutic exercise:* It is crucial to consider the potential side effects, such as drowsiness or sedation, that can affect the ability to engage in physical activity. Furthermore, it is essential to monitor the development of extrapyramidal effects resulting from the interaction between the antipsychotic and exercise, and adjust the exercise plan accordingly to ensure the safety and effectiveness of the treatment.

(d) *Treatment of sialorrhea and dystonia:* In certain cases of sialorrhea and dystonia, botulinum toxin may be an effective treatment option, as it can reduce excessive saliva production and alleviate muscular dystonia in selected areas. Botulinum toxin works by blocking the release of acetylcholine at nerve endings, which relaxes muscles and reduces excessive saliva production in sialorrhea and improves dystonia. Side effects of botulinum toxin are generally mild and include pain at the injection site, temporary muscle weakness and, in rare cases, allergic reactions.

- *Key considerations when prescribing therapeutic exercise:* It is important to consider the effect of toxin injection on muscle function. Depending on the site of toxin application, certain movements and specific exercises may require precautions to avoid interference or potential complications.

Experimental Stage Drugs

1. **Immunotherapy with antibodies targeting the alpha-synuclein protein:** Alpha-synuclein protein plays a critical role in Parkinson's disease by abnormally accumulating in nerve cells and forming protein aggregates known as Lewy bodies, which are characteristic of the disease. Immunological approaches aim to use antibodies to specifically target and eliminate these abnormal alpha-synuclein accumulations.

   (a) *Promising benefits:*

   - Reduce the accumulation of alpha-synuclein protein in the brain.
   - Slowing or halting disease progression.

2. **Cell therapy based on cell use and/or modification:** This approach involves using cells to replace or repair damaged brain cells in Parkinson's patients. It may involve introducing stem cells or genetically modified cells to produce and release neurotrophic factors (substances that promote the growth and survival of nerve cells) to protect and support affected neurons.

   (a) *Promising benefits:*

   - Restore neuronal function and neurotransmitter production.
   - Halt or reverse neurological decline.

3. **Gene therapy, which involves genetic modification:** Gene therapy aims to correct or replace faulty or altered genes that contribute to the development of Parkinson's disease. In the context of this disease, gene therapy could be used to increase the production of neurotrophic factors or reduce the synthesis of toxic proteins such as alpha-synuclein.

   (a) *Promising benefits:*

   - Reduce neuronal toxicity and protect neurons.
   - Slowing or halting the progression of Parkinson's disease.

Beware of Deficits in Dynamic and Static Stability

Dynamic and static stability are among the abilities that are most commonly impaired in Parkinson's disease patients, predisposing them to higher morbidity and mortality due to the risk of falls. Balance is affected differently at each stage of the disease (stages I, II, III, IV, V, and VI). As Parkinson's disease progresses, the loss of cholinergic inputs to the thalamus increases, leading to the death of dopaminergic neurons and affecting cortical circuits, causing changes in postural tone, increased muscle and joint stiffness, bradykinesia, dyskinesia, and ultimately loss of dynamic and/or static stability [4].

Therapeutic Objectives to Improve Dynamic and Static Stability

Below are some important aspects of stability that need to be strengthened and addressed in people with Parkinson's disease. Figures 4.6 to 4.17 and Table 4.1 present therapeutic exercises designed to improve static balance, anticipatory responses, dynamic stability, and postural alignment.

To Improve Static Stability in the Bipedal Stance Through Sensorimotor and/or Proprioceptive Exercises

Examples:
See Fig. 4.6.

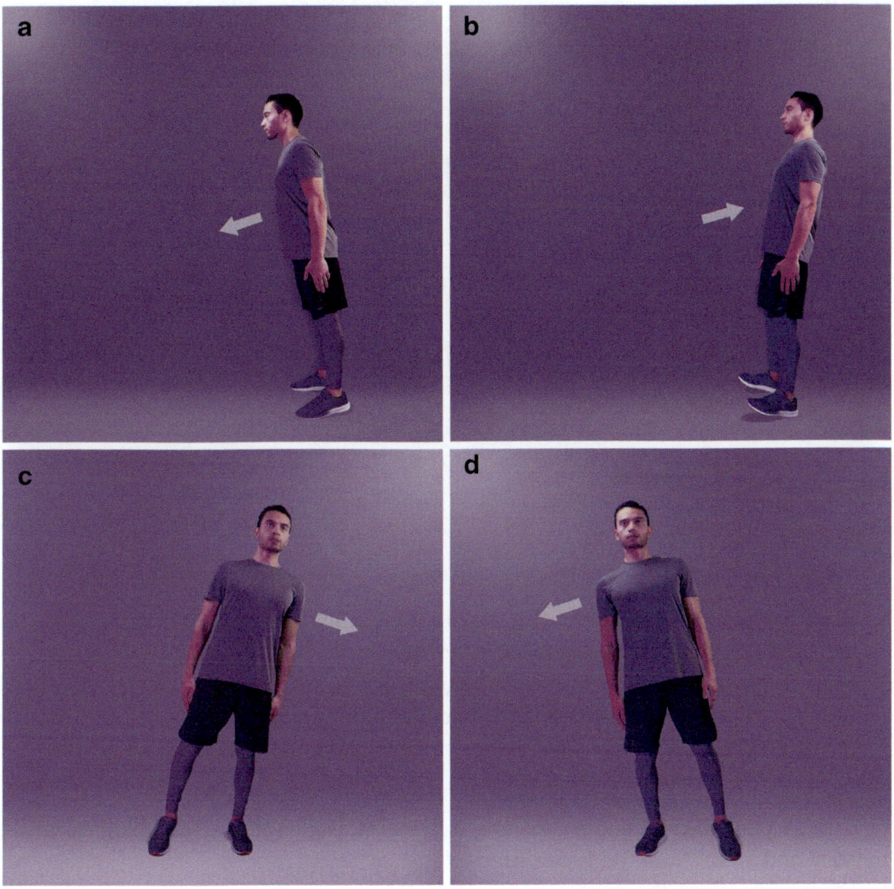

Fig. 4.6 Exercise to regain stability in the bipedal stance

(a) **Forward tilt:** Lean forward slightly and quickly regain stability (this can be achieved by taking a step forward or returning to the starting position with the torso upright).
(b) **Back ward tilt:** Lean back slightly and quickly regain stability (this can be achieved by taking a step back or by returning to the starting position with the torso upright).
(c) **Left lateral tilt:** Lean slightly to the left and quickly regain stability (this can be achieved by taking a left side step or returning to the starting position with the torso upright).
(d) **Right lateral tilt:** Lean slightly to the right and quickly regain stability (this can be accomplished with a right-side step or by returning to the starting position with the torso upright)

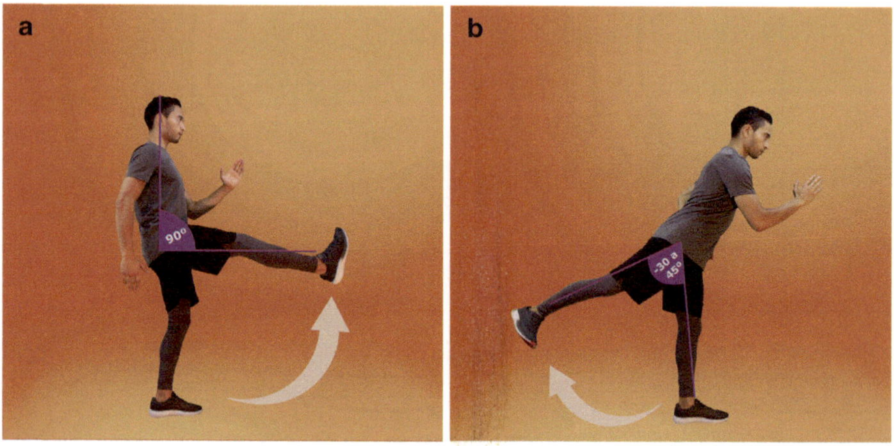

Fig. 4.7 Single-leg balancing

See Fig. 4.7.

Steps to perform the exercise:

- **Step 1:** Balance on one leg with the other leg fully extended, flexing the hip to a 90° angle. Proceed immediately to Step 2.
- **Step 2:** Balance on one leg with the other leg fully extended, aiming to extend the hip to about −45° if possible. Immediately return to Step 1 with a forward leg balance. Continue to alternate between forward and backward balancing.

See Fig. 4.8.

Tree Pose, also known as Vrksasana in Sanskrit, is a yoga pose that helps improve balance and strength in the lower limbs.

Steps to perform the pose:

- Stand upright with feet together and arms at your sides.
- Shift the weight to the right foot and rotate the left knee outward (hip outward rotation), placing the sole of the left foot on the inside of the right thigh. If it is not possible to place the foot on the thigh, it can rest on the calf or ankle, avoiding the knee.
- Hold the hands at the center of the chest in a prayer position (Namaste) or extend them above the head.
- Keep your eyes on a steady point in front of you to maintain balance.
- Maintain this position for several deep breaths, maintaining both balance and focus.
- Repeat the process on the opposite side.

Note:

- Remember to maintain a steady breath and not to worry if it is difficult to maintain balance at first. With practice, improvement in Tree Pose is possible.

See Fig. 4.9.

Steps to perform the exercise:

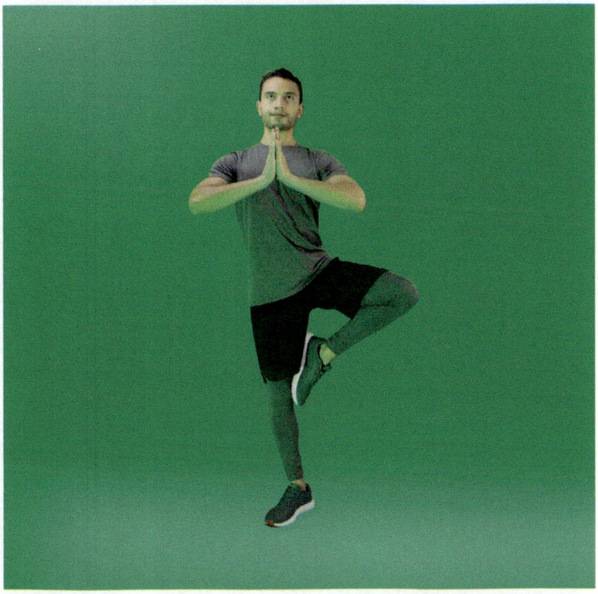

Fig. 4.8 Tree pose

(a) **Step 1**

- Starting position: Stand in a bipedal stance with your right foot straight ahead and your left foot positioned so that the heel of your right foot touches the tip of your left foot.
- Hold an object (such as a marker) with your left hand and keep your eyes on it throughout the exercise.
- With arm fully extended, flex left shoulder to 90°.

(b) **Step 2**

- Maintain balance in starting position.
- Lower left arm to 45° of shoulder flexion.
- Continue to follow the object with your eyes.

(c) **Step 3**

- Maintain balance in starting position.
- Perform 90° of left shoulder flexion and keep arm extended.
- Adduct the left shoulder horizontally and rotate the torso slightly in the same direction.
- Follow the object with your eyes.

(d) **Step 4**

- Maintain balance in starting position.
- Abduct the left shoulder horizontally and rotate the torso slightly in the same direction.
- Continue to follow the object with your eyes.

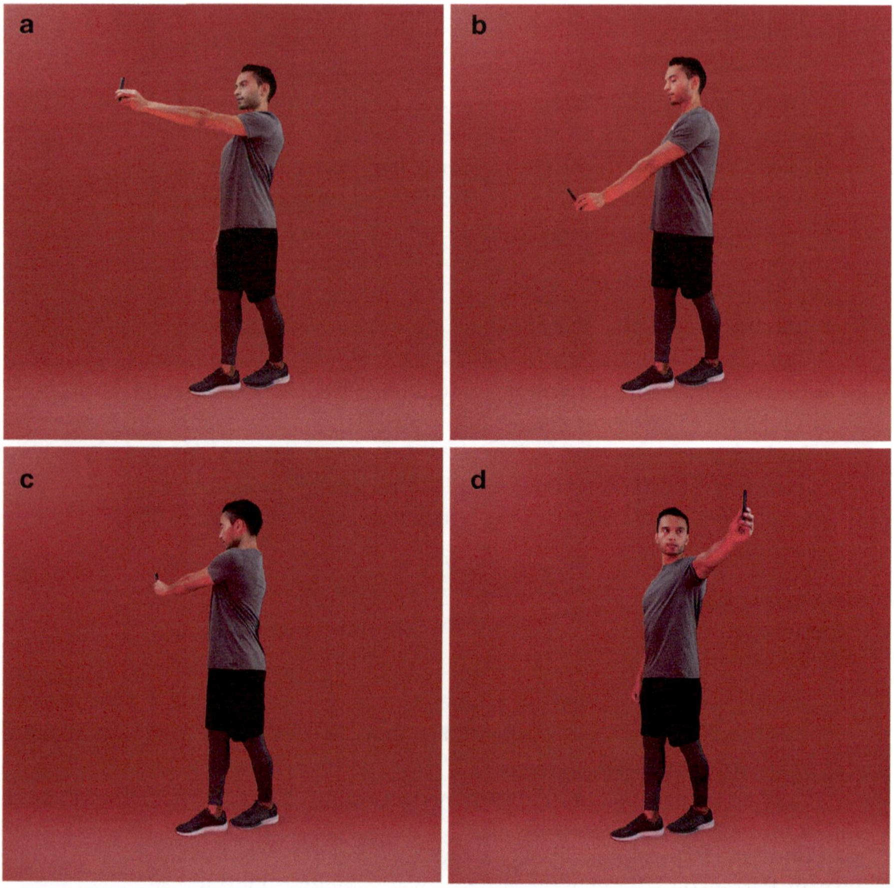

Fig. 4.9 Vision vs. static stability exercise

To Improve Anticipatory Responses and Postural Adjustments Before Starting to Walk

Examples:

See Fig. 4.10.

$\vec{F}$ = Refers to the force vector, with both magnitude and direction.

Steps to perform the exercise:

- Stand barefoot on a flat surface, making sure to keep your feet apart to maintain a stable base of support.
- Focus your attention on the right first toe.
- Consciously activate the intrinsic or internal muscles of the foot, especially those associated with the plantar arch.

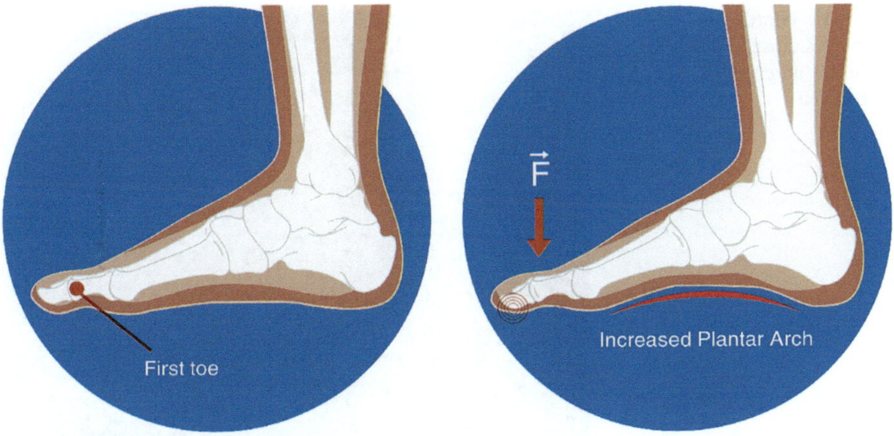

Fig. 4.10 Proprioception of the first toe

- Perform an isometric contraction by pressing down on the ground with the base of the right first toe, creating an upward force and holding the position for approximately 10–30 s.
- During the pressure, there will be activation of the plantar arch muscles and corresponding elevation of the arch structure.
- After activation, allow the foot to return to its neutral position in a controlled manner.
- Repeat with the left foot.

Note:

- This exercise can be performed in either a bipedal or seated position and can even be incorporated into walking, focusing on the pressure of the first toe in the final support phase of each step.
- Remember that this exercise focuses on awareness and activation of the intrinsic muscles of the foot, specifically the flexors and abductors of the first toe. Improving the proprioception of these muscles promotes better foot function and a more balanced posture.

See Fig. 4.11.

This exercise of starting walking with eyes closed after a posterior-anterior imbalance is a proprioceptive challenge that helps improve body awareness, stability, and balance in situations where vision is not available. It is important to perform it safely and gradually, adapting the difficulty to your individual abilities and limitations.

Steps to perform the exercise:

- Stand in a bipedal stance with feet shoulder-width apart.
- With eyes closed, tilt your body slightly forward, creating a controlled posterior-anterior imbalance. Focus on your internal balance and body awareness in space without relying on vision.

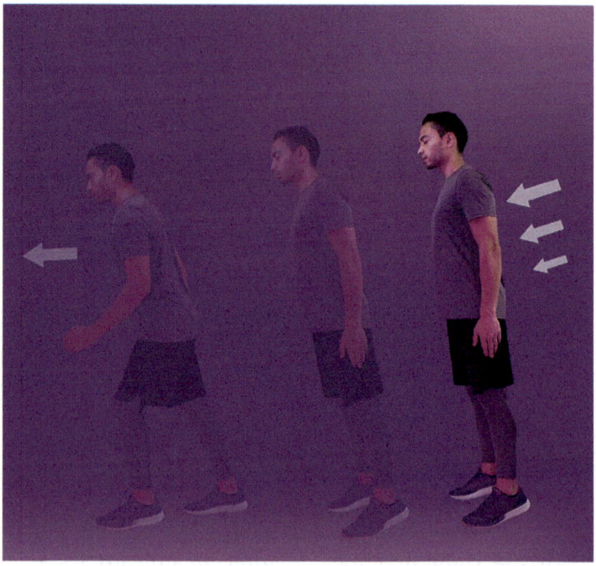

Fig. 4.11 Starting to walk with eyes closed after a posterior-anterior imbalance

- Maintain balance as long as possible and immediately take a step forward to prevent falling.
- Begin to walk slowly, keeping your eyes closed. As you walk, focus on feeling the sensations and making the necessary body adjustments to maintain balance and stability.
- If you feel your balance is compromised or you become unsure, slowly stop and open your eyes to regain stability before continuing.

Note:

- Make sure you have enough free and safe space to walk.
- It is recommended that the exercise be performed on a soft surface or with a person who can support the weight in case the person performing the exercise falls.
- As you gain more practice and control of the exercise, it is recommended that an outside person perform the posterior-anterior imbalance by providing a gentle push.
- If you feel your balance is compromised or you become unsure, slowly stop and open your eyes to regain stability before continuing.

See Fig. 4.12.

Steps to perform the exercise:

The exercises involve closing the eyes for progressively longer periods of 10, 15, 30, 45, 60 s or more, depending on the practitioner's level of readiness, while changing the base of support.

There are many ways to perform this exercise. Below are five options in hierarchical order of difficulty (from easiest to most difficult).

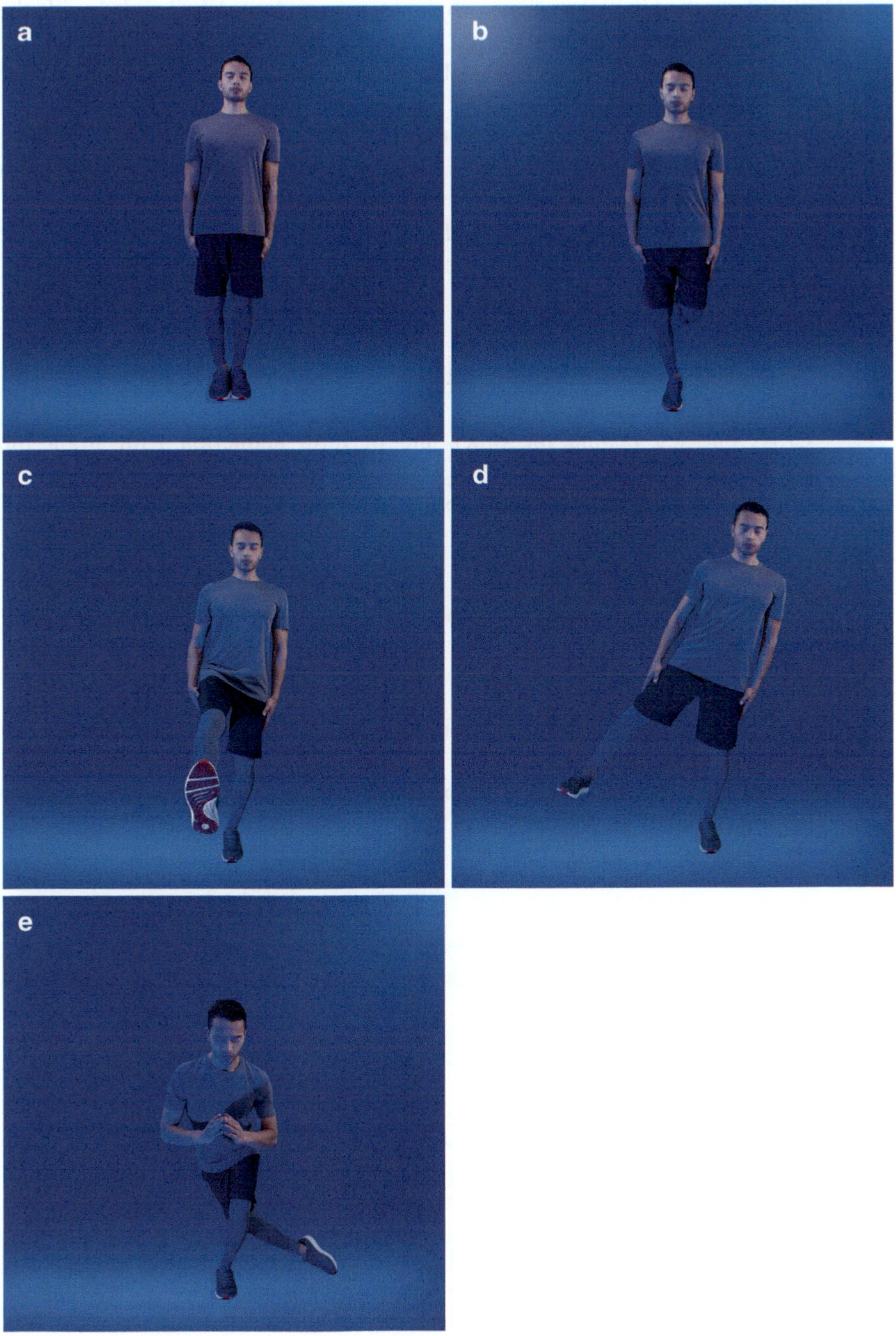

Fig. 4.12 Static stability in bipedal stance with closed eyes

(a) **Option 1:** In the bipedal stance, with the torso upright and the hands beside the body, maintain balance and stability.
(b) **Option 2:** In unipedal balance, with the torso upright and hands beside the body, maintain balance and stability.
(c) **Option 3:** In unipedal balance, with the torso upright and the hands next to the body, perform hip flexion with the extended leg to the maximum possible point and maintain balance and stability.
(d) **Option 4:** In unipedal balance, with the torso upright and hands beside the body, perform hip abduction with the extended leg as far as possible and maintain balance and stability.
(e) **Option 5:**

- In unipedal balance, slightly flex the supporting leg, trunk, and hip.
- Place both hands in front of body.
- Cross one leg behind the other and perform adduction with slight hip extension.
- Finally, maintain balance and stability.

See Fig. 4.13.

(a) 360° turn to the left
(b) 360° turn to the right.

Steps to perform the exercise:

- Stand in bipedal stance with feet shoulder-width apart, maintaining an upright and balanced posture.
- Close your eyes to remove visual information during the exercise and focus on stability and balance control.

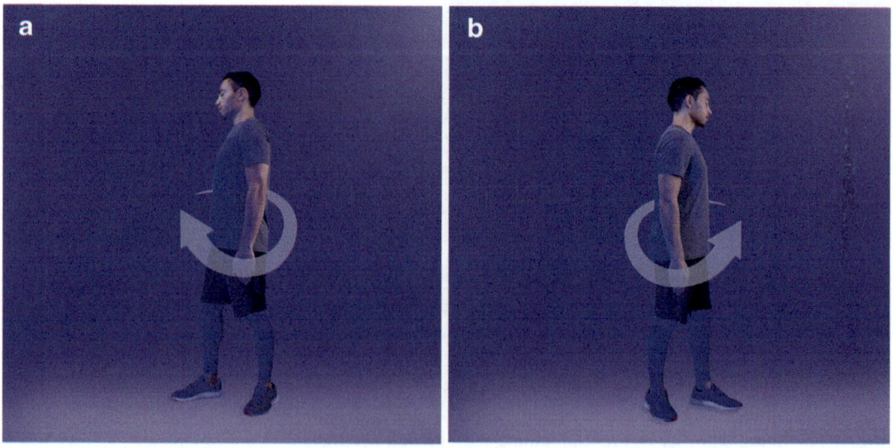

Fig. 4.13 Dynamic stability in bipedal stance through 360° turns with eyes closed

- Choose a direction in which to perform the turns, either to the left or to the right. You can start with whichever direction feels more comfortable or alternate between the two with each repetition of the exercise.
- With your eyes closed, begin to turn slowly in the chosen direction. Initiate the turn by gently moving your foot and leg in that direction.
- Perform full 360° turns, maintaining a steady and smooth rhythm. Throughout the turn, be aware of sensations and adjust your posture and movement to maintain balance. Feel how the weight is distributed on your feet and how the muscles and joints respond.
- After completing a 360° turn, gradually stop and return to your original bipedal stance. Take a moment to regain balance and stability before repeating the exercise. You may rest as long as necessary between repetitions.
- Repeat the process, alternating the direction of rotation or rotating to the same side.

Notes:

- You can mentally count to make sure you complete a full turn.
- It is important to concentrate and be careful during this exercise, as closed eyes can affect spatial perception. If at any time you feel dizzy, excessively unbalanced, or uncomfortable, stop the exercise and seek assistance to maintain stability.

See Fig. 4.14.
Steps to perform the exercise:

- In the bipedal position, maintain an upright stance with feet in a neutral position.
- Step forward with right foot. Make sure your right heel touches the ground first.
- Step forward with your left foot and place it in a straight line just in front of your right foot.
- Continue this motion pattern, alternating feet and maintaining a straight path.

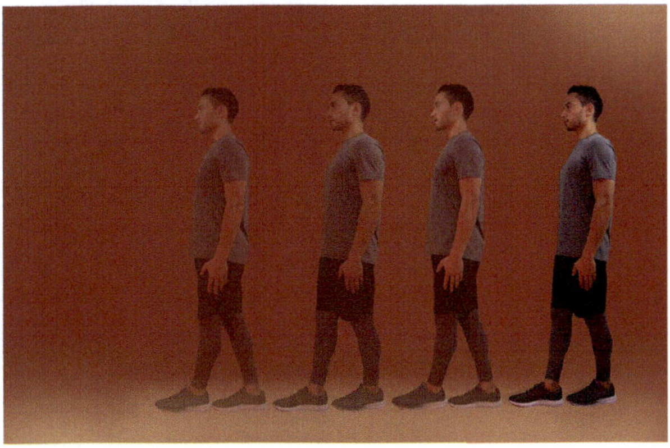

Fig. 4.14 Walking in a straight line

Note:

- Throughout the exercise, keep your eyes forward and maintain a balanced posture.
- Be sure to maintain a steady and smooth stride, ensuring that each step touches the ground from heel to toe.
- If necessary, use your arms to maintain balance and rhythm during the exercise.
- The duration of the exercise can be adjusted to meet the individual needs of the patient or as part of a broader exercise program.
- It is important to remember that this exercise should be performed in a safe and open space with a level surface free of obstacles.

Contribute to the Improvement of Dynamic Stability When Walking or Changing Direction

Therapeutic exercises that stimulate rapid responses to loss of balance are highly beneficial, particularly those stimuli that change the patient's dynamic stability from posterior to anterior.

Examples:

See Fig. 4.15.

Steps to perform the exercise:

The exercise is performed on a floor marked with a quadrant of four squares. The goal is to perform a stationary skip or march (alternating hip flexion), while moving quickly from one side of the quadrant to the other in different directions.

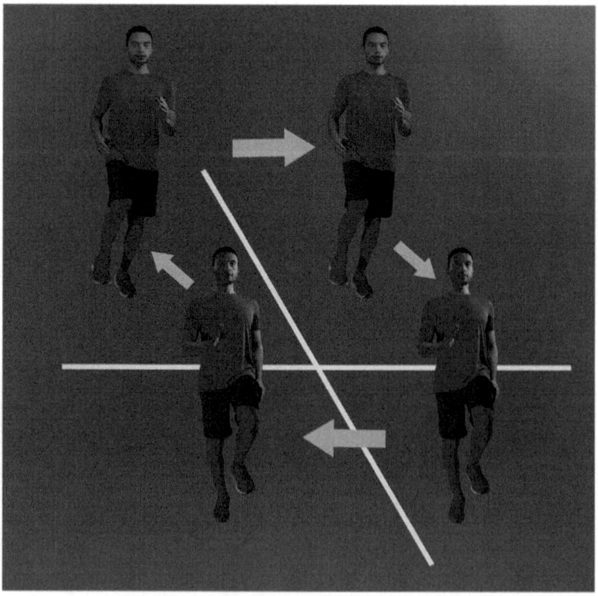

Fig. 4.15 Walking on the quadrant

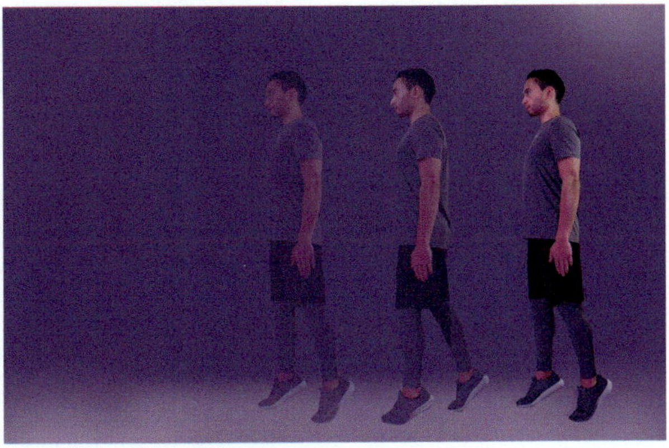

Fig. 4.16 Toe walking

- Begin by standing on one side of the quadrant.
- Begin the movement with stationary skipping.
- Use stationary skipping to move from one quadrant to another in a clockwise direction.

Note:

- Maintain a steady and fluid pace, avoiding pauses or stops between quadrant squares. The goal is to move quickly and continuously from one side to the other.
- As the exercise becomes more comfortable, try increasing the speed and height of the knees to intensify the workout. You can also vary the type of exercise, such as jumps, turns, etc.
- Remember to maintain proper breathing throughout the exercise.

See Fig. 4.16.

Steps to perform the exercise:

- Stand with feet shoulder-width apart and arms relaxed at sides of body.
- Raise the heels off the floor, supporting yourself only on the tips of your toes or metatarsals. Keep leg and foot muscles active and contracted.
- Begin to walk forward, placing one foot in front of the other. Be sure to keep the heels always lifted, relying only on the metatarsals for support.
- Continue walking on tiptoe for the desired distance or recommended time, depending on your fitness level.

Note:

- Avoid arching your back or hunching your shoulders.
- Perform smooth and progressive movements, avoiding sudden or rapid movements that may compromise stability.
- To increase the intensity of the exercise, you can walk on your toes in different directions, such as sideways or backward.

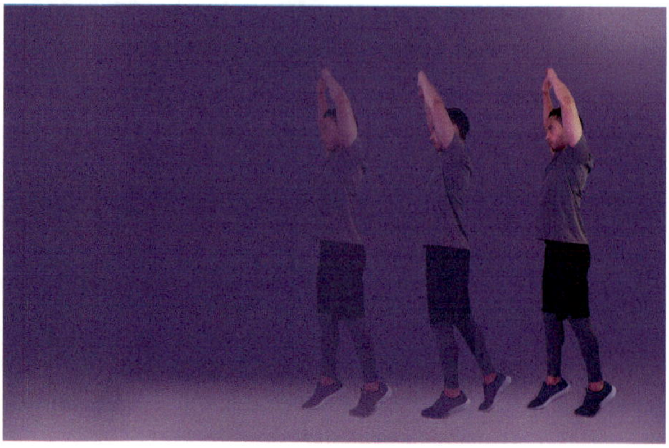

Fig. 4.17 Tiptoeing with 180° shoulder flexion

- It is important to note that if you experience pain or discomfort during the exercise, you should stop. In addition, it is always advisable to warm up the muscles before performing the toe walk.

  See Fig. 4.17.
  Steps to perform the exercise:

- Bipedal stance with feet shoulder-width apart and shoulders flexed 180°.
- Lift the heels off the ground, supporting yourself only on the tips of your toes or metatarsals. Keep leg and foot muscles active and contracted.
- Begin to walk forward, placing one foot in front of the other. Be sure to keep the heels always lifted, relying only on the metatarsals for support.
- Continue walking on tiptoe for the desired distance or recommended time, depending on your fitness level.

  Note:

- It is recommended that you engage your glutes and abdomen to improve stability during the exercise.
- Avoid arching your back or hunching your shoulders.
- Perform smooth and progressive movements, avoiding sudden or rapid movements that may compromise stability.
- To increase the intensity of the exercise, you can walk on your toes in different directions, such as sideways or backward.
- It is important to note that if you feel any pain or discomfort during the exercise, you should stop. In addition, it is always recommended to warm up the muscles before performing the toe walk.

To Contribute to the Improvement of Gait Phase Changes

Providing a useful tool for the therapeutic approach to these conditions: The guide (Table 4.1) is used as a reference to assess, teach, and adapt pathological gait phases, especially in patients with neurodegenerative diseases such as Parkinson's disease.

Table 4.1 Gait phases

	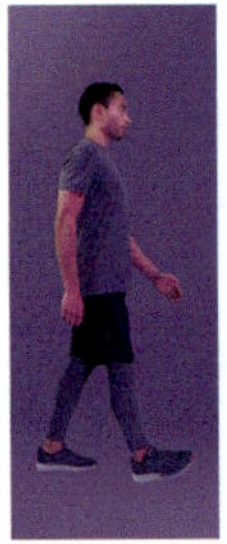	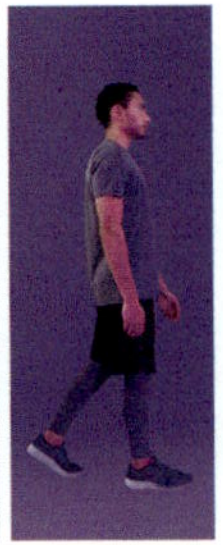	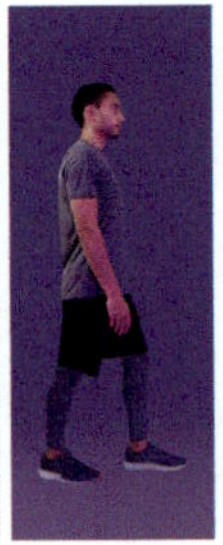	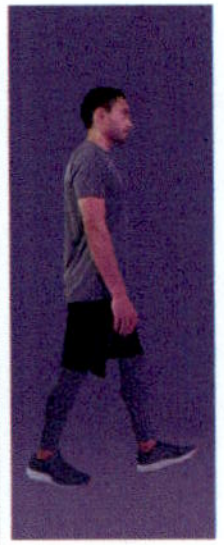	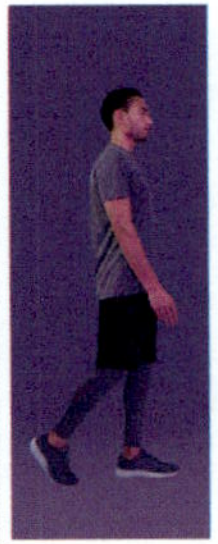	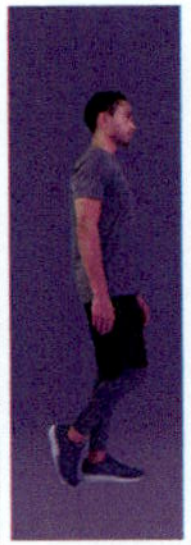	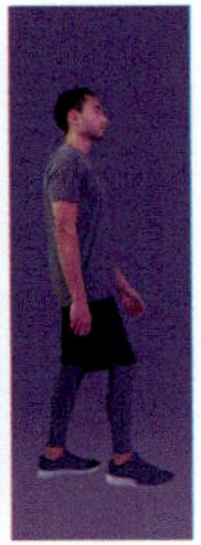	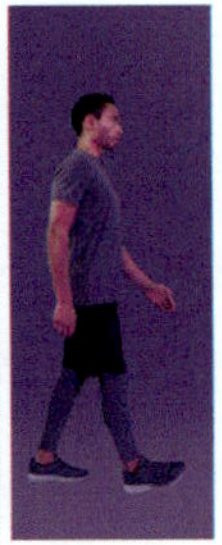
Gait phases	Initial contact	Load response	Midstance	Terminal stance	Pre-swing	Initial swing	Mid-swing	Terminal swing
Percentage of gait	0%	0–12%	12–31%	31–50%	50–62%	62–75%	75–87%	87–100%
Ankle mobility	0°	5°–10° of plantarflexion	5° of dorsiflexion	10° of dorsiflexion	15° of plantarflexion	5 of plantarflexion	0°	0°
Knee mobility	0°–5° of flexion	20° of flexion	0°–5° of flexion	0°–5° of flexion	40° of flexion	60°–70° of flexion	25° of flexion	0°–5° of flexion
Hip mobility	20° of flexion	20° of flexion	0°	−20° of flexion	−10° of flexion	15° of flexion	25° of flexion	20° of flexion
Active muscles	– Quadriceps femoris – Anterior tibialis – Gluteus medius and maximus – Hamstring muscles	– Quadriceps femoris – Anterior tibialis – Gluteus medius and maximus – Abductor magnus – Tensor fasciae latae – Posterior tibialis – Peroneus longus	– Gastrocnemius – Soleus	– Gastrocnemius – Soleus – Flexor digitorum longus – Flexor hallucis longus – Posterior tibialis – Peroneus longus – Peroneus brevis	– Gastrocnemius – Soleus – Rectus femoris – Adductor longus	– Extensor hallucis longus – Flexor hallucis longus – Sartorius – Iliacus – Anterior tibialis	– Semimembranosus – Semitendinosus – Biceps femoris – Anterior tibialis	– Quadriceps femoris – Semimembranosus – Semitendinosus – Biceps femoris – Anterior tibialis

(continued)

Table 4.1 (continued)

	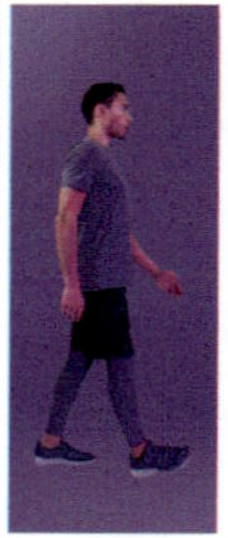	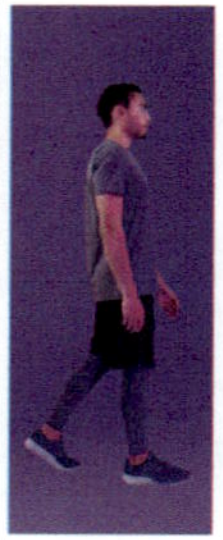	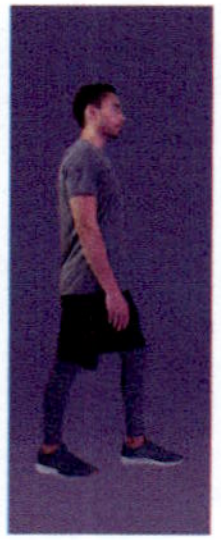	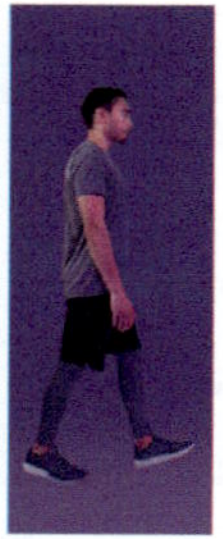	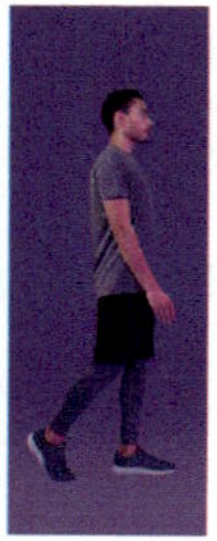	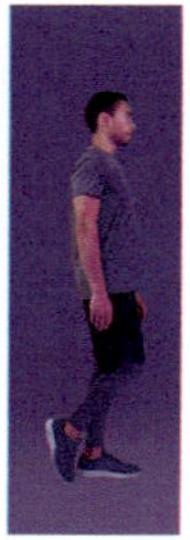	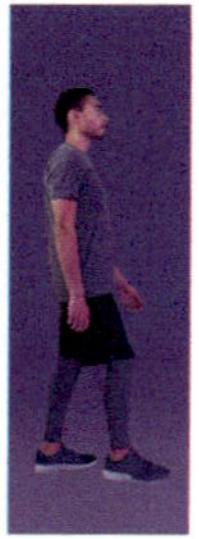	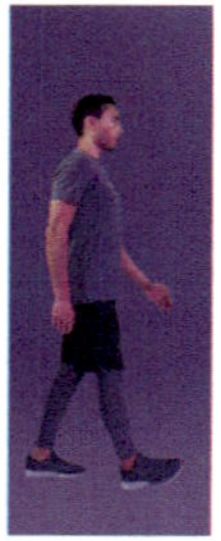
Gait phases	Initial contact	Load response	Midstance	Terminal stance	Pre-swing	Initial swing	Mid-swing	Terminal swing
Phase characteristics	The heel makes initial contact with the surface.	– Impact is absorbed by the knee and ankle. – Load and stability are transferred to the hip.	– The tibia moves forward. – Center of gravity shifts forward.	– There is dorsiflexion of the ankle, lifting the heel off the ground.	– Passive knee flexion to 40° occurs. – Plantar flexion of the ankle occurs.	– The knee flexes to a minimum of 60° to achieve sufficient foot clearance from the ground.	– Hip flexion is gradually increased to 25°. – Ankle dorsiflexion is performed and returns to neutral.	– The knee extends. – Preparation for the initial contact phase takes place.

° = Degrees

To Improve Postural Alignment

Patients with Parkinson's disease may have postural abnormalities such as camptocormia (a rare condition that causes chronic low back pain due to excessive kyphosis of the spine, usually due to weakness of the paravertebral muscles) and/or PISA syndrome (a postural abnormality in which the spine deviates laterally and flexes significantly, occurring during walking or standing).

Therefore, it is important to evaluate posture. This allows us to identify and correct any imbalances or misalignments in the body. Some of the benefits and reasons to evaluate posture include:

- *Injury prevention:* Poor posture can put extra pressure on certain areas of the body, increasing the risk of musculoskeletal injuries. By evaluating and correcting posture, you can reduce tension and imbalance that can lead to long-term injury.
- *Improved physical performance:* Proper posture allows for better physical performance in a variety of activities. Maintaining proper body alignment helps optimize biomechanics, resulting in increased movement efficiency, improved stability, and increased strength.
- *Pain relief:* Assessing and correcting posture can help relieve pain by reducing tension and stress in muscles and joints.
- *Improved appearance:* Correct posture improves physical appearance. Good posture conveys confidence, provides a more streamlined appearance, and promotes a more positive image.
- *Improved overall health:* Posture affects not only the musculoskeletal system, but also respiration, digestion, and other body systems. Proper posture allows for more efficient breathing and improved circulation, which can benefit overall health.
- *Body awareness:* Assessing posture helps us develop greater awareness of our bodies and how we position them in space. This allows us to identify poor postural habits and make conscious adjustments to maintain a healthier posture over time.

Below is a guide to assessing and correcting posture in both standing (see Figs. 4.18 and 4.19) and sitting positions (see Fig. 4.20).

Standing posture assessment:

1. *Necessary elements:*
    - To create the plumb line, use a strong and brightly colored rope or string, such as red or green. The length of the rope should be sufficient to exceed the height of the person. You will also need a small, heavy object, such as a matchbox, pool ball, or golf ball, tied to one end of the rope. This creates the necessary plumb line for measuring and evaluating posture.

- *Note:* The plumb line is used as an imaginary line to identify the optimal anatomical structures of a person in the frontal and sagittal planes. Its purpose is to determine whether an anatomical segment is in balance or symmetry (aligned with the plumb line) or in imbalance or asymmetry (not aligned with the plumb line). Its main purpose is to evaluate the alignment of the body and to detect possible deviations or asymmetries.

- A nail, tack, hook, ceiling anchor, or portable support to attach the rope with the plumb line at the other end.
- A bubble or spirit level.
- A camera and/or cell phone.
- A tripod or someone to take the picture.

2. *Procedure for setting up and assembling the elements:*

- Find a large area in your home where the person can stand.
- Choose a support to hold the free end of the plumb line, such as a ceiling anchor, portable tripod, or creative alternative (nail, tack, hook, etc.).
- Position the anchor point and the plumb line midway between the person and the camera.
- Assemble the plumb line by attaching a heavy object to the bottom end of the rope and securing it with a knot.
- Measure the length of the rope from the anchor point until the plumb line is 2.5 cm from the ground.
- Cut the rope to this measurement, making sure it is taut and forms an exact vertical line due to gravity.
- Tie the opposite end of the rope to the chosen support.

3. *Procedure for recording posture data:*

- The surface on which the subject is standing must be leveled to obtain accurate posture data. The use of a bubble level is recommended to check the accuracy of the surface.
- It is preferable for the person to wear tight-fitting clothing or undergarments to facilitate visualization of the postural guides without distraction.
- The person should stand behind the plumb line, facing it (to assess the frontal plane), and to the side of it (to assess the lateral plane).
- The plumb line should form a vertical line that divides the body into two hemispheres, left and right, in the frontal plane and divides the body into anterior and posterior hemispheres in the lateral plane.
- The subject should maintain his or her habitual standing posture, relaxed and with arms extended.
- Three full body photographs should be taken using a tripod or with the support of an assistant:

  - One anterior frontal plane photograph.
  - One photograph of the right sagittal plane.
  - One photograph of the left sagittal plane.

4. *Photographic errors:*
   - Image misalignment: Proper image alignment is critical to avoid misinterpretation when evaluating posture. Use a spirit level or tripod to assess the vertical and horizontal alignment of the camera.
   - Insufficient camera height: Place the camera at waist level to obtain an optimal image and avoid distortion in the assessment.
   - Improper framing: Avoid frames that are too wide or too narrow, which can prevent accurate posture assessment.
   - Lack of centered image: Ensure that the subject is properly centered in the frame using a perspective grid. Many cameras or cell phones have technical features that automatically create a photographic grid.
   - Incorrect foot positioning: Avoid misaligned or unevenly spaced feet in the front and side planes.
5. *Create the body map grid:*
   - Print the photograph on a letter or legal-sized sheet of paper, making sure that the print covers all or most of the sheet.
   - Draw a grid on the sheet from one end to the other. Horizontal and vertical lines should be drawn 2 cm apart. It is recommended to use a squad ruler to ensure that the lines are exactly horizontal and vertical.
6. *Posture assessment procedure:*
   - After constructing the body map grid, conduct a comparative analysis of postural changes using the frontal and sagittal plane postural assessment guide and Figs. 4.18 and 4.19. Systematically evaluate potential variations within each anatomical region and indicate any observed postural changes in the frontal and lateral planes by marking an “X” in the appropriate column of Figs. 4.18 and 4.19.
7. *Frontal plane postural assessment guide:*
   - *Anatomical landmarks:* The frontal plane plumb line should pass through the center of the body and through certain anatomical points that divide the body into two symmetrical hemispheres (left and right) to determine proper postural alignment; these anatomical points are listed below:
     - Medial to the nasal septum.
     - Medial to the philtrum or labial groove.
     - Medial to the mental region.
     - Medial to the manubrium, body, and xiphoid process of the sternum.
     - Medial to the epigastric, umbilical, and suprapubic regions.
     - Medial to the symphysis pubis.
     - Between each lower extremity.

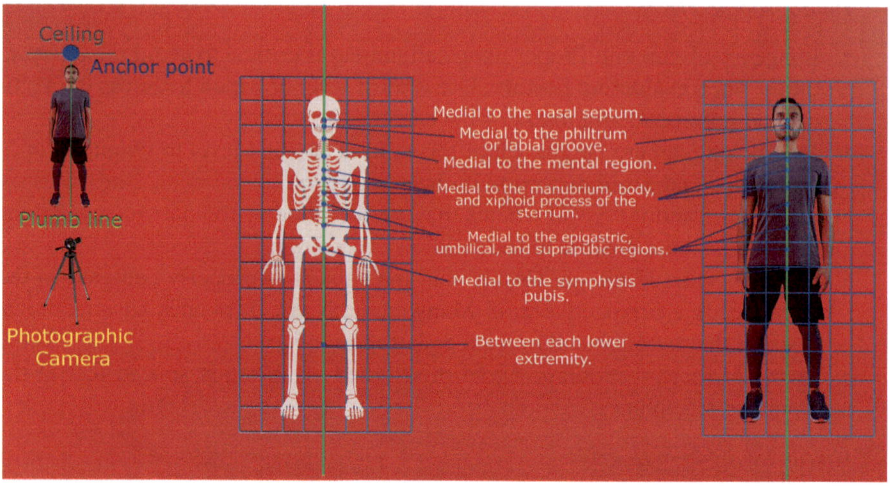

Body areas and characteristics to be assessed	Present on the right side. (Check x)	Present on the left side. (Check x)
Lateral tilt of head and neck		
Head and neck rotation		
Shoulder elevation and abduction		
Shoulder depression and adduction		
Elevation of one side of the hip		
Depression of one side of the hip		
Knee valgus		
Knee varus		
Internal rotation of the hip		
External rotation of the hip		
Tibial malleolus medial tilt		
Lateral tilt of the lateral malleolus		

Fig. 4.18 Reference of an aligned posture in the frontal plane

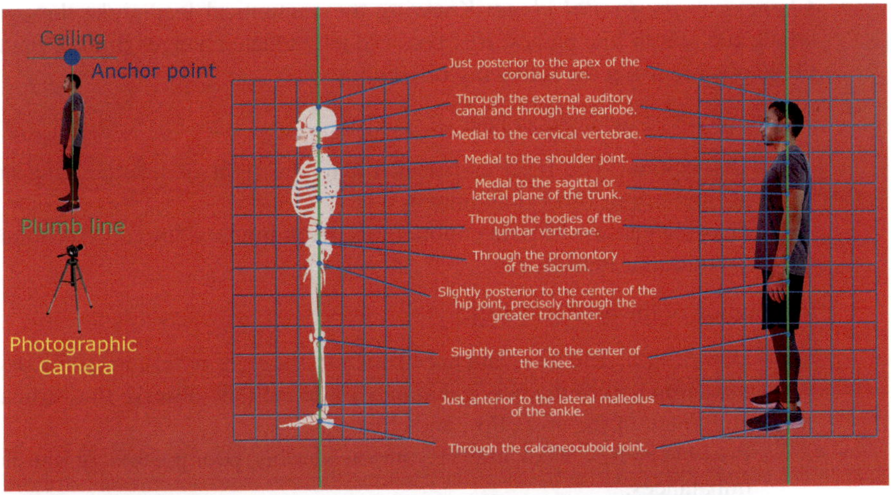

Left side		
Body areas and characteristics to be assessed	**Present on the right side (Check x)**	**Present on the left side (Check x)**
Cervical Anteversion		
Cervical retroversion		
Cervical Hyperkyphosis		
Cervical Hiperlordosis		
Wing Shoulder		
Lumbar Hyperkyphosis		
Lumbar hyperlordosis		
Anterior projection of the pelvis		
Posterior Pelvic Projection		
Pelvic rotation		
Knee hyperextension		
Right side		
Body areas and characteristics to be assessed	**Present on the right side (Check x)**	**Present on the left side (Check x)**
Cervical Anteversion		
Cervical retroversion		
Cervical Hyperkyphosis		
Cervical Hyperlordosis		
Wing Shoulder		

Fig. 4.19 Reference of an aligned posture in the lateral plane

- *Changes in the frontal plane:* Knowing the anatomical landmarks through which the plumb line passes, it is possible to evaluate changes in the frontal plane posture using the following references:
  - Lateral tilt of the head and neck:

    Description: The head and neck tilt to the right or left, creating an asymmetry in vertical alignment.
    Possible causes: Muscle contractures, neck injuries, improper posture, or muscular imbalances.
  - Rotation of the head and neck:

    Description: The head and neck rotate to the right or left, resulting in a misalignment of the cervical spine. To detect this, observe the vertical alignment of the nose, lips, and chin.
    Possible causes: Neck injuries, muscle spasms, poor posture, or muscle imbalances.
  - Shoulder elevation and abduction:

    Description: The shoulder lifts and moves away from the body, creating a higher position of the shoulder joint.
    Possible Causes: Muscle contractures, shoulder injuries, muscular imbalances, or poor posture.
  - Shoulder depression and adduction:

    Description: The shoulder lowers and moves closer to the body, resulting in a lower position of the shoulder joint.
    Possible causes: Muscle weakness, muscle imbalance, shoulder injury, or poor posture.
  - Elevation of one side of the hip:

    Description: One hip is higher than the other, creating an asymmetry at the pelvic level. Observe the level of the anterosuperior iliac crest to identify this.
    Possible causes: Muscular imbalance, leg length discrepancy, hip injury, or poor posture.
  - Hip depression:

    Description: One hip is lower than the other, creating an asymmetry in the pelvic plane.
    Possible causes: Muscle imbalance, leg length discrepancy, hip injury, or poor posture.

- Knee valgus:

  Description: The knees tend to tilt medially, bringing the leg bones closer together, especially in the knee area. To identify this characteristic, observe if the knees show a noticeable inward tilt, creating a lower limb position that visually resembles these symbols: > < .
  Possible causes: Muscle imbalances, weakness in the hip abductor muscles, knee injuries, or poor posture.

- Knee varus:

  Description: The knees tend to tilt outward, causing the leg bones to separate more, especially in the knee area. To identify this characteristic, observe whether the knees have a noticeable outward tilt, creating a lower limb position that visually resembles these symbols: <>.
  Possible causes: Muscle imbalances, weakness in the hip adductors, knee injuries, or poor posture.

- Internal hip rotation:

  Description: The hip rotates inward, causing an internal position of the thigh and foot.
  Possible causes: Muscle imbalance, weakness of the external hip rotator muscles, hip injury, or poor posture.

- External hip rotation:

  Description: The hip rotates outward, resulting in an external position of the thigh and foot.
  Possible causes: Muscle imbalance, weakness of the internal hip rotator muscles, hip injury, or poor posture.

- Medial inclination of the tibial malleolus:

  Description: The tibial malleolus (protrusion of the ankle on its inner side) moves inward or medially, causing a medial tilt of the ankle or pronation of the foot.
  Possible causes: Muscle imbalances, ankle injuries, poor posture, or changes in foot alignment such as flat feet.

- Lateral inclination of the fibular malleolus:

  Description: The fibular malleolus (external or lateral prominence of the fibula bone of the ankle) is displaced outward, causing a lateral tilt of the ankle. It is known as a cavus foot or supination foot.
  Possible causes: Muscular imbalances, ankle injuries, poor posture, or changes in foot alignment.

8. *Sagittal or lateral plane postural assessment guide:*

- *Anatomical landmarks:* The plumb line in the lateral plane should pass through certain anatomical points that divide the body into two symmetrical zones (anterior and posterior) to determine that the posture is aligned:
  - Just posterior to the apex of the coronal suture.
  - Through the external auditory canal.
  - Through the earlobe.
  - Medial to the cervical vertebrae.
  - Medial to the shoulder joint.
  - Medial to the sagittal or lateral plane of the trunk.
  - Through the bodies of the lumbar vertebrae.
  - Through the promontory of the sacrum.
  - Slightly posterior to the center of the hip joint, precisely through the greater trochanter.
  - Slightly anterior to the center of the knee.
  - Just anterior to the lateral malleolus of the ankle.
  - Through the calcaneocuboid joint.
- *Changes in the lateral or sagittal plane:* Knowledge of the anatomical areas through which the plumb line passes allow evaluation of changes in the lateral plane using the following items:
  - Cervical anteversion:

    Description: The head and neck tilt forward, resulting in a forward position of the cervical spine.
    Possible causes: Muscle imbalances, weakness in neck extensor muscles, poor sitting posture, reading, cell phone use, or repetitive heavy lifting.

  - Cervical retroversion:

    Description: The head and neck tilt backward, resulting in a retracted cervical spine posture.
    Possible causes: Muscle imbalances, weakness of the neck flexor muscles, neck injuries, improper use of posture correctors, or persistent poor posture.

  - Cervical hyperkyphosis:

    Description: The cervical spine has an exaggerated posterior convex curvature, resulting in a hunched posture of the upper back and neck.
    Possible causes: Muscle imbalances, weakness in neck extensor muscles, poor sitting posture, or repetitive lifting of heavy objects.

- Cervical hyperlordosis:

  Description: The cervical spine has excessive anterior convex curvature, resulting in a more prominent position of the cervical region.
  Possible causes: Muscle imbalances, weakness of the cervical flexor muscles, neck injuries, or sustained poor posture.

- Winged scapula:

  Description: The scapula (shoulder blade) protrudes outward, creating a "wing" appearance on the back of the shoulder.
  Possible causes: Muscle imbalances, weakness in the serratus anterior muscle, shoulder injuries, or nerve damage that controls the scapular muscles.

- Lumbar hyperkyphosis:

  Description: The lumbar spine has a posterior convex curvature, resulting in a hunched posture in the lower back.
  Possible causes: Muscle imbalances, weakness in the lumbar extensor muscles, poor sitting posture, or repetitive lifting of heavy objects.

- Lumbar hyperlordosis:

  Description: The lumbar spine has excessive posterior concave curvature resulting in greater posterior prominence of the sacrum.
  Possible causes: Muscle imbalances, weakness of the lumbar flexors, back injuries, or prolonged poor posture.

- Posterior pelvic tilt:

  Description: The pelvis and sacrum tilts forward, resulting in a lumbar hyperkyphosis.
  Possible causes: Muscle imbalances, weakness in the abdominal and gluteal muscles, pregnancy, poor posture, or improper standing and sitting habits.

- Anterior pelvic tilt:

  Description: The pelvis and the sacrum tilts backward, resulting in a lumbar hyperlordosis.
  Possible causes: Muscle imbalances, weakness in the abdominal and gluteal muscles, back injuries, poor posture, or improper standing and sitting habits.

- Pelvic rotation:

  Description: The pelvis rotates to one side, creating an asymmetry in the alignment and position of the hips.
  Possible causes: Muscle imbalance, leg length discrepancy, hip injury, poor posture, or improper movement patterns.

- Knee hyperextension:

  Description: The knees extend beyond the straight position. This causes excessive extension of the knee joint.
  Possible causes: Muscle imbalances, weakness in the knee flexor muscles, knee injuries, poor posture, or movement patterns.
  When performing the assessment, it is important to be aware of posture and correct poor postural habits. However, it is important to remember that not all postural changes are solely due to musculoskeletal habits or disorders. In some cases, they may indicate underlying pathologies such as tumors, autoimmune diseases, and deformities.
  It is important to keep in mind that this evaluation provides an overview of posture but does not replace a professional evaluation. If changes or problems related to posture are detected, it is recommended that a healthcare professional, such as a physical therapist or orthopedic surgeon, be consulted. They will be able to make a more accurate assessment and provide appropriate treatment based on each person's individual needs.

Sitting posture assessment:
See Fig. 4.20.

(a) Sit in the chair with your buttocks fully supported by the seat and your feet firmly on the floor or on an adjustable footrest, if available.
(b) Keep the spine erect and in a neutral position, avoiding slouching or rounding of the back. The shoulders should be relaxed and in a straight line with the pelvis.
(c) Distribute weight evenly over both buttocks and avoid crossing legs, which can affect balance and pelvic alignment.
(d) The thighs should be parallel to the ground and the knees bent at about 90°. Make sure there is enough space between the edge of the seat and the back of your knees.
(e) Place feet flat on floor or on adjustable footrest with ankles at right angles and feet slightly apart.
(f) If necessary, use lumbar cushions or supports to maintain the natural curve of the lower back and provide additional support.
(g) Avoid hunching or slouching. Maintain an open posture and keep your arms relaxed along your body or resting on the desk surface as needed.

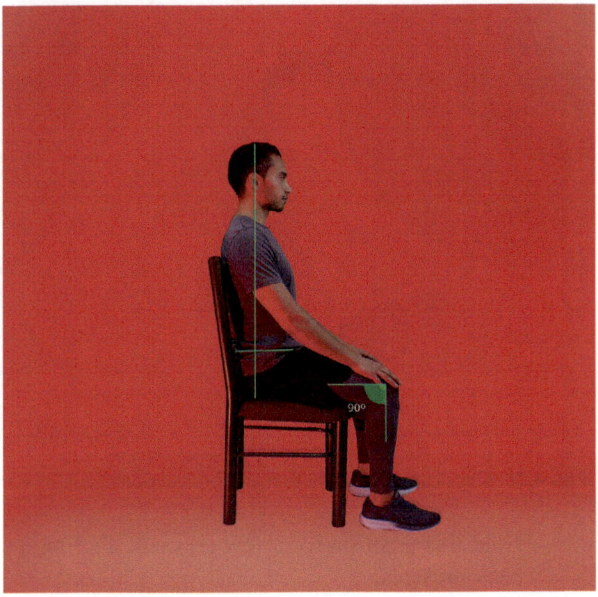

Fig. 4.20 Stable sitting posture

Note:

- Remember the importance of regular breaks, minor posture adjustments, and frequent movement to prevent muscle stiffness or fatigue. Because there is no single "correct" standing or sitting posture, the main problem is to maintain a single posture for a long period of time.

To Increase Axial Tone (Muscles and Soft Tissues of the Head, Neck, and Trunk)

The axial tone usually is altered in people with neurodegenerative diseases. The following figures (4.21 to 4.25) illustrate methods for enhancing axial muscle tone through the implementation of flexibility and strength training exercises.

Examples:

See Fig. 4.21.

Steps to perform the exercise:

- Cervical retraction:
  - Sit in a comfortable position with the spine straight.
  - Keep the head in a neutral position, facing forward.
  - Slowly slide the head back as if the chin is approaching the neck from front to back.

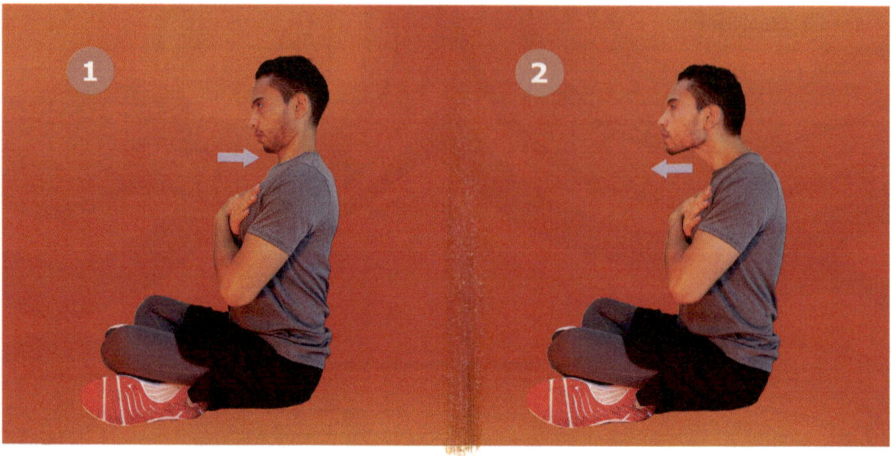

Fig. 4.21 Cervical spine retraction and protraction

  - Hold this position for a few seconds, feeling a stretch in the neck and upper back muscles.
  - Return to neutral and repeat several times.

- *Cervical protraction:*
  - Sit comfortably with spine straight.
  - Keep the head in a neutral position, facing forward.
  - Gently slide the head forward, pulling the chin forward and away from the body.
  - Hold this position for a few seconds, then return to neutral.
  - Repeat this motion several times.

  Note:

- Remember to perform these exercises in a smooth and controlled manner, avoiding sudden or painful movements.

  See Fig. 4.22.

Cervical lateral tilt is a neck movement that involves tilting the head laterally to the left or right. It is important to perform these movements in a smooth and controlled manner to avoid injury or discomfort.

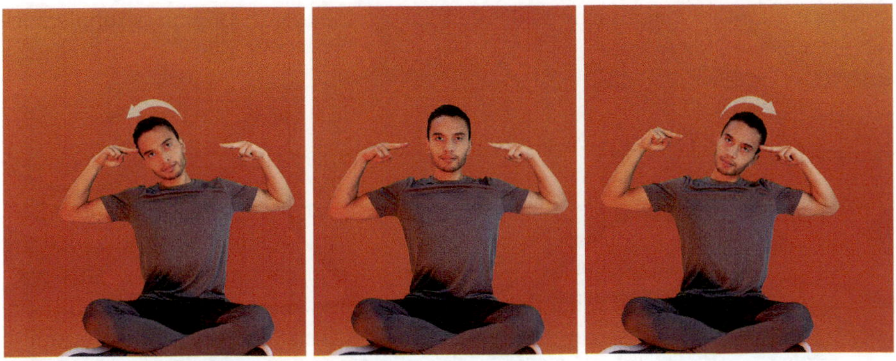

Fig. 4.22 Cervical lateral tilt

- *Starting position:*
  - Sit with spine straight and shoulders relaxed.
  - Raise the arms by flexing them and bringing the tips of the index fingers toward the ear canals (as shown in the center of Fig. 4.23). This will serve as a guide to perform the movement correctly and avoid confusion with a lateral tilt of the neck.
- Shift the neck by moving the chin to the left and/or right, without tilting the head to one side, until the tip of the index finger touches the tragus or concha of the ear, that is, toward the opening of the ear canal.
- *Repetitions:* Perform 5–10 repetitions of each movement, maintaining a smooth and controlled rhythm.
- *Breathing:* Maintain a deep and relaxed breathing throughout the exercise.

- See Fig. 4.24.

  Steps to perform the exercise:

(a) **Step 1:** The person assumes a prone quadruped position, with hands aligned with shoulders and knees aligned with hips, resting their hands and knees on the floor.
(b) **Step 2:** From this position, the person flexes their hip, knee, and trunk to lift one leg forward. The dorsal and cervical areas are flexed, as in humpback or hyperkyphosis.
(c) **Step 3:** The person extends their hip, knee, dorsal and cervical area to lift one leg backward. The person keeps their foot dorsiflexed throughout the exercise.

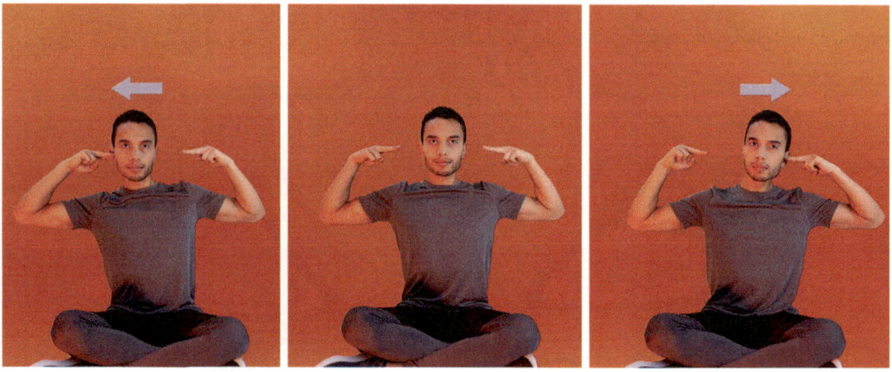

Fig. 4.23 Cervical translation

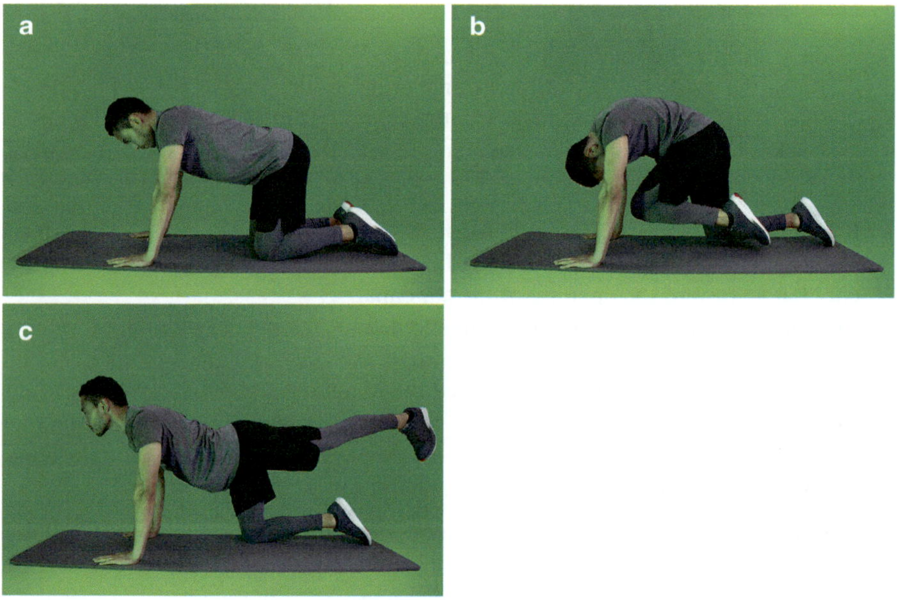

Fig. 4.24 Exercise in prone position with alternating leg extensions

Notes:

- After maintaining the posture for a brief pause, the individual lowers the leg and replicates the motion with the opposite leg, seamlessly alternating between them.
- *Repetitions:* Aim to execute 10–15 repetitions for each leg, although it is advisable to adjust the count based on the individual's requirements and physical prowess.
- *Breathing:* Sustaining a smooth and uninterrupted breathing pattern throughout the exercise is crucial, discouraging any inclination to hold one's breath.

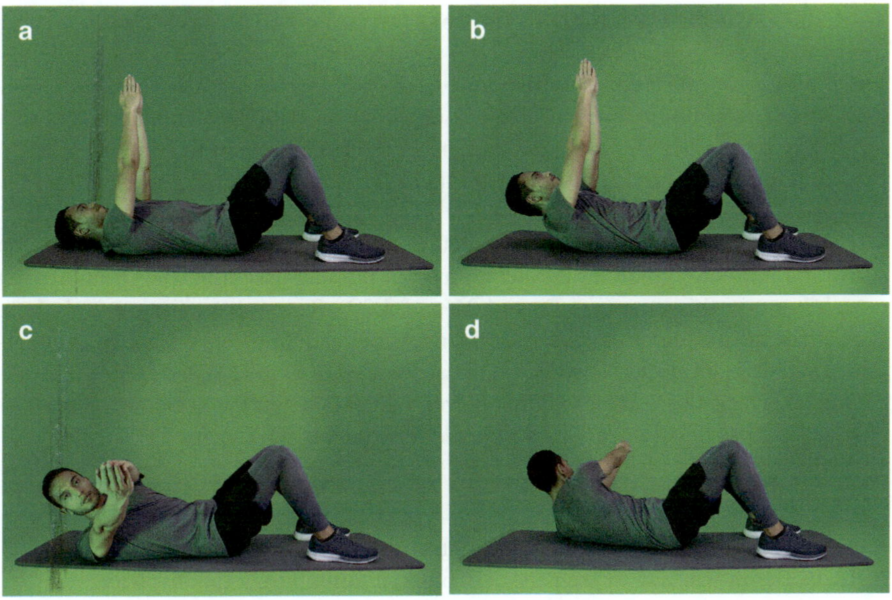

Fig. 4.25 Supine cubitus trunk rotation

See Fig. 4.25.

Steps to perform the exercise:

(a) **Step 1**:

- Lie supine on your back on the floor.
- Bend both legs and widen them slightly more than your hip-width.
- Bend your shoulders to a 90° angle, bring your arms in front of you, and clasp your palms together.

(b) **Step 2:**

- Gently bend the torso, lifting the neck and shoulder blades off the ground.
- As you bend the torso, breathe out and engage the transversus abdominis muscle, pulling your belly button towards your lower back.
- Tighten your gluteal muscles.

(c) **Step 3:** While keeping the trunk flexed and maintaining the position, rotate the trunk to the right by contracting the transversus abdominis and gluteus muscles.

(d) **Step 4:** Maintain trunk flexion and position while contracting the transversus abdominis and gluteus muscles. Rotate the trunk to the left.

Note:

- *Number of repetitions:* Perform 10–15 repetitions per side, or adjust the number based on the individual's needs and physical ability.
- *Breathing:* Maintain fluid and consistent breathing throughout the exercise, avoiding holding your breath.

To Reduce Muscle Hypotonia to Improve Dynamic and Static Stability

The presence of muscle hypotonia in the cervical region is directly related to challenges in performing turns and changes of direction with precision and dexterity, especially those involving neck movements. The critical role of the neck muscles in providing firm support and critical stability to the head in full motion should not be overlooked.

Exercises involving changes in direction and spatial orientation that focus on activating and strengthening the neck muscles play an essential role in improving muscle tone in this area (see Figs. 4.26 and 4.27). These exercises not only help strengthen the muscular structures of the neck, but also improve the ability to maintain dynamic stability while walking and static stability while standing. If the cervical muscles lack sufficient strength, control, and balance of the neck during turns or changes in direction, sudden or ineffective movements will occur.

Examples:

See Fig. 4.26.

- *Starting position:* Stand in a comfortable upright position.
- *Gait:* Begin walking in your usual manner, maintaining a steady pace.
- *Neck rotation:* While walking, gently rotate the neck to the left and then to the right without forcing the movement.
- *Different directions:* In addition to rotating the neck from left to right, circumduction movements can be made forward and backward, keeping the movement smooth and controlled.
- *Continuity:* It is recommended that the neck movements be maintained continuously throughout the gait, alternating between the different directions.
- *Safety and comfort:* The person should ensure that the exercise is performed in a safe environment and that they are comfortable during the gait and neck rotations.
- *Duration:* The duration of the exercise may vary depending on the physical condition of the individual, but is recommended to be as follows:

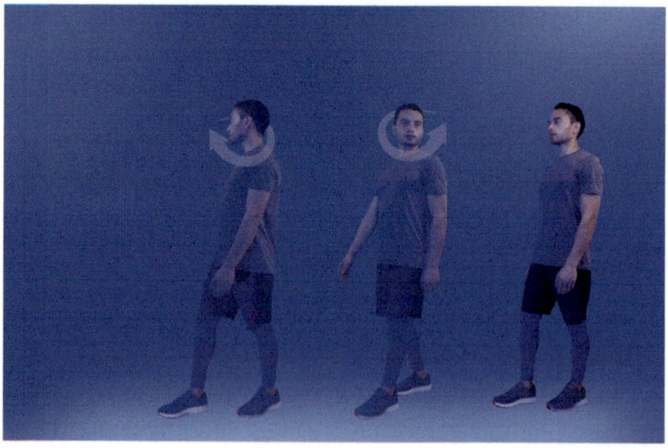

Fig. 4.26 Gait with neck rotation in different directions

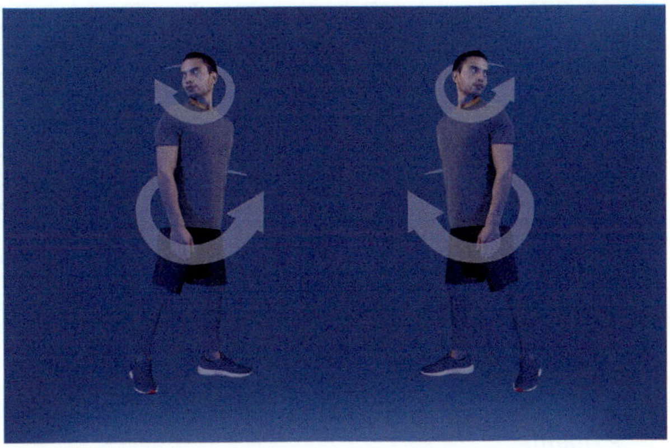

Fig. 4.27 Turning to one side and looking in the opposite direction

- Repetitions: 1 repetition of 3 min.
- Sets: 3–4.
- Density:
- Rest between sets: 1 min.
- Rest between repetitions: 30 s.

See Fig. 4.27.

- The person performs full body rotations to one side that cover a range of 360° while keeping the gaze and neck in the opposite direction of the rotation.
- *This* exercise involves coordinating body and neck movements in opposite directions to improve stability and spatial proprioception.
- It is recommended that the exercise be performed in a controlled manner, in a space free of obstacles or dangerous objects, and without forcing the limits of movement to avoid injury.

To Incorporate Training Methods and Devices That Stimulate Muscle Coactivation

Muscle coactivation refers to the simultaneous activation of agonist and antagonist muscle groups in the performance of a given action or movement. In other words, it involves the coordinated contraction of opposing muscles to produce stability, control, and efficiency in movement. Incorporating training methods and devices that stimulate muscle coactivation is essential to improving the quality and performance of movement and preventing injury. Muscle coactivation training promotes greater control and stability in the joints, allowing for more precise and efficient movement.

There are several training methods and tools that can be used to stimulate muscle coactivation. Some examples include stability exercises, such as the use of unstable surfaces or resistance band work (see Fig. 4.28), which require the activation of multiple muscle groups to maintain balance and control. Isometric resistance exercises (see Fig. 4.29), in which a static position is maintained while the antagonist muscles are activated, can also be used.

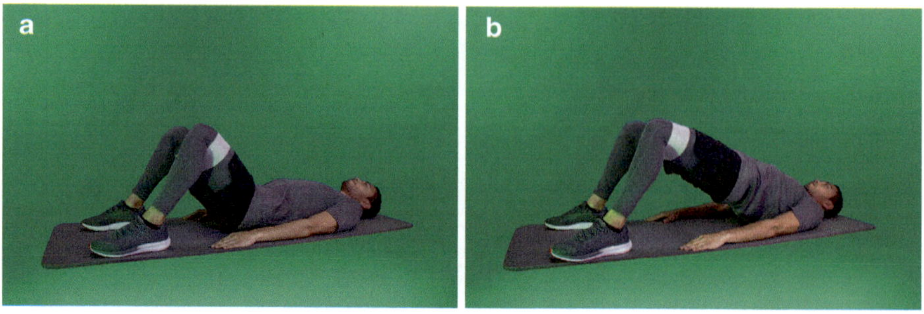

Fig. 4.28 Supine hip extension with elastic tubing

Examples:
See Fig. 4.28.

(a) **Step 1:**

- *Positioning the elastic band:* Wrap the theraband around your thighs, just above the knees. Make sure the band is tight but comfortable.
- Starting position: Lie on your back on a flat surface. Bend your knees while keeping your feet flat on the floor and perform a slight external rotation of your hips, achieved by pointing your toes outward.

(b) **Step 2:**

- *Activate the abdominal and gluteal muscles:* Before starting the movement, contract the abdominal and gluteal muscles to stabilize the pelvis and lower back.
- *Hip extension:* Keeping the abdominal and gluteal muscles engaged, push off the floor with the heels and extend the hips by lifting the buttocks off the floor. The elastic theraband provides additional resistance during hip extension.
- *Pause and Contraction:* At maximum hip extension, pause briefly and focus the contraction on the glutes. Hold this position for a few seconds.
- *Controlled return:* Slowly return the glutes to the floor, maintaining control of the movement and preventing the elastic theraband from losing tension.

Note:

- *Repetitions:* Perform 12–25 repetitions of the exercise or according to your fitness level and ability.
- *Breathing:* Maintain a steady and controlled breath throughout the exercise. Exhale as you extend your hips and inhale as you return to starting position.
- *Resistance adjustment:* If the resistance of the elastic theraband is too high, you can adjust to a lower resistance. If you need more resistance, you can move the theraband closer to the knees over the thighs and using a higher resistance band.
- This exercise helps strengthen the gluteal muscles and posterior leg chain, improving stability and performance in everyday activities that require hip extension.

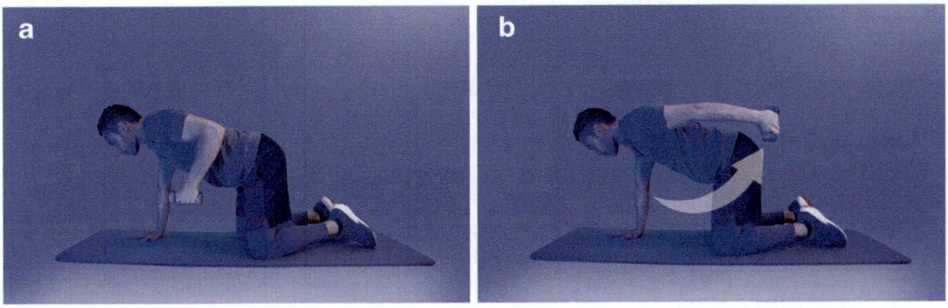

Fig. 4.29 Triceps activation exercises

- See Fig. 4.29.

  Steps to perform the exercise:

(a) **Step 1:**

  - Starting *position: Begin* in a quadruped position, with hands on floor in line with shoulders and knees in line with hips.
  - Hold a dumbbell in one hand, bend arm and direct elbow to side of body.
  - *Body alignment:* Keep back straight, abdomen contracted and shoulders stable and relaxed.

(b) **Step 2:**

  - With the elbow flexed to the side, extend the arm by bringing the dumbbell back and up. The extension of the arm should be controlled and the contraction should be felt in the triceps.
  - *Pause and contraction:* At the point of maximum arm extension, pause and contract the triceps for 8 seconds.

  Note:

- *Repetitions:* Perform 12–15 repetitions of the exercise on each side. The number of repetitions can be adjusted according to your fitness level and ability.
- *Breathing:* Exhale as you straighten the arm and inhale as you bend the arm.
- *Adjust resistance:* If the dumbbell is too heavy or too light, you can adjust the weight according to your needs by using different size dumbbells.
- *Safety:* Be sure to perform the exercise in a smooth and controlled manner, avoiding sudden movements or forcing the elbow joint.

Competing Interests The author have no conflicts of interest to declare that are relevant to the content of this chapter.

References

1. Fahn S, Elton RL. Unified Parkinson's disease rating scale (UPDRS). Encyclop Clin Neuropsychol. 2017;2:1–3.
2. de Bie RMA, Clarke CE, Espay AJ, et al. Initiation of pharmacological therapy in Parkinson's disease: when, why, and how. Lancet Neurol. 2020;19:452–61. https://doi.org/10.1016/S1474-4422(20)30036-3.
3. Armstrong MJ, Okun MS. Diagnosis and treatment of Parkinson disease: a review. J Am Med Assoc. 2020;323:548–60. https://doi.org/10.1001/jama.2019.22360.
4. Mancini M, Nutt J, Fay H. Balance dysfunction in Parkinson's disease basic mechanisms to clinical, primera. London: Elsevier; 2020.

Chapter 5
Guide to Effective and Efficient Training

Initial Questions
- What are the key elements that contribute to the effectiveness and efficiency of an exercise program?
- Can you identify tools, resources, and/or methods that increase the effectiveness and efficiency of therapeutic exercise in patients with neurodegenerative diseases?
- How does independence of movement influence the treatment of patients with neurodegenerative diseases such as Parkinson's disease?

Enhance Therapeutic Exercises with the Motor-Cognitive Dual-Task Training Method

Neurodegenerative diseases, such as Parkinson's disease, are characterized by impairments in both mobility and cognition. In terms of mobility, patients may experience difficulties that manifest as symptoms such as tremors, muscle stiffness, and restricted movement. In terms of cognitive impairment, these diseases can also affect cognitive function, including memory, concentration, decision making, and information processing.

Changes in mobility and cognition are closely linked in patients with neurodegenerative diseases such as Parkinson's. For example, muscle stiffness may be associated with difficulty making decisions, while restricted movement may affect concentration and information processing, or vice versa. In addition, the ability to perform two tasks simultaneously, such as a cognitive task and a motor task, is reduced in these patients, making it difficult to perform everyday activities that require coordination between these two functions.

When faced with a dual task, such as walking while talking, patients with neurodegenerative diseases tend to show increased variability in their gait and balance

C. A. A. Mejía, *Therapeutic Exercise for Parkinson's Disease and Related Disorders*, https://doi.org/10.1007/978-3-031-62119-2_5

due to divided attention. These risks underscore the gap between motor and cognitive skills that individuals with neurodegenerative diseases face.

Therefore, training that addresses both conditional and coordinative physical skills along with cognitive skills through the motor-cognitive dual-task training method has a positive impact on patients' independence and quality of life [1, 2].

This comprehensive approach to dual-task training, as outlined by Fritz et al. [1] and Xiao et al. [2] benefits patients with neurodegenerative diseases such as Parkinson's in the following ways:

- Rehabilitation, improvement, and readaptation of correct gait patterns.
- Increased mental flexibility (the ability to adapt and switch between different mental tasks or concepts), processing speed (how quickly the brain can analyze and respond to information), along with a 31% reduction in errors on a serial subtraction task, especially when trained using dual-task methods through virtual reality training.
- Increased walking speed and stride length.
- Reduction in the amount of effort required by a patient to perform a dual task while walking, indicating an improvement in the ability to perform dual tasks while walking.
- Improve static and dynamic balance and stability.
- Prevent the risk of falls.
- Improved proprioception and motor coordination.
- Significant decrease in Movement Disorder Society Unified Parkinson's Disease Rating Scale score (higher score indicates more severe symptoms) after 8 weeks of training.
- Reduction in episodes of gait freezing.
- Contributes to the improvement of motor skill automatization, allowing more efficient performance of motor tasks without conscious attention.
- Increased brain activity in areas such as the parietal cortex, premotor cortex, cerebellum, precuneus, and prefrontal cortex.
- Facilitates neuroplasticity.
- Promote effective and efficient brain synapses.
- Increase the release of beneficial neurotrophic factors.

The prescription of training using the motor-cognitive dual task training method should be considered a fundamental component in the treatment of Parkinson's patients. To achieve this, it is important to consider the following protocol and recommendations:

- *Integrate motor and cognitive tasks*: It is important to combine a motor activity with a cognitive task or vice versa. These activities may be simple or complex. A simple task involves the performance of one specific motor or cognitive task, while a complex task involves the simultaneous performance of two or more motor or cognitive tasks. An example of a simple cognitive task would be mental addition, while a complex task would be talking while performing mental calculations. An example of a simple motor task would be walking, while a complex task would be walking while turning.

- *Progression from simple to complex*: Training should begin with simple tasks and gradually progress to more complex tasks.
- *Clear goals for motor and cognitive tasks*: It is essential to have a clear understanding of the goals of the proposed motor and cognitive tasks. These goals should be tailored to the patient's daily needs and the skills that need improvement.
- *Use a variety of sensory stimuli*: It is recommended to include sensory stimuli such as auditory, visual, olfactory, gustatory, and kinesthetic stimuli in the training. This helps to enrich the experience and stimulate different senses.
- *Incorporate pleasurable activities*: To maintain patient interest and motivation, it is beneficial to incorporate fun activities such as the use of exergames, virtual reality, and group tasks, among others.
- *Improve the method*: To improve the effectiveness of dual tasking, various tools and approaches can be incorporated, such as:
  - *Action observation and motor imagery*: This approach involves observing an action and then mentally visualizing oneself performing it from different attentional perspectives. This method can improve dual-task performance by combining observation with mental visualization.
  - *Physical training using transcranial stimulation*: This involves the use of a transcranial stimulation device during physical training. This technique can improve cognitive performance on dual tasks and the results of physical fitness tests such as the Timed Up-and-Go.
  - Water therapy in conjunction with dual tasks.

In conclusion, when prescribing motor-cognitive dual-task training for Parkinson's disease patients, it is essential to combine motor and cognitive tasks, gradually increase their complexity, define specific goals, use a variety of sensory stimuli, add pleasurable elements, and enhance the training to optimize therapeutic outcomes.

Prescribing Exercises to Enhance Active Transfers

Parkinson's disease is a neurodegenerative disease that presents a significant challenge: the progressive loss of the ability to perform active and autonomous transfers. The term "transfer," as defined in the International Classification of Functioning, Disability, and Health, refers to the ability to move a person's body actively (with autonomy and independence), passively (where someone else always performs the movement for the patient), or mixed (where the patient receives partial assistance from another person). These transfers include basic position changes, such as moving from a sitting position to lying in bed, moving from one chair to another, moving from a wheelchair to a bed or another seat, and moving to the toilet or into a vehicle.

These activities are essential to daily living and their deterioration poses a significant challenge to people with Parkinson's disease and their caregivers [3].

From this problem arises the urgent need to prescribe exercises and/or training sessions focused on improving active transfers in patients with Parkinson's disease or other neurodegenerative diseases. These exercises aim to train the patient in the active transfers that they need to perform in their daily life, designing tasks ranging from the simplest to the most complex. In addition, the patient's physiological profile, stage of disease development, pharmacological treatment, and specific goals will be considered [4].

Echemendía del Valle et al. [4] present an example of a therapeutic exercise program designed to improve strength and facilitate active transfers in patients suffering from neurodegenerative pathologies or who have experienced strokes. The program is structured as follows:

- Total duration: 2 months.
- Daily sessions: 2.
- Duration of each session: 2 h.
- Repetitions:
  - For trunk muscles: 10–30 repetitions.
  - For other muscle groups: 10–15 repetitions.
- Density:
  - Rest time between sets: 2 min.
  - No rest time between repetitions.
- Intensity:
  - Intensity is determined in advance through an assessment of maximum strength using a 10-repetition maximum test. Intensity is set at around 60% of the 10-repetition maximum and is reevaluated weekly to make adjustments based on the patient's progress.
- Instruments used:
  - A variety of tools and equipment are used, including dumbbells, stationary bicycles, climbers, balance trainers, wall pulleys, multi-force equipment, and horizontal presses.
- Program Stages: The training program is divided into three progressive stages in load and intensity as shown below:
  - First stage (general preparation):

    Objectives:

    - Improve joint range and mobility.
    - Normalize muscle tone.
    - Increase muscle strength.
    - Perform passive and/or mixed transfers.

Exercises:

- Passive, active, assisted, and resisted mobilizations of the upper and lower limbs.
- Shoulder exercises with dumbbells (abduction, adduction, horizontal adduction).
- Elbow exercises with dumbbells (flexion and extension).
- Trunk exercises (flexion and extension).
- Hip exercises with overload (flexion, extension, abduction, adduction).
- Knee exercises with overload (flexion and extension).
- Mechanical therapy with various equipment.

– Second stage (special preparation):

Objectives:

- Neuromuscular reeducation of affected muscle groups.
- Perform active and/or mixed transfers.
- Contribute to improving endurance capacity through mitochondrial oxidative and glycolytic pathways.

Exercises:

- Transfer training to and from the chair.
- Work on the mattress or bed (turns and incorporations).
- Transfer training from sitting to walking.
- Four-point work patterns.

– Third stage (functional preparation):

Objectives:

- Achieve independent walking or with technical aids.
- Perfect active transfer patterns.
- Contribute to improving endurance capacity through mitochondrial oxidative, glycolytic, and phosphagen pathways.

Exercises:

- Static and dynamic walking patterns within parallel bars.
- Walker or Canadian crutch training.
- Climbing up and down stairs.
- Marching in place with leg lifts.
- Stationary bicycle.
- Climbing machine.
- Treadmill.
- Walking without crutches.
- Walking on uneven terrain.
- Active position changes such as turns and incorporations in bed, car, or seat.
- Changes in direction.
- Obstacle course walking training.

This therapeutic approach aims to provide patients with an effective and personalized intervention to improve their strength and active transfer capabilities within the context of their specific neurological conditions.

Other Points to Consider When Prescribing Exercise for Parkinson's Patients

- Evaluate the patient beforehand to determine his or her level of motor control and ability to plan an appropriate intervention that considers the limitations to be overcome or addressed.
- Consider the principles of training, especially those of individuality and progression, when selecting exercises and activities to avoid frustrating the patient.
- Perform activities that are fun and familiar to the patient, avoiding complex or unusual tasks that may be difficult to understand.
- Incorporate dynamics, exercises, or movements related to the patient's daily life and repeat them daily in preparation for new tasks or challenges.
- Consider the patient's history of physical activity when designing the intervention.
- Avoid performing interventions when the patient is in a bad mood or unwilling.
- Use a soft tone of voice and avoid imposing tones with very high volume to avoid causing discomfort or rejection in the patient.
- Respect the patient's personal space, avoid invading the patient's work area, and act gently and calmly if it is necessary to intervene.
- Address the patient by name and establish a dialogue by directly looking the patient's eye level.
- Remember that the patient may be in a constant state of confusion and may not always behave as expected.
- Ensure the patient's safety by making sure the procedure area is unobstructed and well lit.
- Be flexible in planning the intervention and try new exercises based on evidence and professional experience.
- Establish routines with repetitive activities but vary minor aspects as the patient may remember some of them due to body memory.
- Consider the timing of the intervention and assess the patient's mood and energy to adjust the plan.
- Use materials that are safe in size, shape, and use when performing exercises with materials.
- Give the patient verbal and nonverbal commands to facilitate understanding and imitation.
- Avoid judging the patient during the session and allow activities to unfold naturally, recognizing unplanned goals that may be beneficial.
- Include pelvic floor exercises to help manage sphincter dysfunction, especially urinary incontinence, which is common in people with Parkinson's disease.

Competing Interests The author have no conflicts of interest to declare that are relevant to the content of this chapter.

References

1. Fritz NE, Cheek FM, Nichols-Larsen DS. Motor-cognitive dual-task training in persons with neurologic disorders: a systematic review. J Neurol Phys Ther. 2015;39:142–53.
2. Xiao Y, Yang T, Shang H. The impact of motor-cognitive dual-task training on physical and cognitive functions in Parkinson's disease. Brain Sci. 2023;13(3):437.
3. World Health Organization. Clasificación internacional del funcionamiento de la discapacidad y de la salud: CIF: versión abreviada, Versión abreviada. 1st ed. Organización Mundial de la Salud; 2001. https://iris.who.int/handle/10665/43360
4. Echemendía del Valle A, Sentmanat Belisón A, Yumila Noa Pelier B, Gómez Pérez R. Programa de ejercicios para las transferencias y la marcha en los pacientes lesionados medulares. Rev PODIUM Rev Ciencia Tecnol Cult Física. 2022;17:876–91.

Chapter 6
Conventional Therapeutic Exercises: Explanation, Examples, Effects and Dosage

Initial Questions

- How can the combination of different active therapeutic methods be used in the treatment of neurodegenerative diseases, especially Parkinson's disease, to achieve more effective results in the management of motor and non-motor signs and symptoms?
- What is the scientific support for conventional therapeutic exercise and how does this support translate into tangible improvements in the condition of patients with neurodegenerative diseases?
- To what extent can the appropriate dosage of the load for each therapeutic method and medium influence the results obtained, and how can these interventions be personalized to meet the specific needs of each patient with neurodegenerative diseases such as Parkinson's?

Below is a description of a series of methods and means of conventional therapeutic training, aimed at prescribing movement in a dosed manner based on scientific evidence for patients with Parkinson's and related disorders.

Physical Activity

Among the protective factors against Parkinson's disease, which include genetic factors, psychosocial factors, lifestyle, diet, and medications, continuous engagement in physical activity (PA) stands out. A study conducted by Loprinzi et al. [1] of Parkinson's patients who underwent moderate to vigorous PA sessions showed that continuous PA was associated with the following benefits:

- Improvement of cognitive abilities in adults with Parkinson's disease, specifically information processing, attention, memory, and learning.

C. A. A. Mejía, *Therapeutic Exercise for Parkinson's Disease and Related Disorders*, https://doi.org/10.1007/978-3-031-62119-2_6

- Regulation of BDNF and insulin-like growth factor.
- Facilitation of neurogenesis, neuroplasticity, and new blood vessel formation or angiogenesis.

Effects of Physical Activity

According to various studies such as those by Aho et al. [2], Albani et al. [3], Bhalsing et al. [4], Cusso et al. [5], Fayyaz et al. [6], Galimberti and Scarpini [7], Khalil et al. [8], Landers et al. [9], Shalash et al. [10], Shih et al. [11], van Uem et al. [12], and Wassenaar and Zimmermann [13], the effects of PA are:

- Neuroprotective effects: PA increases neural plasticity and gray matter in specific brain areas, such as the frontal and lateral lobes, associated with diseases such as Alzheimer's, Parkinson's, and cognitive impairment.
- Reduction of age-related brain atrophy.
- Increased angiogenesis, which promotes the formation of new neuronal synapses.
- Increased dopamine secretion in the basal ganglia, especially in the dorsal and ventral striatum.
- Increased levels of neurotrophins, which promote the maintenance, proliferation, and differentiation of neurons.
- Reduction of proinflammatory bacterial lipopolysaccharides associated with Parkinson's and Alzheimer's disease.
- Increased bacterial production of short chain fatty acids, reducing inflammation associated with Parkinson's and Alzheimer's disease.
- Increased peripheral levels of BDNF, which is associated with cognitive function, neurogenesis, plasticity, and neuronal survival.
- Prevention of the risk of developing Parkinson's disease through moderate PA.
- Reduction and/or delay of Parkinson's neuropathology.
- Moderation and availability of dopamine transporter proteins.
- Reduce neurotoxicity in bilateral dopaminergic pathways, improve neuroplasticity, and increase BDNF levels.
- Improve spatial cognition and cognitive executive functions.
- Prevention of dementia and cognitive impairment in Parkinson's disease.
- Improve sleep quality and mood.
- Improve gait, balance, and muscle strength.
- Prevention of osteoporosis and cardiovascular disease common in sedentary Parkinson's patients.

- Reduce pain perception and sensation by activating neural pathways associated with nociceptive signal reduction.
- Reduced dependence on pharmacotherapy.
- Reducing the mortality rate due to falls and loss of balance, while preventing the fear of future falls.

It is important to note that these effects may be more or less pronounced depending on when PA is initiated. In other words, the earlier PA is incorporated into a person's life, the lower the risk and the more beneficial the biological, psychological, and social effects on the patient's quality of life.

Methods and Means for PA Practice

High-Intensity Treadmill Training (HITT)

A review and study conducted by Armstrong and Okun [14] and Schenkman et al. [15] found that HITT in individuals with Parkinson's disease reduced motor symptoms and signs, such as increased walking speed, reduced freezing of gait episodes, and improved dynamic balance.

The HITT proposed by Schenkman et al. [15] includes specific load parameters, as described below:

- *Total intervention duration*: 26 weeks.
- *Intensity*: The goal is to reach 80–85% of the maximum heart rate (MHR) during exercise. Intensity is gradually increased from week 1 to week 8 to achieve the target MHR percentage. In addition, it is recommended that the first 2 weeks be supervised at a health center by professionals trained in first aid. This heart rate can be achieved by adjusting the treadmill speed and/or incline.
- *Volume*:
  - Session phases:

    Warm-up: 5–10 min
    Main phase: 30 min at % of target MHR
    Cool down: 5–10 min

  - Frequency: 4 days per week
- *Biological monitoring elements*: Heart rate monitor

There are parameters from resistance training that are useful as guidelines for prescribing HITT, as shown in Table 6.1:

Table 6.1 Methods and adaptations for resistance training prescription in HITT, information adapted from Pallarés and Morán Navarro [16]

Zone	Objectives and adaptations	Training methods that foster its development	Intensity												Volume				Density	
			% MAV		%VO2 max		%HRR		%MHR		%AT		[Lact-] mmol L^{-1}		T′ of total session	T′ rep.	N° rep.	N° series	T′ of recovery between reps	T′ of recovery between series
Threshold for transition to activation of glycolytic metabolic pathways	Increasing the physiological ability to endure prolonged efforts that activate oxidative mitochondrial metabolic pathways close to the threshold of glycolytic metabolic pathways. – Promoting glycogen oxidation. – Enhancing systolic volume, cardiac output, blood volume, and pulmonary diffusion. – Adaptations at the nervous system level. – Increased peripheral circulation and capillarization.	Continuous variable 1	75	90	75	90	75	90	80	95	85	100	2	4	30–60 min	>5 min	–	–	–	–
		Continuous variable 2	85	95	85	95	85	95	90	95	100	110	4	6	20–40 min	3–5 min	–	–	–	–
		Extensive long interval	85	95	85	95	85	95	90	95	90	105	3	5	45–60 min	2–8 min	6–9	–	2–5 min or until HR falls below 60% of MHR or 120 bpm.	–

Explanation of the abbreviations used in Table 6.1:

- ***HITT = high-intensity treadmill training.***
- ***% MAV = percentage of maximum aerobic velocity***: It is a term used in the field of sports performance, especially in endurance sports such as running, cycling, or skiing. MAV is the theoretical minimum speed required to achieve maximum oxygen consumption (VO2max). In other words, it is the speed at which the body operates at the maximum of its mitochondrial oxidative metabolic capacity (aerobic). MAV is like the starting point at which your body reaches its maximum capacity to absorb and efficiently use oxygen during exercise.
When you reach MAV, you are in what is called the "beginning of the plateau" of VO2max. VO2max is the maximum amount of oxygen your body can use during intense exercise. The "plateau" is a part of the performance curve where VO2max peaks and remains stable for a while before declining. MAV marks the beginning of this plateau on the performance curve, which means that you are exercising at a high enough intensity to reach your maximum oxygen consumption, but you are not yet at the peak of that capacity. The typical unit of measurement for MAV is kilometers per hour (km/h) or meters per second (m/s), depending on user preference or the specific context of the exercise or activity.
Let us say a patient's MAV when running 2 km is 8 km/h. We want to calculate 80% of this MAV to determine that this patient should jog at 80% intensity above their MAV. To find 80% of the MAV, we simply convert the percentage to a decimal and multiply it by the MAV:

$$80\% \text{ of MAV} = 8\,\text{km/h} \times 0.8 = 6.4\,\text{km/h}$$

So, 80% of MAV in this case would be 6.4 km/h. This means that for a specific exercise requiring an intensity equal to 80% of the patient's MAV, the jogging velocity should be 6.4 km/h.
- ***% VO2max = percentage of maximum oxygen consumption***: Percentage of maximum oxygen consumption, or VO2max, is the maximum amount of oxygen a person can use during intense physical exercise. It is expressed in milliliters of oxygen per kilogram of body weight per minute (ml kg^{-1} min^{-1}) and is considered a crucial indicator for evaluating an individual's physiological status. VO2max is related to various central and peripheral aspects of the body, like lung function, cardiac output, blood volume, muscular capillarity, diffusion capacity, and mitochondrial activity.
VO2max is heavily influenced by genetic factors and can be measured through several methods, including maximal and submaximal tests performed commonly on a treadmill or stationary bike. While maximal tests are accurate, they can be costly and pose health risks, especially in people with heart problems. Submaximal approaches and those unrelated to exercise are less accurate but more economical and less risky. Therefore, the use of submaximal tests in the clinical setting is suggested as a method for estimating VO2max. It is important to note that these tests may not provide the same level of accuracy as maximal tests, but they are a viable alternative in certain situations.

- ***% HRR = percentage of heart rate reserve***: Heart rate reserve is calculated by subtracting resting heart rate from maximum heart rate. This measure is used to adjust heart rate during physical exercise to maintain adequate and sustained effort, and to program training intensity. The term "heart rate reserve" is commonly used instead of 'reserve beats' to avoid misunderstandings and standardize its use.
  For instance, consider a 30-year-old person with a resting heart rate (RHR) of 70 beats per minute (bpm) and an estimated maximum heart rate (MHR) of 190 bpm. This person aims to train at 70% of their MHR.
  - We calculate the HRR:

$$\text{HRR} = \text{MHR} - \text{RHR}$$

$$\text{HRR} = 190 - 70\text{bpm}$$

$$\text{HRR} = 120 \text{ bpm}$$

  - We calculate the training heart rate (THR) as 70% of the MHR. THR represents the number of ventricular contractions of the heart achieved during exercise or training. It is recommended to measure this value in real-time using recording devices such as a heart rate monitor or electrodes. To calculate THR, we use the following formula:

$$\text{THR} = \left(\text{HRR}^{*}\%\text{of exercise intensity expressed as a decimal}\right) + \text{RHR}$$

  Substituting the values into the formula:

$$\text{THR} = \left(120 \text{ bpm}^{*} 0.70\right) + 70 \text{ bpm}$$

$$\text{THR} = 84 \text{ bpm} + 70 \text{ bpm}$$

$$\text{THR} = 154 \text{ bpm}$$

  Therefore, for this 30-year-old individual, a THR of 70% would be approximately 154 bpm.
- *%MHR = percentage of maximum heart rate*: %MHR is the highest number of ventricular contractions that the heart can achieve during intense exercise until exhaustion, expressed as a percentage. This value depends on various factors, including age, gender, ethnic origin, level of physical activity, and other biopsychosocial factors.

This indicator is crucial in training programs and exercise monitoring as it allows for personalized adaptation of training intensity. It determines exercise intensity in beats per minute (bpm), enabling assessment of a person's level within a specific intensity zone.

For instance, if an individual has a maximum heart rate of 200 bpm and intends to use the variable continuous training method 2, which requires maintaining the target range of % MHR between 90% and 95%, they should maintain their training heart rate within the range of 180–190 bpm.

To calculate the working heart rate within the target % MHR range (90–95%), you can use the formula:

$$\text{Training heart rate} = \text{maximum heart rate} \times \%\text{MHR}$$

Where % MHR is expressed as a decimal (e.g., 90% is entered as 0.90). Applying the formula with the values given in the previous example:

$$\text{Training heart rate} = 200\ \text{bpm} \times (0.90) = 180\ \text{bpm}$$

$$\text{Training heart rate} = 200\ \text{bpm} \times (0.95) = 190\ \text{bpm}$$

- *%AT = percentage of anaerobic threshold (activation of glycolytic metabolic pathways)*: The % AT or the activation threshold of glycolytic metabolic pathways is the exercise intensity point at which lactic acid production surpasses its elimination, resulting in a significant increase in blood lactate concentration. This change describes a shift from primarily utilizing the mitochondrial oxidative metabolic system (commonly referred to as aerobic) to the glycolytic system (known as anaerobic) for energy production. Various terms, such as maximum lactate steady state, Mader's aerobic-anaerobic threshold, Kindermann's anaerobic threshold, Keul and Stegmann's individual anaerobic threshold, Sjödin and Jacobs' blood lactate accumulation onset, and Orr's ventilatory threshold 2, are used to describe this phenomenon. The activation threshold of glycolytic metabolic pathways is typically reached at 80–95% of VO2 max, which is theoretically equivalent to a blood lactate concentration of 4 mmol·L$-^{1}$ (lactate concentration in millimoles per liter), indicating high-intensity effort.
- *[Lact-] mmol·L^{-1} = lactate concentration in millimoles per liter*: This measurement is used to quantify the amount of lactate present in a blood sample or other biological fluid. Lactate is a by-product of glycolytic metabolism, and its concentration in the blood may increase during intense exercise or in situations where oxygen delivery to tissues is lower than normal. Measurement of lactate concentration is important in evaluating exercise performance and monitoring the metabolic status of patients, as elevated levels may indicate muscle fatigue, lactic acidosis, or metabolic problems.
- *T' = time*
- *Rep. = repetitions*
- *N° = number*
- *min = minutes*

- *HR = heart rate*: Refers to the number of times the heart beats per minute. It is measured in beats per minute (bpm) and is a key indicator of cardiovascular system activity. Heart rate can vary depending on age, level of physical activity, health status, and other factors.
- *MHR = maximum heart rate*: Refers to the maximum number of ventricular contractions performed by the heart, reached in a maximal intensity effort with high muscular involvement until exhaustion. Maximum heart rate is the highest that a person can reach during intense exercise and depends on factors such as age, gender, ethnic origin, level of physical activity, and other biopsychosocial factors.
- *bpm = beats per minute*

Examples of HITT

- Variable slope and speed training: This type of training involves regularly and randomly changing the speed and incline of the treadmill to mimic the variability of outdoor running conditions. For instance, the patient might run at a 5% incline at 6 mph for 1 min, then switch to a 2% incline at 4 mph for 2 min before returning to the 5% incline.
- High-intensity intervals: This is a type of training in which short periods of high intensity are alternated with longer periods of low intensity to allow for recovery. For example, a session could include 30 s of sprinting at a very high speed, followed by 60 s of walking at a slower speed. This would be repeated several times during a session.
- Continuous high-intensity training: In this type of training, the patient runs at a high and constant speed throughout the entire session. The duration and speed of the session can vary depending on the patient's capacity, but the goal is to maintain a high intensity throughout the training.

Perturbed Treadmill Training

Perturbed treadmill training for Parkinson's patients involves introducing changes to the treadmill surface, such as obstacles or changes in speed, so that the patient must adjust their movement and balance unexpectedly. This form of training significantly improves gait speed in patients with mild to moderate Parkinson's disease. A study conducted by Klamroth [17] found that 10 min of perturbed treadmill training using a tilting platform with inflatable tires (see Fig. 6.1) positioned under the treadmill (which is designed to raise one or another part of the treadmill while the subject runs or walks on it, with harnesses attached to the body to prevent falls) improved dynamic stability, gait variability, and speed in patients with Parkinson's disease.

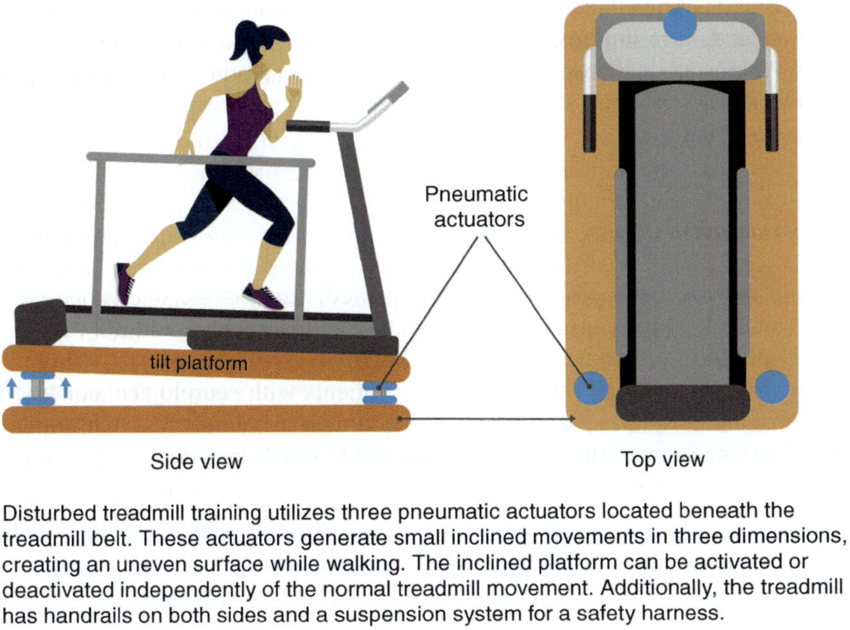
Pneumatic
actuators
tilt platform
Side view
Top view
Disturbed treadmill training utilizes three pneumatic actuators located beneath the treadmill belt. These actuators generate small inclined movements in three dimensions, creating an uneven surface while walking. The inclined platform can be activated or deactivated independently of the normal treadmill movement. Additionally, the treadmill has handrails on both sides and a suspension system for a safety harness.

Fig. 6.1 Diagram of the treadmill adapted from Klamroth [17]

Examples of Perturbed Treadmill Exercises

- Walking on the treadmill while small vibrations are introduced to the treadmill surface.
- Walking on the treadmill while introducing a series of obstacles (such as wooden blocks) for the patient to overcome.
- Walking on the treadmill while the incline changes, forcing the patient to adjust their posture and movement to maintain balance.

It is important to emphasize that disturbed treadmill training should be supervised by a health-care professional trained in the technique, as it is a more complex and potentially risky exercise than simple treadmill walking.

Aquatic or Suspension Treadmill Training

Aquatic or suspension treadmill training has proven to be highly beneficial for cardiovascular, metabolic health, and fall prevention in patients with Parkinson's disease when compared to conventional treadmill training. The hydrostatic pressure in the aquatic environment leads to chest expansion and an increase in cardiac output. Furthermore, the aquatic environment significantly reduces the risk of falls due to its safety.

The benefits of treadmill training in the aquatic environment, whether in suspension or on land, have similar effects on the biomechanics, akinesia, and gait festination of Parkinson's patients. This is why the WHO (World health organization) recommends short walks, lasting 20–30 min, for Parkinson's patients as supplementary exercise [18].

Other Treadmill Training Methods

Currently, new technologies are being employed, such as the one proposed by Motek Medical, which consists of an interactive virtual reality treadmill called the CAREN platform (computer-assisted rehabilitation environment) [19]. This platform aims to assist in gait rehabilitation for patients with neurological conditions. CAREN is an advanced system designed for human movement research, training, and evaluation. Some of the benefits and uses of CAREN include:

Benefits:

- *Human movement research*: Allows for comprehensive studies on human movement under various conditions and environments.
- *High-performance training*: Offers high-performance gait and balance training programs using virtual and augmented reality.
- *Evaluation of emerging technologies*: Allows testing of emerging movement rehabilitation technologies, such as prosthetics and exoskeletons, in immersive and challenging environments.
- *Clinical valuation and training*: Facilitates clinical assessment and functional training of patients by efficiently collecting precise data.

Uses:

- *Motion analysis*: Captures and analyzes human movement in real time, providing detailed data for research and clinical assessment.
- *Gait and balance training*: Designs customized training programs to improve gait and balance in simulated and challenging environments.
- *Functional assessment*: Enables functional assessments in environments that mimic real-life scenarios, providing valuable information for therapy and rehabilitation.
- *Assistive technology evaluation*: Allows for the evaluation of assistive technology performance in human movement, such as prosthetics and exoskeletons, before clinical implementation.

Occupational Therapy

Occupational therapy is a valuable therapeutic tool for people with Parkinson's disease, allowing them to become more independent in their daily lives and preventing disability through a variety of techniques, methods, and resources. This therapy facilitates the effective and efficient performance of daily tasks such as leisure activities, sports, work, social relationships, and self-care. Occupational therapy has a positive impact on many aspects of human well-being, addressing biological, psychological, and social aspects. Therefore, it is considered a profession with biopsychosocial benefits that contributes significantly to the overall well-being of Parkinson's disease patients. Through occupational therapy, patients can improve their quality of life, develop functional skills, and better adapt to the daily challenges associated with Parkinson's disease. It is a comprehensive therapeutic discipline that addresses the individual needs of each patient and focuses on maximizing their independence and active participation in society [20].

This profession has been and continues to be useful to Parkinson's patients as it has proven to be an ally in the management of both motor and non-motor symptoms of the disease. Its benefits range from adapting safe spaces for patients, implementing technological devices to facilitate daily living, improving mobility, and integrating educational programs that contribute to a healthier lifestyle [21].

The review by Foster et al. [22] suggests that occupational therapy is useful for people with Parkinson's disease in the following ways:

- Evaluate and train instrumental activities of daily living to increase the independence and functionality of Parkinson's disease patients.
- Performing a comprehensive assessment and diagnosis of the person with Parkinson's disease before planning any therapeutic intervention.
- Use coaching techniques to help patients modify health habits and behaviors to promote better self-care.
- Stimulate the patient through group and heterogeneous activities tailored to the different cognitive and motor abilities of the target group.

Effects of Occupational Therapy

According to Foster et al. [22], Kirwa [20], and Tofani et al. [21], the effects of occupational therapy on the management of Parkinson's disease are varied and significant:

- Occupational therapy, combined with physical and speech therapy, has been shown to significantly improve the independence of Parkinson's patients.
- The use of occupational therapy alongside brain stimulation and virtual reality has been shown to be effective in promoting patient independence.
- Improved joint mobility and control of postural balance are observed in both static and dynamic conditions.
- Occupational therapy helps reduce the risk of falls in patients.
- There is evidence of improved cognitive abilities, including increased duration of focused attention and improved memory.

- Occupational therapy promotes physical activity and benefits endurance through mitochondrial oxidative pathways, as well as improving flexibility and gait patterns.
- It contributes to the rehabilitation needed to maintain or improve fine motor skills, such as writing.
- Occupational therapy plays an important role in the emotional well-being of Parkinson's disease patients.
- It facilitates adherence to medication, which is essential for proper disease management.
- It enhances social participation, especially when occupational therapy activities, methods, and resources are delivered in heterogeneous groups, considering the level of cognitive and motor disability of the patients.

Exercises, Programs, and Dosage

REHACOP (Rehabilitation Cognitivity Program for Psychosis)

The REHACOP program was developed by a team from the University of Deusto and aims to facilitate clinical intervention in patients with psychosis, who often have deficits in attention, memory, social skills and learning difficulties, which are also common in people with Parkinson's disease. This program is available for professionals and can be obtained through the official website of the University of Deusto. For more details, it is recommended to refer to the article published by Ojeda del Pozo et al. [23].

REHACOP consists of 8 modules that address different aspects: attention, learning and memory, language, executive functions, social cognition, social skills, activities of daily living and psychoeducation. The program consists of two sets of files, one for the patient to interact with and complete, and another for the professional to use as a guide for conducting therapeutic sessions for each module.

Interventions with the REHACOP program can be conducted either individually or in a group setting, with a minimum duration of 12 weeks. Sessions take place three times a week and last 1.5 h each. The total duration of the program is 5 months.

The comprehensive and structured approach of REHACOP provides professionals with a valuable tool to address cognitive and social deficits in patients with Parkinson's disease, with the goal of improving their quality of life and promoting independence in daily living.

Sensory Stimulation Using Cues Combined with Electrotherapy and Proprioception Exercises

For effective intervention, it is recommended that the program has a minimum duration of 4 weeks, with a total of three sessions per week. Each session should last approximately 1 h on average. This time and frequency will ensure adequate progression and provide sufficient opportunity to work on the therapeutic goals in a steady and consistent manner.

Example:

Multilateral sumo squat with elastic band and muscle electrostimulation (see Figs. 6.2 and 6.3):

- **Objective**: To contribute to the improvement of dynamic stability through temporal and spatial stimulation exercise and resistance strength training.
- **Equipment**:
  - Electrostimulator and adhesive electrodes
  - One theraband
  - Eight plastic plates or colored cones for exercise
- **Diagram of the exercise** (Fig. 6.2):

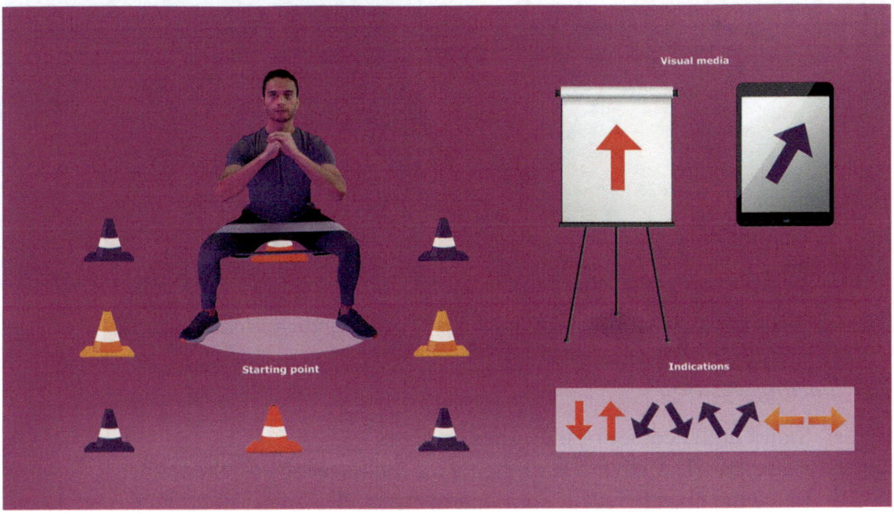

Fig. 6.2 Diagram of the exercise (multilateral sumo squat with elastic band and muscle electrostimulation)

- The purpose of each color is to serve as a visual guide, to take a step in that direction from the starting point, and to always return to the starting point during the exercise.
- To give the visual commands, the professional must show a sign indicating the direction and/or the color of the cone; for this purpose, he/she can use:
  - Arrow diagrams printed or drawn on sheets to indicate direction and color.
  - Slides on a digital screen (such as a tablet, mobile phone, or television) showing the arrows with the corresponding direction and color (Fig. 6.3).

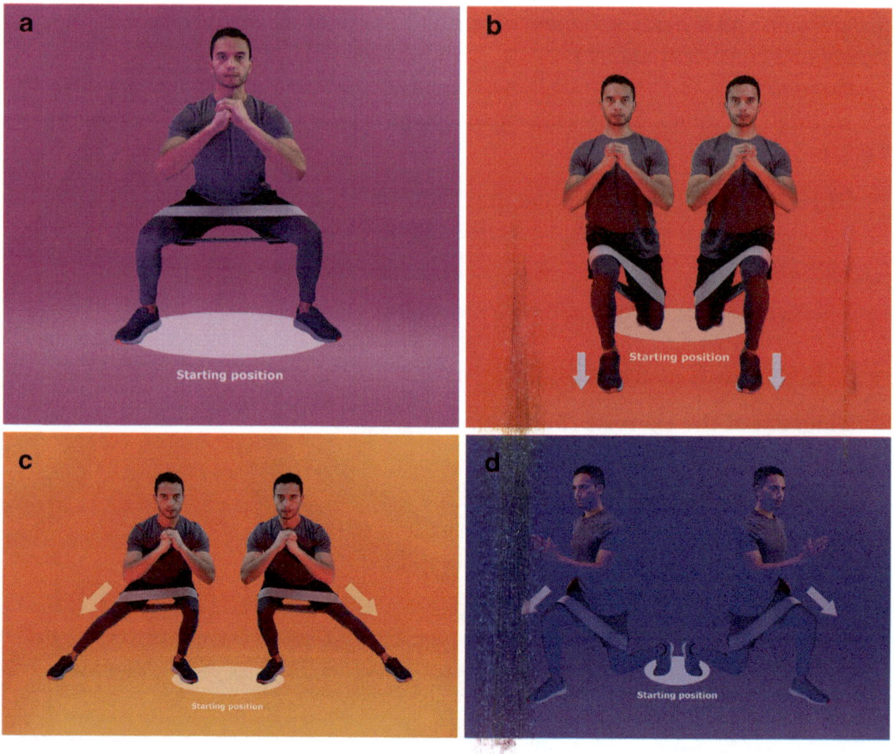

Fig. 6.3 Multilateral sumo squat with elastic band (exercise progressions and steps)

(a) ***Starting position***:

- Stand in the center of the cones or plates.
- Place the elastic band over the top of the kneecaps on the thighs.
- Place the muscle electrostimulation electrodes on the quadriceps and gluteal muscles (gluteus medius, maximus, and minimus). It is recommended to use large electrodes that cover a large area to avoid discomfort at the conduction points. The size depends on the area to be treated and the desired intensity of muscle stimulation.
- Keep your legs wide apart and squat down. Bend your knees to a maximum of 90°.
- Perform an external hip rotation with the toes pointing outward.
- The goal of each cone or plate is to serve as a guide for lateral, forward, backward, or diagonal movements.

(b) ***Red cone (front and back)***:

- Maintain the starting position.
- When the visual command appears in red and the arrow indicating the direction of the step (viable options: forward or backward), perform a lunge step.
- Return to starting position.

(c) ***Orange cone (left and right side)***:

- Maintain the starting position.
- When the visual command appears in orange and with the arrow indicating the direction of the step (possible options: left or right), perform a lateral step by extending the leg and maintaining knee flexion with the opposite leg.
- Return to starting position.

(d) ***Purple cone (upper and lower left and right diagonal)***:

- Maintain the starting position.
- When the visual command appears in purple with the arrow indicating the direction of the step (options: diagonal left and/or right), perform the movement.
- Return to starting position.

- **Type of Cueing stimulus**:
  - **Auditory cues (instructions given to the patient)**: Use verbal commands rather than visual cues. For example: "Take a step to the top left diagonal," "Take a step to the blue color."
  - **Visual cueing**: Use printed diagrams or slides that show the patient the arrow direction and color.
  - **Kinesthetic cueing**: Muscle electrostimulation.
- **Technical aspects of training**:
  - **Training method**: Neurosensory training.
  - **Load control/instrument used to control load**: Movement speed (speed at which slides or graphs are presented)/slides or graphs.
  - **Dosage for active muscle electrostimulation**:

    Session duration: 10 min.
    Frequency: 50–75 Hz.
    Pulse duration: 200–400 μs (microseconds).
    Intensity: The highest intensity that can be tolerated without harm to the patient. According to the review by Bispo et al. [24], an intensity between 60 and 100 mA is suggested.

  - **Dosage for exercise**:

    Volume:

    Repetitions (each repetition corresponds to each step in the direction of the arrow and color): 40.
    Sets: 5.

    Intensity: Intensity can be adjusted based on theraband resistance, muscle electrostimulation intensity, and the speed at which graphs or slides are presented.

Density (rest intervals ***between sets and repetitions. Values are given in the ratio of "loading phase*: *recovery phase")***:

Between repetitions: N/A
Between sets: 1:2

- **Exercise modifications**:

Basic level:

Option 1: Start from a standing position without maintaining an isometric squat.
Option 2: Perform the exercise without the theraband.

Advance level:

Option 1: Do the exercise on one leg balance and do jumps instead of steps.
Option 2: Use a Theraband with strong resistance and maintain a squat position with 90° flexion throughout.

Transcranial Direct Current Stimulation (tDCS) Alongside Occupational Therapy

tDCS is a noninvasive method of stimulating cortical and subcortical areas of the brain by applying mild cathodal and anodal electrical currents to the skull. The effects of tDCS are broad, including improved cerebral neuroplasticity, communication skills, proprioception, memory, pain management, migraine, fibromyalgia, chronic fatigue, neuralgia, and multiple executive cognitive functions. For application, a helmet with integrated electrodes (known as fixed-layout high-definition tDCS) is placed on the head, or individual electrodes are placed on the skull (known as variable-layout tDCS); both systems are controlled by an electrical stimulator.

In terms of dosage, a minimum of eight sessions is suggested, alternating between occupational therapy interventions (1-h session duration) and tDCS (20-min session duration). Another option is to combine occupational therapy and tDCS simultaneously.

Quantitative Parameters of tDCS

- Intensity: The intensity varies according to the current flow and ranges from 0.5 to 2 mA (sufficient to excite the cerebral cortex).

- Density: The amount of current or flow through an area is known as current density. Typically, for neuromodulation, it varies from 0.08 to 0.20 A/m^2.
- Frequency: A minimum of five sessions is suggested, but all varies according to the individual response of each patient and the condition being treated.
- Stimulation duration: Neuroplasticity is directly related to stimulation duration, but excessive duration leads to side effects. Therefore, multiple tDCS sessions are performed to minimize the risk to the patient. A session typically lasts 10–20 min.
- Position: Position varies depending on the purpose of the treatment and the objective direction of current flow. A standardized guide for equitable placement of extracranial electrodes is the International 10–20 EEG System for Electrode Placement.
- Electrode size: Varies from 25 to 35 cm^2. Larger electrodes result in a lower maximum current density per surface area.
- Side effects: Side effects are mild to moderate, ranging from mild headache, warmth at the stimulation site, tingling, muscle spasms, to seizures, dizziness, and possible hearing loss (if proper ear protection is not used).
- Contraindications: Epilepsy, abdominal or inguinal hernia, cardiac pacemakers, skin irritations or burns on the scalp, high uric acid levels, magnetic implants near the stimulation site, bullet fragments, severe cardiovascular, pulmonary, hepatic, and renal pathologies, among others.

Example:

tDCS activation alongside strength and stretching exercises (For a better understanding, see Figs. 6.4, 6.5, 6.6, 6.7, 6.8, and 6.9):

The example was based on the Souza et al. [25] and Straudi et al. [26] reviews.

- **Objective**:
  - Reduce symptoms and perception of low back pain through active tDCS in conjunction with therapeutic exercises focusing on strength and static active flexibility.
  - Enhance static stability through active tDCS combined with therapeutic exercises emphasizing strength and static active flexibility.
- **Elements**:
  - tDCS
  - Electrode-equipped helmet
- **Location of tDCS according to the international 10–20 system** (Figs. 6.4 and 6.5; Table 6.2):

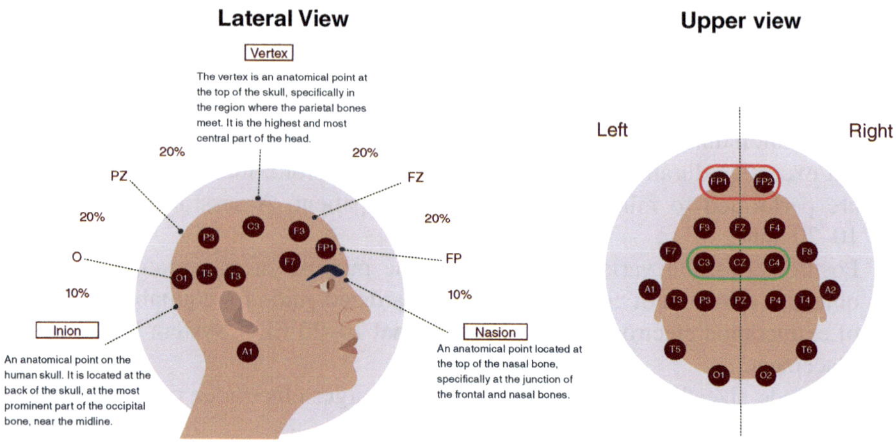

Fig. 6.4 Active tDCS

- F = frontal
- FP = frontopolar
- C = central
- P = parietal
- O = occipital
- A = Auricular,
- T = temporal
- Z = midline (zero line)
- Even numbers = 2, 4, 6, 8 are the electrodes located in the right hemisphere
- Odd numbers = 1, 3, 5, 7 are the electrodes located in the left hemisphere

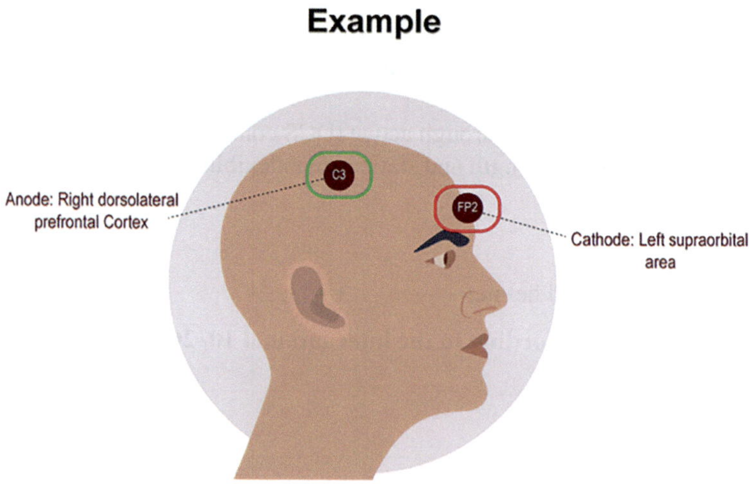

Fig. 6.5 Example of tDCS for sensorimotor functions.

Anode electrode placement: Over the primary motor cortex (C3, CZ, and C4)

Cathode electrode placement: Contralateral area to the anode over the supraorbital or frontopolar region (FP1 or FP2)

Table 6.2 Electrode placement in each cerebral area

Cerebral area	Left hemisphere	Midline	Right hemisphere
Frontopolar	FP1		FP2
Frontal	F3	FZ	F2
Fronto temporal	F7 C3	CZ	F8 C4
Mid and parietal temporal	T3 P3	PZ	T4 P4
Posterior and occipital temporal	T5 O1		T6 02

- **Type of exercises to perform with tDCS**:
  - *tDCS along with strength exercises* (Figs. 6.6 and 6.7):

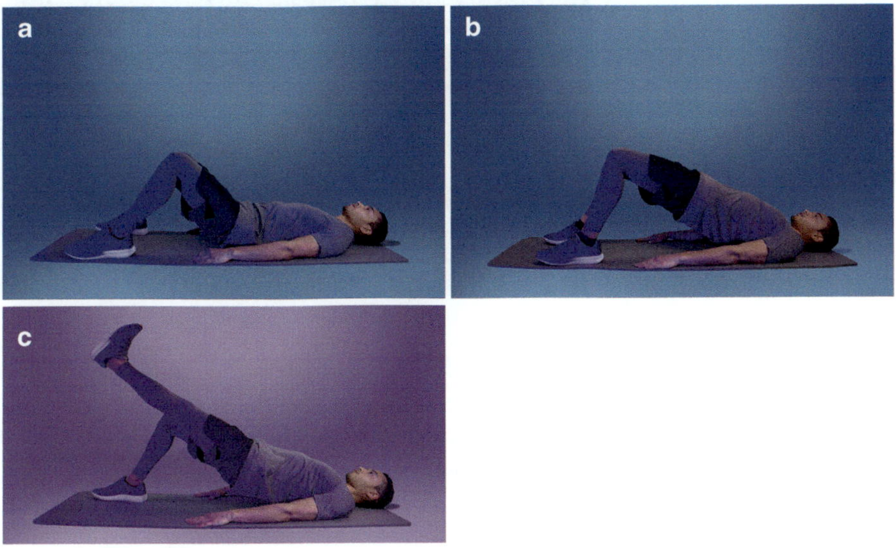

Fig. 6.6 Bridge exercise with one or two legs

Steps to perform the exercise:

(a) ***Starting position***:

- Place the electrodes according to the parameters of the International 10–20 System for tDCS and the goals to be achieved.
- Lie on your back (supine position) with both legs flexed at 120° (avoid flexing at 90°). Keep your feet slightly wider than hip width and rotate your hips outward with your toes slightly outward. Relax and extend arms out to sides of body.
- Additionally, engage the abdominal muscles by pulling the navel down to the lumbar vertebrae and contract the glutes.

(b) Raise hips off floor to hip extension and hold this position for 6 s, then slowly lower your hips and return to the flexed position. Repeat as many times as required.

(c) ***Alternative to step b***: You have the option to perform the exercise using only one leg, which serves as a more challenging alternative.

Note: Avoid lifting or extending your hips too much and keep your abs always engaged. You should feel the exercise primarily in your glutes.

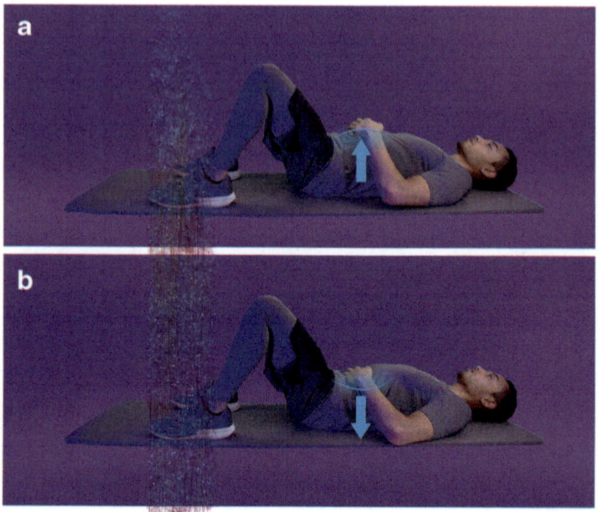

Fig. 6.7 Abdominal hollowing

Steps to perform the exercise:

(a) ***Step 1***:

- Starting position: Lie on your back (supine position) with both legs bent at 90° and feet in contact with the floor.
- Place hands on lower abdomen.
- Inhale deeply and slowly.

(b) ***Step 1***:

- Exhale slowly, pulling your abdomen inward (a guide is to direct your navel toward the lumbar area, essentially pulling it in).
- Hold this position for 6 s while continuing to exhale slowly.
- Repeat the exercise according to the load parameters.

– *tDCS along with flexibility exercises* (see Figs. 6.8 and 6.9):

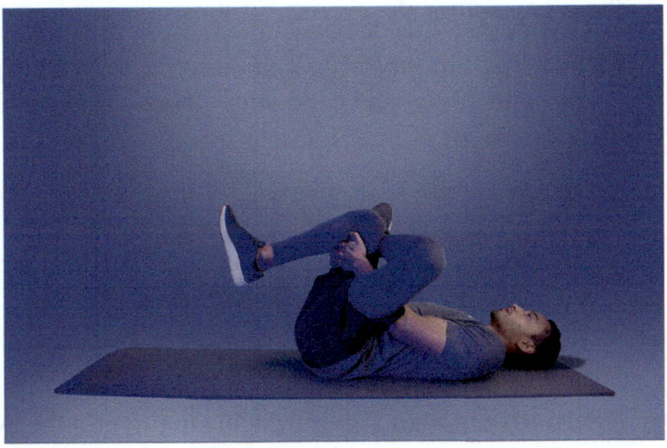

Fig. 6.8 Hip rotator stretch

Steps to perform the exercise:

- *Starting position*: Lie on your back (supine position) with both legs flexed at 90° and feet in contact with the floor.
- Cross one foot over the opposite leg so that one ankle is near to the knee of the opposite leg.
- Place your hands behind the thigh of the opposite leg. Slowly and gradually bring the knee, of that leg, toward your chest. Be sure to include the abdominal area to prevent excessive arching of the lower back in hyperkyphosis and/or hyperlordosis.
- Maintain this position for 30 s.
- Repeat the exercise according to the load parameters.

Note: You should feel the stretch in the buttock of the crossed leg.

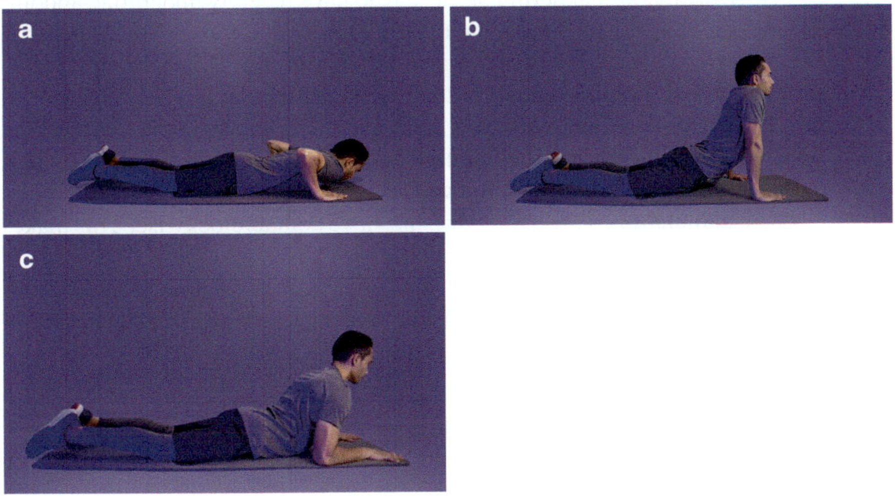

Fig. 6.9 Hip prone extension

Steps to perform the exercise:

- **Step 1**: *Starting position*: Lie on your abdomen (prone position), place your hands on the floor, and bend your elbows (as if starting a push-up).
- **Step 2**:
  - Slowly extend your elbows, lifting only the upper part of your torso. Keep your pelvis and lower limbs relaxed on the floor.
  - Extend your spine, creating an arch. Perform the arch carefully and without experiencing any pain.
  - Hold the position for 30 s.
  - Repeat the exercise according to load parameters.
- **Alternative to Step 2**: It is possible to perform the exercise without fully extending your arms, supporting yourself on your elbows and forearms, to avoid excessive spinal extension if it causes you pain or discomfort.
  Note: If you have a radicular condition, the pain may increase depending on the affected disc area or affected nerves. Consult a professional before performing the exercise.
- **Technical aspects of training**:
  - **Training method**: tDCS (transcranial direct current stimulation) in combination with strength and stretching exercises.
  - **Dosage of load for tDCS**:

    Total treatment duration: 4 weeks
    Session duration: 20 min
    Frequency: 5 times per week consecutively
    Electrode placement:

    - *Anode*:
      - In cases of central or bilateral low back pain, the anode is placed over the primary motor cortex of the dominant hemisphere (C3, CZ, and/or C4), for sensorimotor function stimulation.
      - In cases of unilateral low back pain, the anode is placed over the primary motor cortex contralateral to the hemisphere of the lumbar pain region (C3, CZ, and/or C4), for sensorimotor function stimulation.
    - *Cathode*:
      - The cathode is placed on the contralateral area to the anode, specifically over the supraorbital zone.

    Intensity: 2 mA
  - **Dosage of load for strength exercises**:

    Total treatment duration: 4 weeks
    Frequency: 5 times per week consecutively, following tDCS
    Volume:

- Repetitions: 10 with an isometric phase at the peak of muscle tension. This isometric contraction should be hold for at least 6 s.
- Sets: 5

Intensity: 60% of maximal voluntary muscle contraction
Density (rest intervals between sets and repetitions, values are given as follow "loading phase: recovery phase ratio"):

- Between repetitions: N/A
- Between sets: 1:1

– **Dosage of load for flexibility exercises**:

Total treatment duration: 4 weeks
Frequency: 5 times per week consecutively
Volume:

- Repetitions: 4 per muscle group and hemisphere
- Duration per repetition: 30 s
- Sets: 3

Intensity:

- Level 31–70, according to the perceived effort scale of flexibility (perflex) shown in the Table 6.3:

Table 6.3 Perceived effort of flexibility (perflex), based on Conceição and Dantas [27]

Level	Sensations	Effects	Characteristics
0-30	Normality	Mobility	Plastic, mechanical, and inextensible components do not change.
31-60	Forced	Stretching	Sub maximum deformation of plastic and elastic components.
61-80	Discomfort	Flexing	Lasting modifications of plastic, mechanical and inextensible components.
81-90	Bearable pain	Possible injury	The musculotendinous and connective units are extremely stretched.
91-110	Strong pain	Injury	It surpasses the safe stretching and mobility capacity of the musculoskeletal structures.

Density (rests between sets and repetitions. Values are given as follow "load phase: recovery phase ratio"):

- Between repetitions: N/A (not applicable)
- Between sets: 1:1/2 (1 min of recovery for every 2 min of exercise)

Hand and Forearm Writing and Muscle-Strengthening Exercises

Fine motor skills are affected in the early stages of Parkinson's disease, so it is important to address them at the first sign of Parkinson's symptoms. The skills most often affected are handwriting, micrography, and the use of everyday objects such as utensils or glasses while eating. Therefore, it is important to incorporate activities into the daily routine that stimulate and strengthen fine motor skills.

Activities such as drawing, writing, or diagramming are suggested because these activities require precise control of hand and finger movements. In addition, incorporating games that require fine motor skills, such as video games, construction games, or assembling puzzles, is also beneficial.

It is also important to strengthen the muscles of the forearm and hands, as their strength is directly related to the risk of falling in people with Parkinson's disease. A lower level of grip strength in these areas can increase the risk of falls, so specific exercises to strengthen these muscles should be included in the treatment plan [28, 29].

Regarding the dosage of the load, it is recommended to have four sessions of 30 min each per week throughout the course of the disease. These sessions should focus on grip strength and fine motor skills.

Example:

Writing exercises:

- **Objective**: Improve fine motor skills when writing, drawing diagrams, or handling objects with hands.
- **Elements**:
  - Various pens, markers, or pencils of varying dimensions, textures, and colors.
  - Notebook with writing guides (preferably lined ones).
  - Printed or drawn diagrams (see Figs. 6.10, 6.11, 6.12, and 6.13).
  - Laser pointer.
- **Exercises**:
  - Connect the dots (Figs. 6.10 and 6.11):

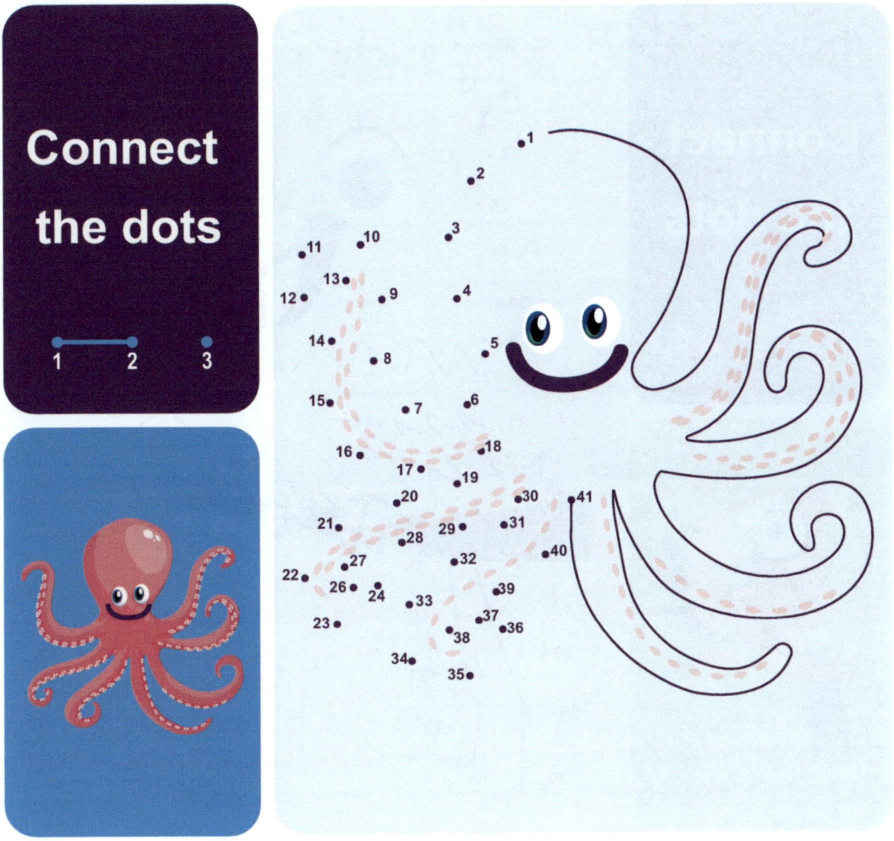

Fig. 6.10 Connect the dots option 1

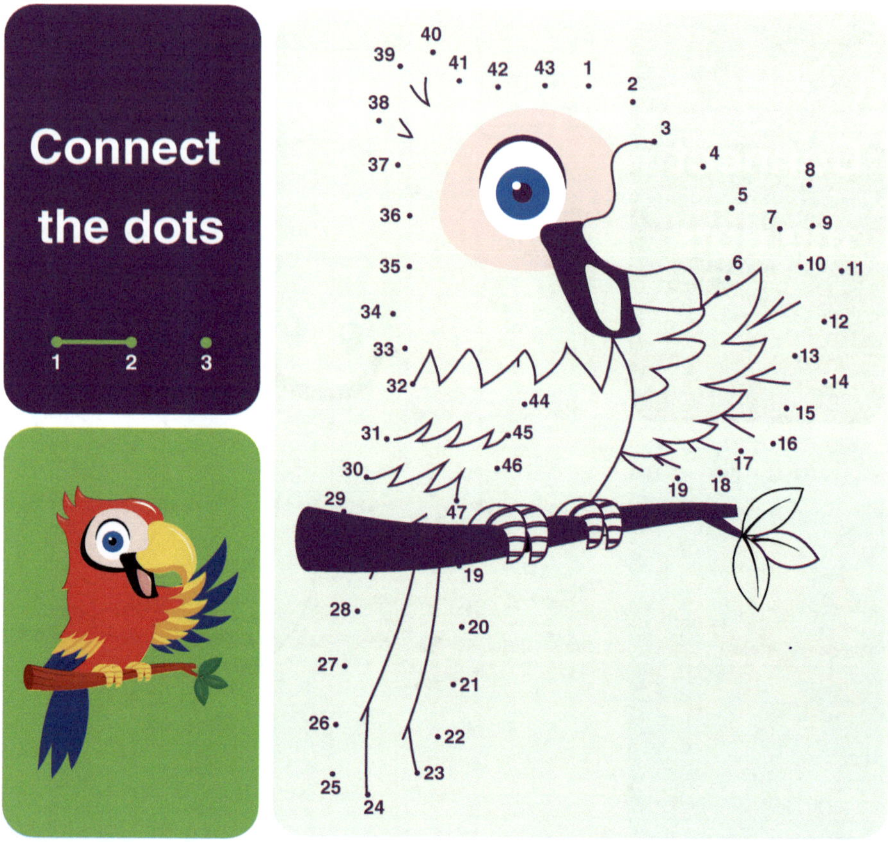

Fig. 6.11 Connect the dots option 2

- **Instructions**:
  - Print diagrams for connecting dots (like the example shown above) in letter or legal paper size.
  - Draw straight lines between dots, ensuring the numerical order of each.
- **Exercise modalities**: Connect lines to complete the numerical dot diagram, following these adiotional challneges:
  - Connect numerical dots from lowest to highest.
  - Connect numerical dots from highest to lowest.
  - Connect numerical dots alternately.
  - Visualize the line between two numerical dots, then close your eyes and trace the connecting line.
  - Connect numerical dots with both dominant and non-dominant hands.
  - Draw dashed lines between dots.
  - Use different colors, thicknesses, and dimensions of the pen or pencil while drawing the lines.

  – While drawing the lines, apply a kinesthetic stimulus to the forearm muscles, such as vibration from a percussion device, muscle electrostimulation, cold, or heat.

- Fine motor coordination exercise (Fig. 6.12):

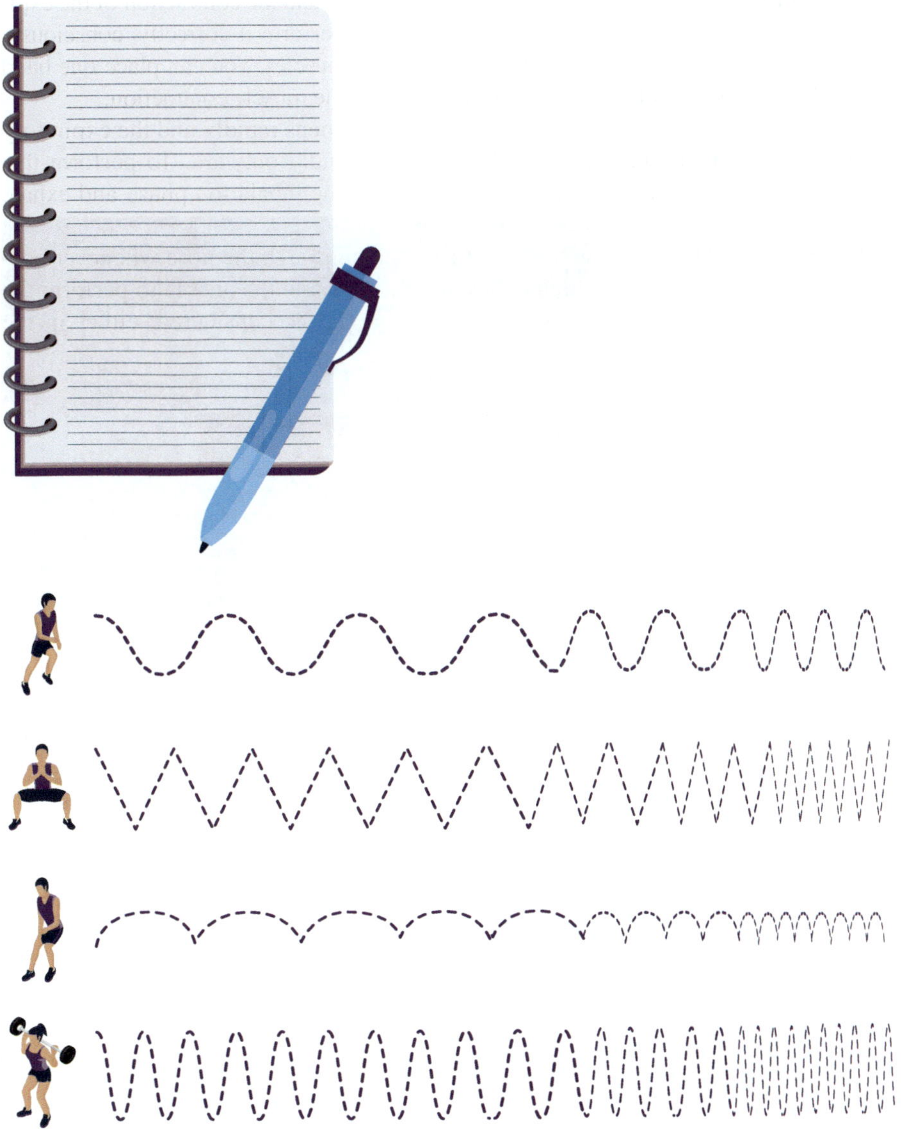

Fig. 6.12 Exercise diagram to enhance fine motor coordination for writing skills

- **Instructions**: Use a notebook for daily writing, with horizontal guides to facilitate writing orientation and diagrams.
- **Explanation**:
  - Use a thick pen to facilitate writing and keep the hand flexor muscles relaxed.
  - Write letters or numbers in cursive and/or regular form, varying dimensions and thicknesses.
  - Write with the nondominant hand.
  - Write in reverse of normal dominant writing.
  - Write based on inspiration or purpose.

- Motor control with laser pointer (Fig. 6.13):

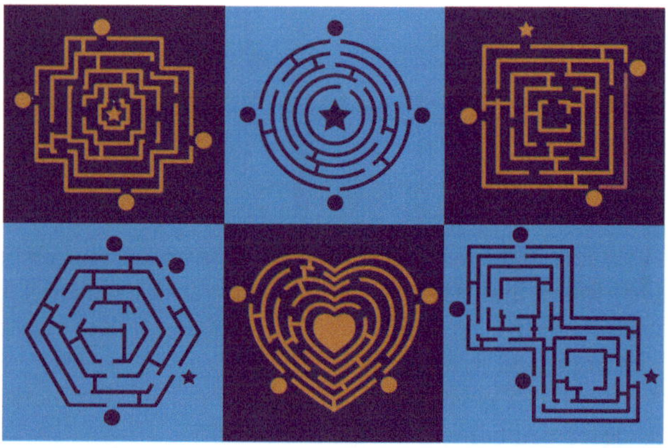

Fig. 6.13 Possible maze diagrams for use with the laser pointer

The following Figs. 6.14, 6.15, and 6.16 show the possible locations for the laser pointer:

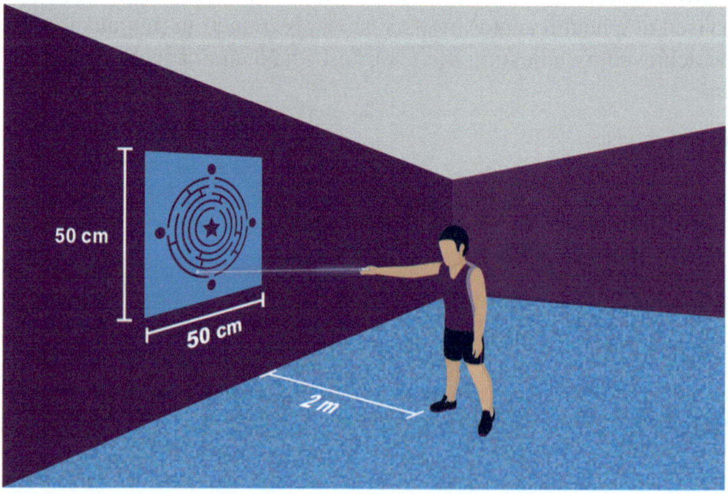

Fig. 6.14 Use of the hands. m = meters. cm = centimeters

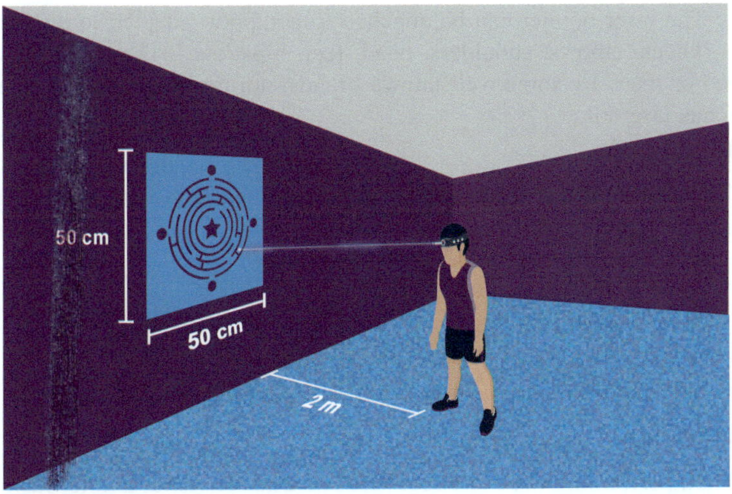

Fig. 6.15 Use of the head. m = meters. cm = centimeters

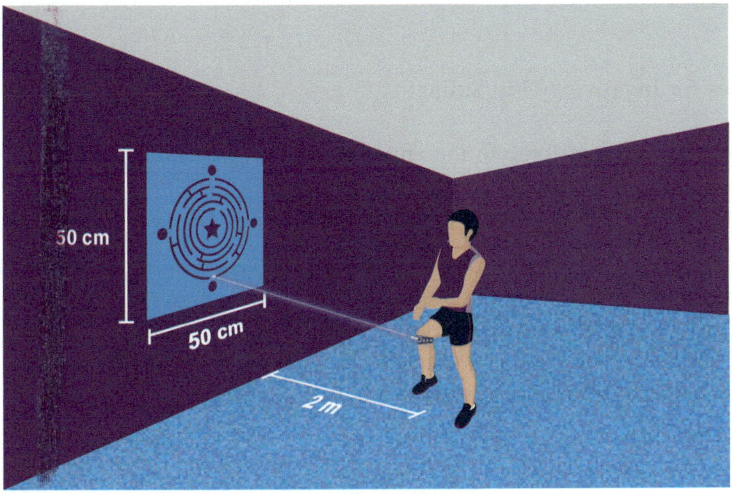

Fig. 6.16 Use of the knees. m = meters. cm = centimeters

- **Instructions**: Print a maze diagram and affix it to a wall or surface at shoulder level. The print size should be large enough for the exercise; suggested sizes are 50 × 50 cm, 50 × 70 cm, and/or 1 m × 1 m, depending on individual patient needs, exercise, and available space.
- **Explanation**:
  - Stand in front of the diagram, two steps away from it.
  - Hold the laser pointer in your hand, turned on, and trace the maze with the laser light, without getting close to it.

Note: The laser pointer can be attached to a support adapted to different body areas (knees, elbows, shoulders, head, feet, hips, etc.). These supports can be crafted or there are some well-known brands, not for advertising purposes, like the focus laser kit.

- **Dosage of load**:
  - Total duration of treatment: Throughout the entire evolutionary or unevolutionary process of the pathology.
  - Session Duration: 30 min
  - Frequency: 4 times per week
  - Volume: Varies according to the number of diagrams utilized
  - Intensity: Varies based on exercise modifications
  - Density (rest intervals): 2 min between exercises
- **Suggestions**:
  - When performing the exercises, focus on one activity at a time, such as writing a letter or making a stroke.
  - If the hand or forearm becomes stiff during the exercise, pause, and perform another activity, then resume the exercise after a few seconds.

Exercises for Improving Grip Strength

- **Objective**: To contribute to the enhancement of grip strength through muscle-strengthening exercises.
- **Elements**:
  - Sand or rice-filled cube, where extended fingers and the entire hand can be inserted.
  - Exerciser for finger extensor muscles.
  - Two heavy dumbbells (alternative: two backpacks with sand, two buckets with water or sand, 2 large water bottles).
- **Exercises**:
- *Sand or rice cube* (Figs. 6.17 and 6.18):
  - *Possible movements to perform* within the sand or rice-filled cube:

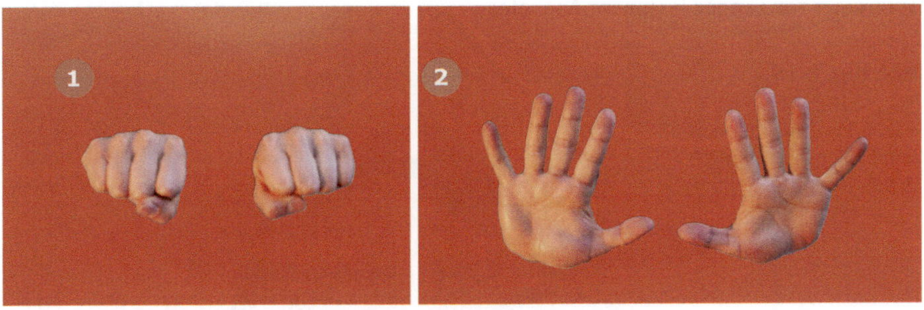

Fig. 6.17 Flexion and extension of the fingers

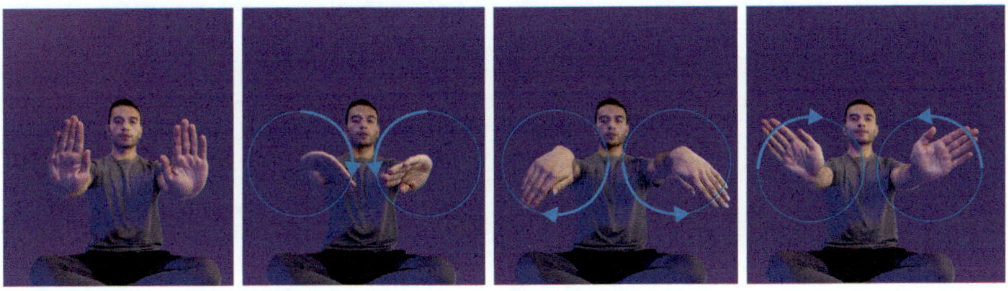

Fig. 6.18 Wrist circumduction

– *Guidelines*: Fill a cube with rice or sand, leaving enough space to fully insert and open the fingers of the hands.
– *Exercise*: Insert the hands into the sand or rice-filled cube and perform the following movements:

  Extend and flex the fingers.
  Open and close the fist.
  Touch the tip of finger number 1 (thumb) with the tip of each finger alternately.
  Perform ulnar and radial deviations of the wrist.
  Perform movements freely.

- **Load Dosage**:
  – Frequency: 4 times per week, with 1 day of rest between each session
  – Volume:

    Repetitions: 30
    Sets: 6.

  – Intensity: Varies based on movement speed and cube content
  – Density (rest intervals): 40 s between sets

Exerciser for Finger Extensor Muscles

See Fig. 6.19.

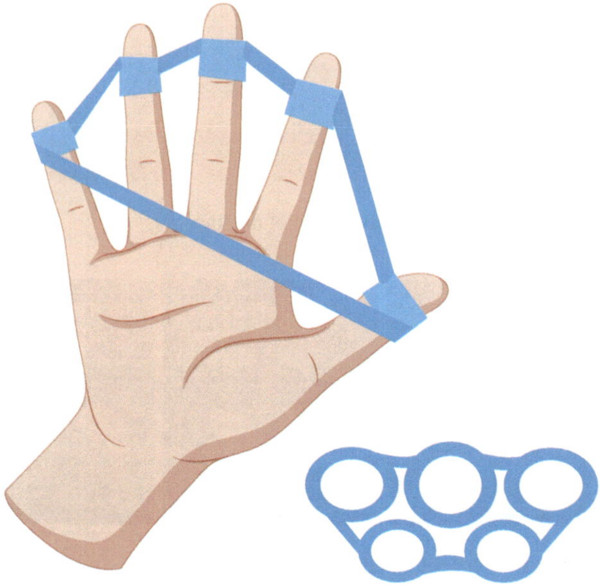

Fig. 6.19 Illustration of a hand extensor training device

- **Exercise**:
  - Place the fingers inside the exerciser.
  - Slowly extend and separate the fingers from each other (abduction), until reaching the maximum point of muscular contraction.
  - Hold the position for 5 s.
  - Relax and repeat.
- **Load dosage**:
  - Frequency: 4 times per week, with 1 day of rest between each session
  - Volume:

    Repetitions: 15
    Sets: 4

  - Intensity: Varies based on movement speed and exerciser resistance
  - Density (rest intervals): 45 s between sets

Farmer's Walk (Fig. 6.20)

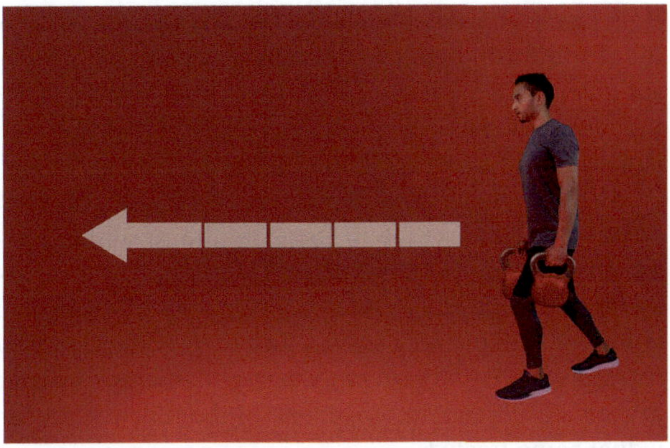

Fig. 6.20 Farmer's walk

- **Exercise**:
  - Stand upright, gripping two heavy dumbbells or objects such as a backpack or bag filled with sand, water-filled bottles, and buckets with sand or water.
  - Move walking from one point to another without releasing the weight. The minimum suggest distance for walking is 10 m.
  - Release the weight and repeat the round.
- **Load dosage**:
  - Frequency: 4 times per week, with 1 day of rest between each session
  - Volume:

    Repetitions (one repetition corresponds to 1 round trip): 4
    Sets: 3

  - Intensity:

    Varies based on movement speed and weight of the carried object
    70–80% of RM (maximum repetitions) is recommended

  - Density (rest intervals):

    Between repetitions: 10–15 s
    Between sets: 1–90 s

- **Suggestions**:
  - Prior to performing the exercises, engage in joint mobility exercises for fingers and wrists.
  - After completing the exercises, perform stretches (neurodynamic, static, or proprioceptive neuromuscular facilitation stretch methods).
  - It is recommended to practice these exercises throughout the entire evolutionary or unevolutionary process of the pathology.

Physical and Occupational Therapy

Both physical and occupational therapy share a common goal: to improve the quality of life for individuals through rehabilitation and to promote independence and autonomy in daily living. Both specialties work closely with other health-care professionals such as physicians, nurses, and psychologists to provide comprehensive patient care.

Although there are differences between the two therapies, the line that separates them is very narrow. Both focus on the rehabilitation of injuries, physical illness, and the improvement of daily living skills. For this reason, it is suggested that both therapies should be considered as the scientific and practical foundation of rehabilitation, complementing each other to provide complete and effective Parkinson's patients care. By working together, both therapies can achieve more effective results in the recovery and improvement of the functionality and quality of life of the individual being treated.

Authors such as Ángel [30], Lear [31], Palazón García et al. [32], and Radder et al. [33] recommend in their studies that both therapies must be practiced for a minimum of 12 weeks, with three sessions of 90 to 120 min per week. By integrating these two therapies, a comprehensive and satisfying rehabilitation can be achieved that addresses both physical function and the ability to perform activities of daily living, thereby improving the patient's quality of life.

Example of a Therapeutic Protocol (Table 6.4)

Table 6.4 Example of a therapeutic protocol

Therapeutic protocol

Objective:
- Maintain joint mobility
- Prevent contractures
- Improve posture and gait
- Relearn and facilitate activities of daily living

Modules

Module of body mobility	Cognitive basic training module	Daily activities module
1. Respiratory exercises involving diaphragmatic and thoracic cavities 2. Mobility of the entire facial musculature 3. Mobility of upper limb joints (including cervical and dorsal spine) 4. Coordination training, dynamic and static balance 5. Seated exercises 6. Bipedal stance exercises 7. Hip dissociation and mobility exercises 8. Motor unlocking exercises **Note:** These exercises should be internalized by the patient to be executed independently in case of freezing of movement episodes.	**Reality orientation activities:** – Focuses on providing the patient with current and everyday information to increase his or her knowledge of the environment. Reminiscence and life review exercises: – Therapeutic techniques are used to improve memory based on lived experience by organizing information in time and space. **Note:** For session planning, it is suggested to follow these steps: • *Reception:* Establish initial contact with the patient to create a trusting environment with the therapist and/or the group. • *Preparation:* Use reality-based questions to prepare the patient for reminiscence and life review activities. • *Development:* Conduct specific activities such as presentations, mapping, role-playing with professions, newspaper readings, and cooking exercises, to encourage memory, attention, language, and social interaction. • *Farewell:* Pay attention to the final moment of contact with the patient to bid farewell positively and personally. • *Evaluation:* Conduct patient assessments, activity evaluations, and therapist self-assessment to determine the effectiveness of therapeutic sessions.	**Feeding:** – Recommendations include closing the mouth before swallowing (to facilitate the swallowing reflex) and using aids such as flexible straws for drinking, bowls with high and non-slip rims, cups and glasses with double handles, and angled utensils. **Transfers:** – Practice changing positions from lying down to other positions such as supine or lateral. – Information on how to properly get out of bed. – Environmental modifications to facilitate transfers, such as using firm mattresses and furniture, adjusting bed height to facilitate lying down and rising. **Clothing:** – Avoid fabrics that create friction; choose loose-fitting clothing with Velcro or elastic fasteners instead of buttons or zippers; and choose shoes with breathable soles, preferably without laces, which support the ankle. **Personal care and hygiene:** – Use grab bars, toilet seat risers, nonslip mats, bathtub seats, and single-lever faucets to improve accessibility and safety.

Dosage of load
- Total duration of treatment: Throughout the evolutionary or degenerative process of the condition
- Session length: 90–120 min
- Frequency: 3 times a week

Suggestions:
- The program should preferably be led by professionals or very specific guidelines for the patient.
- It is recommended to mix the modules when planning the therapeutic sessions.

Dance

The practice of dance has been shown to be beneficial for people with Parkinson's disease, improving motor function, cognition, depression, and quality of life. In addition, patients who participate in dance have shown long-term improvements in balance and mobility. Studies suggest that dance sessions for Parkinson's disease patients should last between 60 and 90 min and be performed 1–3 times per week for a total of 6–12 months [34–36].

The authors propose different types of dances and their subgenres, including:

- **Contemporary dance:** Fluid and expressive movements that emphasize creativity and individual technique.
- **Ballroom dance:** Partner dances with elegant and precise movements, such as tango, waltz, and salsa.
- **Folkloric dance:** Energetic and expressive movements that reflect the culture and traditions of a particular region or country.
- **Creative dance:** Improvisation and individual expression based on music, emotion, and physical sensation.
- **Line dance:** Dancing in a line or circle with a predetermined sequence of steps, such as country and hip-hop.
- **Belly dance:** Soft and fluid movements of the torso and hips, originating in the Middle East and North Africa.
- **Free movement dance:** Improvisation and individual expression without adherence to a specific style or technique.

Virtual Reality Training

Virtual reality training has gained increasing interest in the research and treatment of Parkinson's patients. This innovative technology has shown promise in improving functionality and quality of life for these individuals.

In general, it is suggested that virtual reality training sessions be at least 1 h in length to provide effective stimulation and practice of motor and cognitive skills. These sessions should be structured and tailored to the individual needs of each patient. To optimize the benefits of virtual reality, it is recommended that short breaks of at least 3 min be included between exercises. These breaks allow the patient to rest, regain focus and maintain interest throughout the training program. Regarding the total duration of the program, a minimum of 2 months is suggested to achieve significant results in rehabilitation and improvement of motor and cognitive skills. It is important to emphasize that continuity and consistency in training are fundamental to achieving significant advances in patient functionality.

It is important to recognize that each Parkinson's patient is unique and may respond differently to virtual reality training. Therefore, it is essential to tailor the program individually, considering each person's abilities and limitations.

Virtual Training Sessions

A professional-led virtual training session is an experience in which a specialized therapist and/or coach works with a Parkinson's patient to perform a variety of exercises. These exercises include aspects such as strength, flexibility, endurance, coordination, agility, and speed, enhanced by the integration of virtual reality interaction. During these sessions, the therapist takes an active role, monitoring and dynamically adjusting the exercises to ensure proper execution and alignment with the patient's specific needs. The therapist's presence also facilitates immediate and tailored feedback to the patient, a key factor in improving technique and progress with each session.

It is recommended that these sessions last between 40 and 60 min and that they take place three times a week in order to achieve significant results. Consistency and regularity in training are critical to realizing improvements in functionality and quality of life for Parkinson's patients.

Hatha Yoga

Hatha yoga is an ancient discipline that combines postures, breathing techniques, and meditation to promote overall health and well-being. Hatha yoga practice involves a series of postures that focus on body alignment, muscle strengthening, flexibility, and balance. These postures help improve physical function and mobility, which is particularly beneficial for Parkinson's patients who struggle with motor symptoms such as rigidity and tremors.

Beyond the postures, conscious breathing is an integral facet of hatha yoga. Breathing techniques help to calm the mind and reduce stress, an important benefit for Parkinson's patients who often struggle with the emotional challenges associated with the disease. Meditation also plays a central role in the practice of hatha yoga. Guided meditation during yoga sessions can reduce anxiety, facilitate relaxation, and increase mental focus. This is particularly valuable for Parkinson's patients, as stress and anxiety can exacerbate motor symptoms and impact quality of life.

Research underscores the substantial benefits of regular hatha yoga practice in managing and improving motor symptoms in Parkinson's patients. The combination of postures, conscious breathing, and meditation creates a holistic practice that addresses both the physical and emotional dimensions of the disease.

Group hatha yoga sessions are recommended, as a sense of community and support can be particularly beneficial for Parkinson's patients. Sessions should last at least 1 h and be held twice a week for at least 12 weeks to achieve significant results [37].

Exercise Through Mobile Applications

The use of mobile applications for physical exercise has proven to be an effective tool for improving motor symptoms and quality of life in Parkinson's patients. This modality of exercise offers flexibility and convenience, allowing patients to engage in exercise from the comfort of their home or other preferred location.

It is recommended that exercise sessions last from 30 min to 1 h and be performed consistently over a period of no less than 8 weeks to achieve significant results. Supervision by a trained professional is essential to ensure that the exercises are tailored to the specific needs of each patient and are performed safely and effectively.

It is essential that the application used, takes into account the patient's pathological characteristics and provides exercises that are appropriate to address their specific symptoms and limitations. In addition, the application should facilitate the monitoring and recording of exercise progress, allowing both the patient and the professional to meticulously track progress and modify the program as necessary.

A key factor in the success of the program is personalization. Each Parkinson's patient is unique, so the program must be tailored to the individual's needs and abilities. Personalization allows exercises to be focused on specific areas that require increased attention, providing a more comprehensive and effective approach to disease management.

Muscular Strength Training with Free Weights Combined with Exercises to Activate Mitochondrial Oxidative Pathways

Strength training using free weights and machines in conjunction with mitochondrial oxidative pathway activation (aerobic) exercises provides a regimen tailored to improve both muscular strength capacity and cardiopulmonary endurance in Parkinson's disease patients. This exercise paradigm has potential benefits as it may increase functional capacity and promote independence in performing activities of daily living. In addition, resistance and machine-based training may help prevent the loss of muscle mass and weakness associated with aging and Parkinson's disease.

It is recommended that training sessions last between 60 and 90 min and are performed 2–3 times per week, with the intervention program lasting at least 12 weeks. Throughout the training session, careful consideration must be given to the intensity of the exercise to ensure that it is appropriate for the patient's abilities. The presence of an experienced therapeutic exercise professional is essential to supervise the program, thereby reducing the risk of injury and optimizing the benefits for the patient (Table 6.5).

Table 6.5 Illustration of a muscle-strengthening regimen that incorporates free weights alongside aerobic exercises designed to activate the mitochondrial oxidative pathway

Exercise	Explications	Volume	Intensity	Rests	Suggestions
Dumbbell bench press	Strengthening exercise that primarily targets the pectorals, deltoids, and triceps, while also engaging the core and stabilizing muscles of the shoulders and back.	3–4 sets of 8–12 repetitions (reps.) per set	Moderate load, allowing for the indicated number of repetitions.	1–2 min rest between sets	– Be sure to maintain proper technique to avoid injury. – Adjust the load to your ability and increase it gradually. – Use a training partner or safety equipment if necessary.
Free squat	Strengthening exercise that works primarily the muscles of the legs and buttocks, but also activates the core and stabilizing muscles of the back and hips.	3-4 sets of 8–12 reps. per set	Moderate load that allows you to complete the indicated number of reps.	1–2 min rest between sets	
Rowing exercise	Strength exercise that primarily targets the back, shoulders, and arms, but also activates the core and stabilizing muscles of the shoulders and back.	3–4 sets of 8–12 reps. per set	Moderate load that allows you to complete the indicated number of reps.	1–2 min rest between sets	
Stationary bike	Cardiovascular exercise that works mainly the leg muscles and improves cardiopulmonary endurance.	30 min of moderate or vigorous intensity	Adjust the intensity to the patient's ability.	5 min of active rest at the end of the workout	– Monitor heart rate and blood pressure during exercise. – Adjust intensity and duration according to patient capacity. – Maintain proper posture and smooth pedaling technique.
Treadmill	Cardiovascular exercise that works mainly the leg muscles and improves cardiopulmonary endurance.	30 min of moderate or vigorous intensity	Adjust the intensity to the patient's ability.	5 min of active rest at the end of the workout	

Muscle Electrostimulation

Muscle electrostimulation (ME) is a technique used to prevent muscle wasting, loss of muscle mass, and lack of strength in patients with Parkinson's's disease. It involves the activation of muscle fibers and increased capillarization through controlled electrical stimulation.

ME has been shown to have significant therapeutic and preventive benefits in Parkinson's patients with postural and biomechanical alterations. This technique is widely used for various therapeutic applications. One of the most prominent applications of ME in Parkinson's patients is the rehabilitation of dysphagia by activating the cricothyroid, suprahyoid and buccinator muscles, which helps improve swallowing and control of the muscles involved in this process. In addition, ME is used to prevent falls by strengthening the muscles of the lower extremities, abdomen, and pelvis, thereby improving balance and stability in patients. Another important benefit of ME in the treatment of Parkinson's disease is its use in therapeutic cueing techniques to prevent gait freezing. Precise and controlled electrical stimuli can guide and focus the patient's attention during walking, helping to avoid freezing episodes [38, 39].

There are two ways to perform muscle electrostimulation (ME): passive and active. Passive ME refers to when the muscle contraction is generated solely by the electro stimulator, while active ME combines muscle activation by the device with voluntary contraction of one or more muscles by the patient. There are also emerging trends in the field of ME, such as whole-body muscle electrostimulation [40, 41].

Effects of Muscle Electrostimulation

According to Alouini et al. [42], Bispo et al. [24], Centeno [43], García Arribas [38], María Sánchez [41], and Sweeney et al. [44], the effects of muscle electrostimulation include:

- Reduction of tremor and dyskinesia.
- Improved postural control, balance, and muscle stiffness.
- Pain reduction.
- Improved swallowing by activating muscle fibers involved in the swallowing process.
- Prevention of muscle wasting.
- Strengthens muscles, reducing the risk of falling.
- Improved proprioception.
- Control and normalization of altered muscle tone.

Examples of Some Exercises Used in Active and Passive Muscle Electrostimulation

Active Biceps ME

See Fig. 6.21.

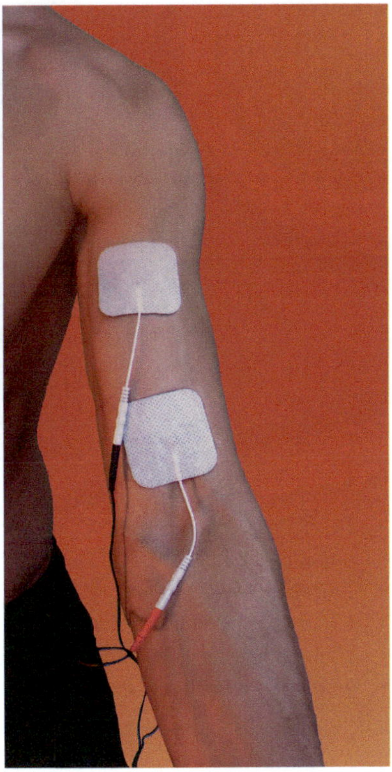

Fig. 6.21 Active biceps ME

- Purpose: This exercise is designed to increase biceps muscle strength.
- Electrode placement: Electrode on the muscular belly of the biceps, combined with voluntary muscle contraction.
- Electrode size: Depending on individual muscle size.
- Volume and other parameters:
  - Repetitions: 10
  - Sets: 3
  - Frequency: 50 H
  - Pulse duration: 250 μs.
  - Density: 1:2
- Intensity: Adjusted to the patient's tolerance

Passive Respiratory ME

See Fig. 6.22.

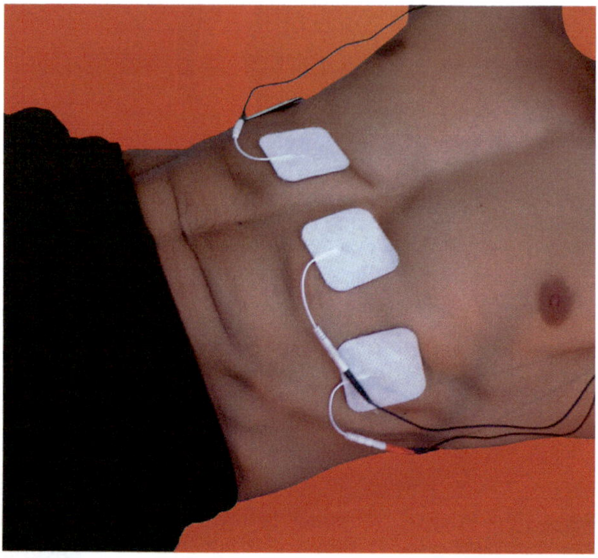

Fig. 6.22 Passive respiratory ME

- Purpose: This exercise is performed to improve respiratory function and lung capacity.
- Duration: 5–10 min.
- Electrode placement: Electrodes placed on intercostal muscles and diaphragm.
- Electrode size: Depending on muscle size.
- Volume and other parameters:
  - Repetitions: 2 (5 min each)
  - Sets: 2
  - Frequency: 20 Hz
  - Pulse duration: 300 μs
  - Density: 2 min rest between repetitions
- Intensity: Adjusted to patient tolerance.

Speech and Language Therapy

According to Berenguer and Yévenes [45], nearly 90% of patients with Parkinson's disease experience speech disorders known as Parkinson's dysarthria. These disorders affect various aspects of speech, which can lead to misinterpretation of the patient's messages and affect their quality of life.

Some of the most common changes include alterations in breathing rate and fluency, prosody, and phonation. These problems can result in soft or loud voices, which are often misinterpreted as mood swings. In addition, poor articulation of words can lead the listener to question a possible cognitive impairment. Dysarthria can also have a significant impact on the patient's mood, as they may experience persistent depression, low self-esteem, frustration, shyness, and social isolation.

Other aspects affected include voice intensity, where hypophonia (low voice intensity) may be mistaken for lack of interest in conversation or the patient's hearing impairment. Voice quality is also affected, often accompanied by hoarseness, leading to misinterpretations such as a cold or infection. In addition, facial expression tends to decrease as the disease progresses, which can affect nonverbal communication and further hinder social interaction.

Current treatment options for dysarthria include dopaminergic pharmacotherapy, transcranial electrical stimulation, neurosurgery, and speech behavior therapy. However, it is important to note that these approaches have limited effects on dysarthria and, in some cases, may cause side effects such as deterioration of vocal articulation and prosody [45] Therefore, speech-language pathology or speech-language pathology aimed at preventing and improving speech and language disorders uses techniques such as Lee Silverman voice treatment (LSVT), respiratory reeducation, video-assisted swallowing therapy (VAST), and music therapy, as described below [45–49].

Lee Silverman Voice Treatment (LSVT)

There are various methods employed in speech behavioral therapy, but our emphasis is on the Lee Silverman voice treatment (LSVT) method due to its Level 1 scientific evidence in the following domains:

- Enhancing vocal volume and intensity.
- Facilitating voice inflection and tone modifications.
- Improving articulation and phonation.
- Boosting facial expression.
- Supporting respiratory and swallowing therapy.

The LSVT method, developed in the 1980s by Dr. Lee Silverman, aims to enhance voice quality and speech intelligibility. The core principle is encapsulated in the motto "think loud—think shout" because increasing vocal volume improves phonation, articulation, prosody, and respiration [49]. The method's results indicate residual effects lasting up to 2 years after a 4-week, 4 times weekly intervention with 60-min sessions [45, 48].

LSVT-BIG, one of the current modifications of LSVT), centers on training a range of large, full-body movements, with BIG signifying the increased range of movement. The objective of LSVT-BIG is to enhance postural balance, walking speed, and everyday activities for the patient. The treatment takes place for a month with 1-h sessions, four times a week, and must be conducted by a certified professional in this therapy [47] (Table 6.6).

Table 6.6 Presents useful exercises under the Lee Silverman voice treatment (LSVT) method

Exercise	Description	Suggestions
Tone exercise	The individual should vocalize an "ah" sound with emphasis on a high note, sustaining it for 3 s. Subsequently, the individual should vocalize an "uh" sound with the emphasis on a low note also lasting 3 s. This exercise should be repeated five times.	Perform the exercise 2 times a day.
Vocal intensity exercise	The person should produce with his/her voice, a high tone, as loud as possible while counting from 1 to 10. Then, gradually decrease the intensity while counting from 1 to 10. Repeat five times.	Perform the exercise 2 times a day.
Vocal articulation exercise	The individual should read a text aloud with an emphasis on consonant pronunciation, and then repeat the same text without any such emphasis. This process should be repeated five times.	Perform the exercise 2 times a day.
Conversation exercise	The person should converse with the professional in charge, while performing physical exercises. The objective is to increase the intensity and duration of the conversation while doing physical activity.	Perform the exercise during therapy sessions.

Breathing Reeducation

Respiratory Reeducation is achieved by training the strength of the main and accessory respiratory muscles. Patients with Parkinson's disease often experience a reduction in this type of strength, resulting in decreased expiratory pressure for voice production. EMST (expiratory muscle strength training) is a program developed by the University of Florida in the United States to strengthen the expiratory muscles, upper respiratory muscles, and digestive muscles. These exercises use equipment that provides resistance to patient-initiated expiratory pressure. Using these devices is simple; it's like lifting weights in a gym, except that the exercise load is controlled by expiration time, device resistance, and the number of repetitions and sets [50].

It is important to note that EMST, which focuses on skeletal respiratory muscles, can have residual effects for up to 8 weeks after completing a consistent training program of 1-h sessions twice a week for 1 month [49].

According to Claus et al. [50] and Zárate [49], EMST benefits Parkinson's patients by:

- Facilitating the production of a strong and quality cough, as it increases expiratory pressure by strengthening the expiratory muscles. This is particularly useful in cases of pneumonia due to aspiration of food or drink, which is common in Parkinson's patients.
- Reduces temporary breathlessness (shortness of breath).

- Improving and making safer the swallowing of food and beverages, thus preventing dysphagia.
- Improve articulation, phonation, and voice tone.

There are other methods of respiratory reeducation, such as forced expiration technique with open glottis, directed cough exercises and global mobilization of the thorax, which will be discussed below.

Breathing Reeducation Exercises

The following exercises demonstrate breathing reeducation by emphasizing the expiratory phase.

Exercises with the EMST Device

There are various EMST devices, but in this case, we will describe as an example the commonly used EMST 150 device (Fig. 6.23) [51].

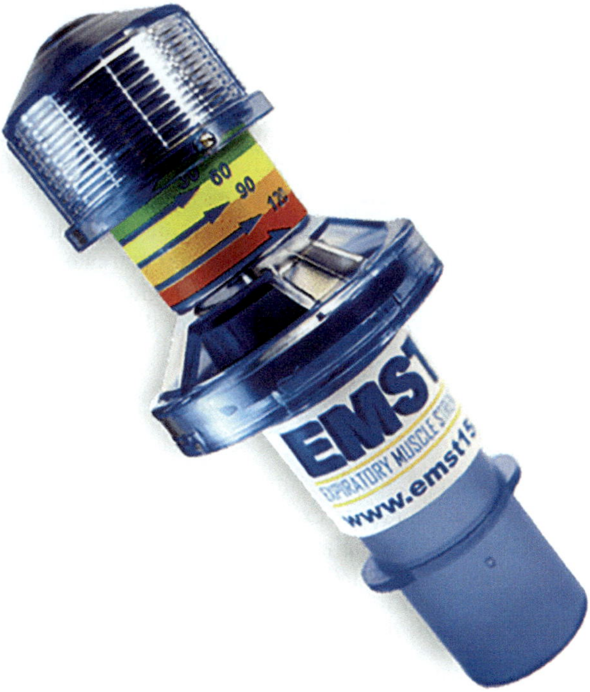

Fig. 6.23 Figure of the EMST 150 device. Taken from [51] [Photo], https://emst150.com/product/emst150/ (The link provided will take you to the official page used as the source for the image below, which provides information about the EMST 150 device and other related features, including its usage and manual)

Instructions for Use EMST Device

- *Precautions*:
  - Do not share the device with others and clean it at least monthly to reduce the risk of respiratory infection.
  - You should not experience pain while using these devices for training.
  - When used on individuals with a tracheostomy, ensure the tracheal cuff is fully deflated, and secretions are properly managed.
  - For patients who have recently had their tracheostomy tube removed, it's crucial that the previous tracheotomy site is completely closed or healed, with approval from the respective physician.
  - History of pneumothorax.
  - Epistaxis.
  - If you have experienced traumatic pneumothorax or a rib fracture, it is important not to use the EMST device until you've fully recovered.
  - In case of cerebrospinal fluid drainage or the need to monitor intracranial pressure.
  - After recent surgery or trauma to the face, mouth, neck, skull, or chest (including cardiac surgery).
  - Esophageal surgery.
  - Active hemoptysis.
  - Lung transplant, lung resection.
- *Contraindications*:
  - Asthmatic individuals with poor symptom perception and recurrent severe episodes or abnormal perception of respiratory difficulty (dyspnea).
  - Patients affected by tympanic membrane perforation or other ear conditions.
  - People with uncontrolled and untreated reflux.
  - Individuals with uncontrolled and untreated hypertension.
  - Pregnant women or those who might be pregnant.
  - Patients with abdominal hernia or those who have recently undergone abdominal surgery.
- *To adjust the tension of the device appropriately for each patient, follow these steps*:
  - To increase the difficulty of exhalation, turn the valve clockwise. This makes it harder for air to exit through the valve.
  - To decrease exhalation difficulty, turn the valve counterclockwise. This makes it easier for air to exit through the valve.
- *Measure your maximum expiratory force by following these steps*:
  - Remove the cap from the device.
  - Insert the mouthpiece into the EMST device.
  - Place the nasal clip over your nose.

- Turn the blue knob on the EMST until the small blue guide at the bottom aligns with the number 30.
- Take a deep breath.
- Place the mouthpiece behind your front teeth.
- Close the mouthpiece tightly with your lips.
- Do not exhale until the mouthpiece is securely in place. You can use your free hand to press the sides of your cheeks against the mouthpiece to help seal your lips around it.
- Exhale through the device as forcefully and quickly as possible using your exhalation muscles. For a better understanding, engage your chest and abdominal muscles as you exhale.
- If the task seemed easy and there was little resistance to the airflow through the valve, increase the complexity by turning the blue knob one full rotation clockwise. Then, repeat the previous procedures.
- If unable to get the air to pass through the device, turn the blue adjustment knob in the opposite direction, a quarter turn, and continue until allowing the passage of air through the valve. This will be your maximum expiratory pressure. For the first week, start with an adjustment one quarter turn below your maximum expiratory pressure.

• *Example of implementation within a 5-week respiratory training program*:

- *Instructions*:

  Remove the cap from the device.
  Insert the mouthpiece into the EMST device.
  Place the nasal clip over your nose.
  Set the valve with the guide at the point of your maximum expiratory pressure.
  Turn the valve ¼ turn counterclockwise. The reason for this is that we should start training our expiratory muscles at 75% of maximum expiratory force.
  Place the mouthpiece behind your front teeth.
  Close the mouthpiece tightly with your lips.
  Take a deep breath.
  Do not exhale until the mouthpiece is securely in place. You can use your free hand to press the sides of your cheeks toward the mouthpiece to help tighten your lips around the mouthpiece.
  Exhale through the device as forcefully and quickly as possible, using your expiratory muscles, engaging your chest and abdominal muscles as you exhale.
  Pause according to the indicated load parameters and repeat.

- *Note*:

  Try to exercise at the same time each day.
  You can perform the exercise sitting or standing, although sitting is recommended.

If you experience dizziness or severe headache, stop immediately and rest.
Record your progress.
Use of the device should not cause extreme fatigue.

- *Dosage*:

  Total duration: 5 weeks. It is worth noting that the only load parameter that varies from week to week is the intensity. It's important to remember that the intensity should be increased gradually by turning the valve a quarter turn clockwise, which corresponds to a 25% increase in work intensity.

  - Week 1:
    - *Volume*: 5 sets, 5 repetitions, 5 times per day, for a total of at least 25 exhalations per day.
    - *Density*:

      Rest between repetitions for at least 15–30 s. Do not skip the rest between repetitions; your muscles need to recover for the next maximal exhalation.
      Between sets: Rest at least 1 min.

    - *Frequency*: 5 times per week.
    - *Intensity*: 75% of maximum expiratory pressure.
  - Week 2:
    - *Intensity*: 75–100% of maximum expiratory force and/or pressure.
  - Week 3:
    - *Intensity*: 100–125% of maximum expiratory force and/or pressure.
  - Week 4:
    - *Intensity*: 125% of peak expiratory force and/or pressure.
  - Week 5:
    - *Intensity*: 125%–150% of peak expiratory force and/or pressure.

  Note: After week 5, you can continue with a maintenance expiratory force program, following the load parameters from week 5 and modifying them from there. As a recommendation, reduce the training frequency to 3 times per week.

- *Reference values for Maximum Expiratory Pressure (MEP): See Table 6.7*

Table 6.7 Reference values for Maximum Expiratory Pressure

Age	MEP Range (cm H_2O)
20–29	$147.3 \pm 11.0^{+,***}$
30–39	$140.3 \pm 21.7^{***}$
40–49	$126.3 \pm 18.0^{***}$
50–59	$114.7 \pm 6.9^{***}$
60–69	$111.2 \pm 10.9^{***}$
70–80	$111.5 \pm 21.0^{***}$

cm H_2O: Centimeters of water column
Data retrieved from [51]. The values are presented as mean ± standard deviation (SD)
$^{+}$Significant effects were found between age groups ($P < 0.05$) in the 20–29, 40–49, 60–69-, and 70–80-years groups
***Significant effects were also observed concerning gender within the age groups ($P < 0.05$)

Forced Exhalation Technique with Open Glottis

The forced exhalation technique with open glottis is used to facilitate secretion removal and improve productive cough, two aspects that are often affected in Parkinson's patients. By performing a rapid and forceful exhalation, secretions are moved from the larger airways to the pharynx. This technique is especially recommended for patients with secretions in the middle and proximal airways.

Technique Instructions

- *Preparation or warm-up*:
  - Sit with your back straight and comfortable.
  - Lift the chin slightly to open the throat.
  - Open mouth.
  - Perform abdominal-diaphragmatic and upper thoracic breaths, maintaining a normal respiratory rate and tidal volume, avoiding activation of accessory muscles. Continue for 1–2 min.
  - Take 3 deep breaths followed by a low volume exhalation with pursed or closed lips.
- *Forced exhalation technique with open glottis*:
  - Take a deep breath.
  - Perform a forced exhalation with the glottis open, contracting the chest and abdominal muscles. As you exhale, visualize yourself fogging a glass or mirror.
  - It is recommended to perform a maximum of 3 consecutive repetitions, always preceded by a deep inhalation.

- *Note*:
  - If someone is assisting you, ask them to place their hands on the front-lateral part of your chest and apply gentle pressure during exhalation to help you exhale with more force.
  - This technique may cause bronchial collapse and is not recommended for patients with bronchial hyperreactivity or recent bronchospasm.
  - It is important to consider that patients with COPD (chronic obstructive pulmonary disease) may have fragile bones due to osteoporosis, so caution should be exercised when applying manual pressure to the chest.
  - Regular monitoring and auscultation of the patient is essential, along with assessment of maximal cough flow, especially in those with neuromuscular disease.
- *Dosage*:
  - *Volume*: 3 sets of 3 repetitions
  - *Frequency*: 3–4 times per week
  - *Rest periods*:

    Between sets: 1 min
    Between repetitions: 10 s

Cough-Directed Exercises

Before performing this technique, it is important that the patient has competent, effective, and autonomous respiratory muscles to perform the three steps that make up this technique. The aim of this technique is to mobilize and expel secretions present in the middle and proximal airways (5th–6th bronchial generation).

Technique Instructions (see Fig. 6.24)

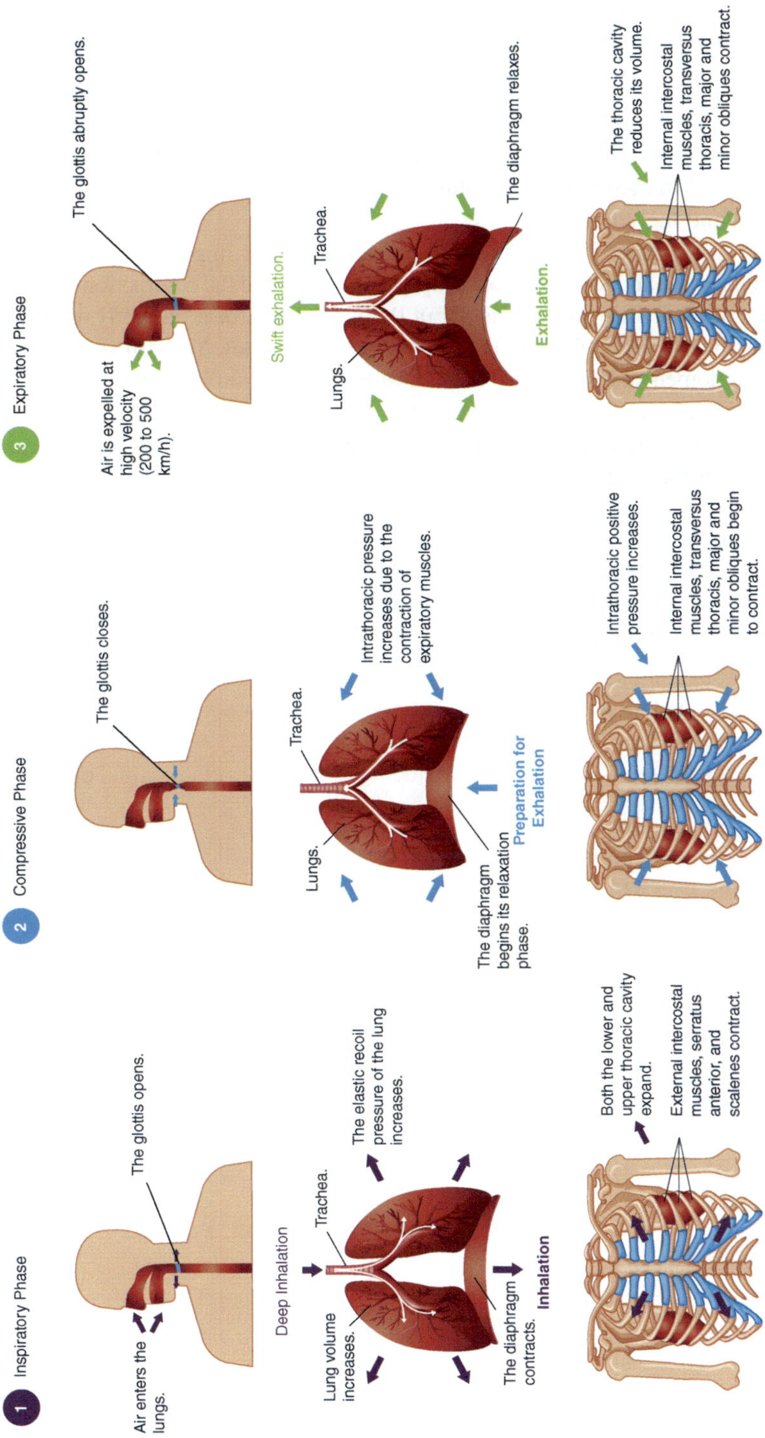

Fig. 6.24 Phases of productive cough

Sit upright or, if unable, recline partially in a supine position to perform the following exercises:

- *Inspiratory phase*: During this phase it is important to open the glottis, contract the diaphragm and some inspiratory muscles to increase the elastic recoil pressure of the lungs. To do this, take a deep breath and expand both the lower and upper chest. Imagine the air reaching your chest, back, abdomen and intercostal muscles and feel them expand.
- *Compressive phase*: In this phase, there is an increase in positive pressure in the chest due to the abduction and opening of the glottis and the contraction of the expiratory muscles. This phase lasts about 0.2 s. To perform it correctly, consciously contract the thoracic, abdominal, and intercostal muscles. You can place one hand on the abdomen and the other on the chest to feel the muscle contraction.
- *Expiratory phase*: During this phase, the glottis opens rapidly and the expiratory muscles contract, causing air to be expelled rapidly outward. To perform this phase, continue to follow the instructions from the inhalation phase and exhale forcefully, mimicking a cough.
  Note: It is recommended that the patient inhale through the nose whenever possible to achieve adequate lung expansion. If the patient is unable to perform the directed cough, an assisted cough technique can be considered, either in the inspiratory or expiratory phase.
- *Dosage*:
  - Volume: 3 sets of 5 repetitions
  - Frequency: 3 times per week
  - Rest intervals:

    Between sets: 1 min
    Between repetitions: 5–10 s

Global Mobilization of the Rib Cage

These exercises are designed to increase mobility and ventilation in the specific target area, with the goal of achieving long-term improvements.

Thoracic Mobility Exercises (Figs. 6.25, 6.26, 6.27, 6.28, 6.29, 6.30, 6.31, 6.32):

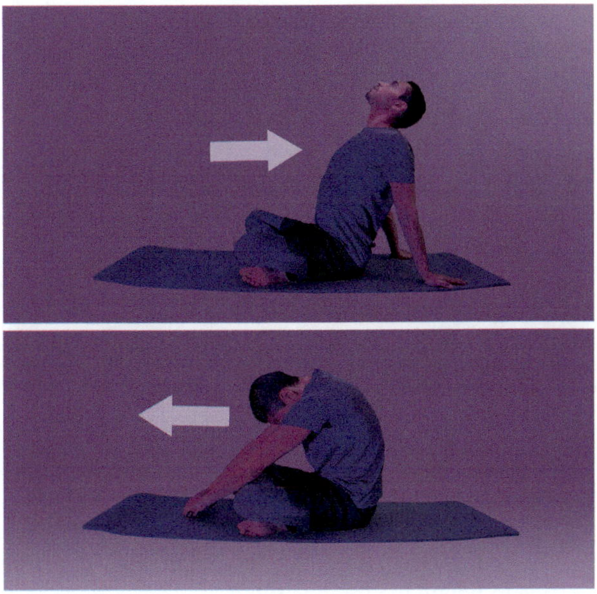

Fig. 6.25 Dorsal and cervical flexion-extension

- Sit on a mat with legs crossed.
- Keep back straight and shoulders relaxed.
- Extend arms backward for support.
- Tilt your head and lower back backward, pushing your chest outward.
- Hold this position for 5 s.
- Slowly return head to starting position.
- Tilt your head forward and flex your pelvis, bringing your chin toward your chest as you extend your arms forward.
- Hold this position for 5 s.
- Slowly return the head to the starting position.

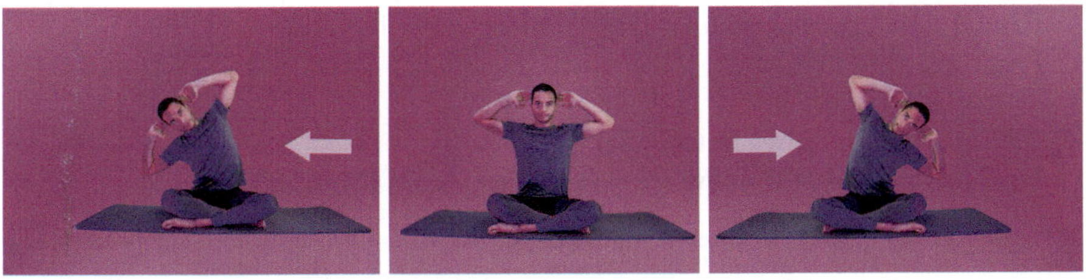

Fig. 6.26 Left and right trunk lateral flexion with elbows bent

- Sit on floor with legs crossed.
- Bend your arms and place your hands behind your head.
- Bend laterally your torso to the left and/or right.
- Hold this position for a few seconds.

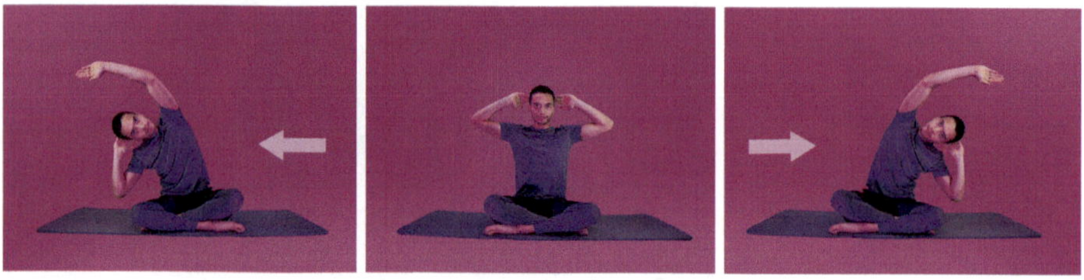

Fig. 6.27 Left and right trunk lateral flexion with one outstretched arm

- Sit on floor with legs crossed.
- Bend your arms and place your hands behind your head.
- Tilt your torso to the left and/or right while extending the arm from the opposite side to where the torso is tilted.
- Hold this position for a few seconds.

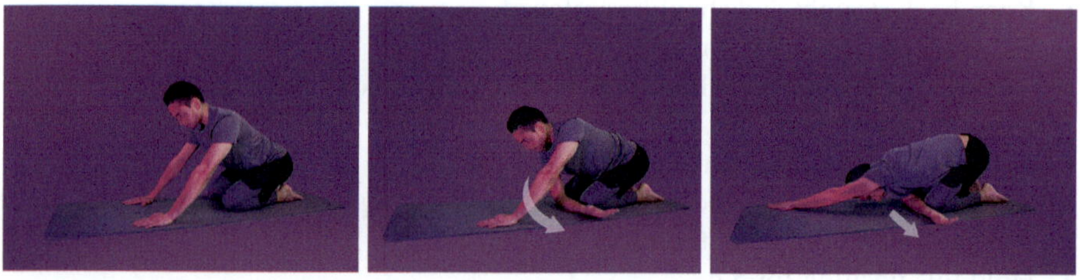

Fig. 6.28 Stretching the latissimus dorsi, minor and major rhomboids

- Kneel on a mat with your hands shoulder-width apart and placed in front of you.
- Extend right arm and adduct right shoulder under left arm.
- Flex hips and torso.
- Extend left arm.
- Tilt the torso sideways to the right.
- Hold this position for a few seconds and repeat on the other side.

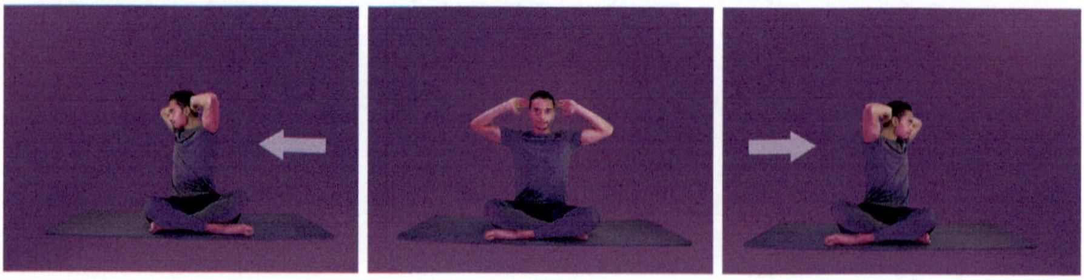

Fig. 6.29 Rotating the torso to the left and right

- Sit on a mat with legs crossed and hands behind head or occiput.
- Rotate the torso to the left.
- Hold this position for a few seconds and repeat on the other side.

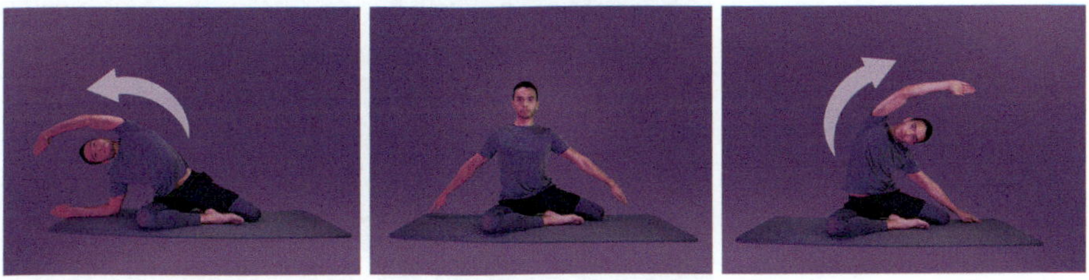

Fig. 6.30 Yoga pose called mermaid or eka pada rajakapotasana

- Starting position:
  - Sit with crossed legs on a mat.
  - Bend your right knee and place it on the floor in front of you. In addition, place the sole of the right foot against the left thigh.
  - Bend the left knee and extend the left hip, moving the leg backward. Ideally, the sole of the left foot should touch the right buttock.
- Extend arms.
- Tilt your torso sideways to the left with your extended arms above your head.
- Tilt your torso sideways to the right with your extended arms above your head.
- Hold this pose for 5–10 deep breaths.

Fig. 6.31 Spine mobility while inhaling

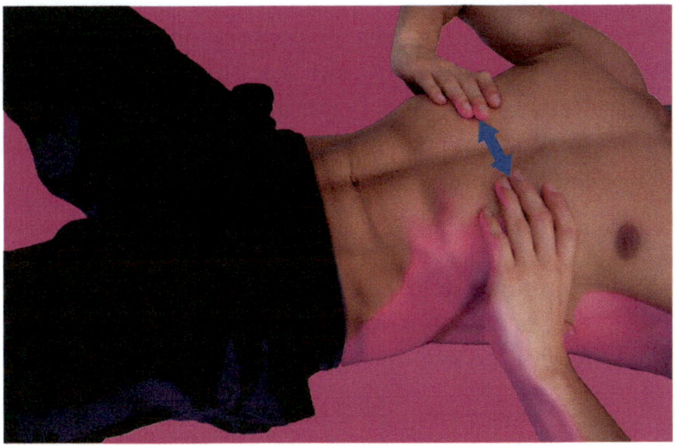

- Lie on your back on the floor.
- Place your hands at the sides of your body.
- Use your hands as an indicator of rib mobility during inhalation.
- Take a deep breath. As you do, there will be a slight separation between your hands.
- This exercise is designed to promote rib expansion during inhalation, which can help improve breathing capacity and costal flexibility.

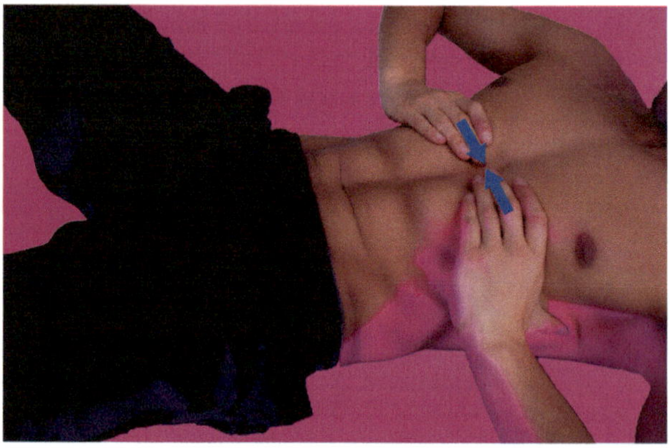

Fig. 6.32 Costal mobility during exhalation

- Lie on your back on the floor.
- Place your hands on the sides of your body.
- Use your hands as an indicator of rib cage mobility during exhalation.
- Exhale slowly. As you do, the distance between your hands will decrease slightly.
- This exercise is designed to promote rib mobility during exhalation, which can help improve respiratory capacity and costal flexibility.
- *Note*:
  - Perform the chest mobility exercises as shown in the illustration.
  - Throughout the exercises, take inhalations and exhalations to facilitate muscle adaptation.
  - Do not force the movements and perform the exercises without holding your breath.
  - You can adjust the inspiratory or expiratory flow, speeding up or slowing down the pace, by working actively and completely.
  - Remember that it is not necessary to always work with the same movement for inhalation and exhalation. To improve breathing control, you can reverse the breathing pattern used.
- *Dosage*:
  - *Volume*: 4 sets of 10 repetitions
  - *Frequency*: 2–3 times per week
  - *Rest intervals*:

    Between sets: 1–2 min
    Between repetitions: 15 s

Video-Assisted Swallowing Therapy—VAST

The VAST method is a technique that combines conventional swallowing and breathing therapies with specific training through interactive videos. These animated videos show patients the anatomical structures involved in swallowing and their functions, as well as a comparison of their own swallowing to a reference video of correct swallowing. After watching the training videos, the patient eats foods provided by the therapist with different consistencies, depending on the type of dysphagia. Finally, feedback videos of the swallowing process are reviewed to identify and correct any difficulties or abnormalities. This process is done regularly to ensure that the patient is progressing and improving their ability to swallow properly [52].

VAST is a method proposed by Manor et al. [46]. The author studied two groups of patients: those with dysphagia without Parkinson's disease and those with dysphagia and Parkinson's disease. Participants underwent 30-min sessions, five times a week, for a total intervention period of 2 weeks. The results showed that the VAST method was beneficial for Parkinson's patients with dysphagia, as it improved swallowing and reduced the presence of pharyngeal residue after ingestion of food or drink. As a result, an improvement in the quality of life of the study participants was observed [46] (Table 6.8).

Table 6.8 Sequence of exercises according to the VAST method

Exercise	Description/diagram	Objective/load parameters/ recommendations
Tongue mobility in various directions	Elevate, protrude, lateralize, and perform circular movements with the tongue around the mouth (Figs. 6.33 and 6.34). 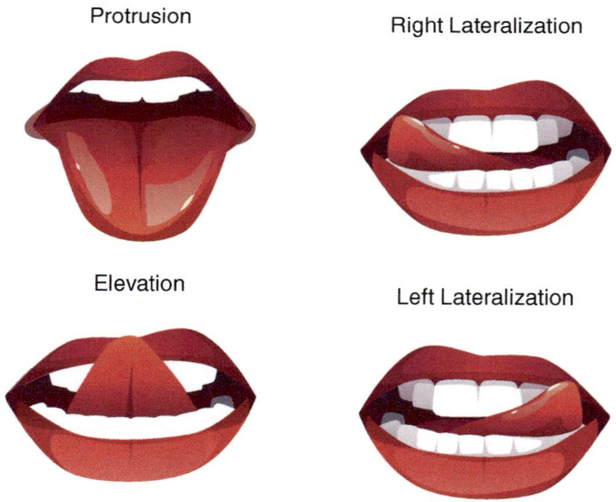 **Fig. 6.33** Movements of the tongue, including elevation, protrusion, and lateralization motions	***Objective***: Strengthen the tongue muscles to improve food bolus formation. ***Load parameters*** • Volume: 5 sets of 10 repetitions • Frequency: 2–3 times per week, 2 times per day • Density: – Between sets: 1 min. – Between repetitions: not applicable

	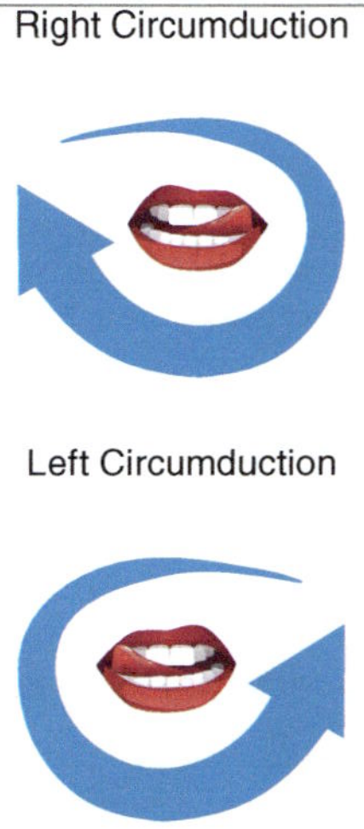 **Fig. 6.34** Circular movement of the tongue	
Soft palate elevation exercise	Elevate the soft palate while vocalizing the expression "ah" (Fig. 6.35). 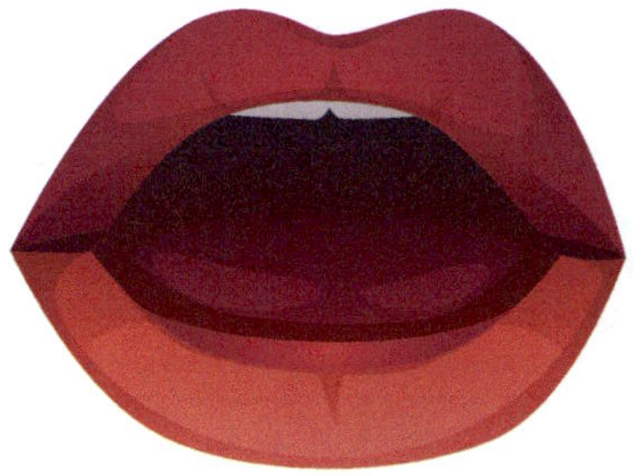 **Fig. 6.35** Soft palate elevation during vocalization of "ah"	***Objective***: Strengthen the muscles that elevate the soft palate to prevent food reflux into the nasopharynx. ***Load parameters*** • Volume: 5 sets of 10 repetitions. • Frequency: 2–3 times per week, 2 times per day • Density: – Between sets: 1 min. – Between repetitions: not applicable

(continued)

Table 6.8 (continued)

Exercise	Description/diagram	Objective/load parameters/ recommendations
Swallowing exercise	This exercise involves practicing swallowing different textures of food. Before performing the exercise, it is important to determine if the patient has specific dysphagia related to certain food consistencies, as there is a risk of aspiration during feeding. It is recommended that a doctor be consulted to assess the need for tests to diagnose the different types of dysphagia the patient may be experiencing. ***Types of dysphagia based on the area affected***: • *Oropharyngeal dysphagia*: Characterized by difficulty moving food from the mouth to the throat. • *Esophageal dysphagia*: Refers to difficulty passing food through the esophagus. • *Functional dysphagia*: Occurs when there is difficulty swallowing or moving food without an apparent structural or medical cause. In many cases, it may be associated with mental disorders. • *Neuromuscular dysphagia*: Indicates the presence of a progressive neurological disorder or neurological damage that interferes with the movement of food through the digestive system. ***Types of dysphagia based on the viscosity of the food***: • *Thin liquid dysphagia*: Refers to difficulty swallowing liquids with a viscosity of less than 50 centipoise. These liquids are similar in consistency to water. • *Thick liquid dysphagia*: Refers to difficulty swallowing liquids with a viscosity between 51 and 350 centipoises. These liquids have a thick consistency like fruit nectar. • *Honey-thick dysphagia*: Is characterized by difficulty swallowing liquids with a viscosity between 351 and 1750 centipoises. These fluids have a consistency like honey. • *Pudding-thick dysphagia*: Involves difficulty swallowing liquids with a viscosity greater than 1750 centipoises. These liquids have a thick consistency like pudding. These viscosity categories are used to tailor liquid consistency to the individual needs of people with dysphagia, allowing them to swallow safely and avoid aspiration problems.	**Objective**: Practice swallowing with different food and liquid consistencies. **Recommendations**: Start with smoother textures and thin liquids, gradually increasing the consistency. It is recommended to consult a specialist doctor beforehand for a diagnostic test to determine if any form of dysphagia is present.

Feedback exercise	Watching a video of one's own swallowing and comparing it to a video of correct swallowing. This video can be recorded while the patient is eating different types of food (solid, liquid, and/or semi-solid), in order to identify possible improper movements or the presence of dysphagia. It is also possible to use frame-by-frame images or video from an esophagogastroduodenal transit study, known as an esophagogram, where we can see live the passage of food and the structures involved in the process.	**Objective**: Identify issues and work on problematic areas to improve swallowing. **Suggestions**: Perform this exercise after each swallowing session. It is recommended to take the videos during the section you plan for the previous swallowing exercises. It is advisable to consult a specialist physician beforehand to undergo a test that can diagnose any form of dysphagia.
Head, neck, and jaw massage	Massage the muscles of the neck, head, and jaw to relax them before and after swallowing. Please note the following warnings. Consult a healthcare professional to determine if these exercises are appropriate for you. ***Caution***: There are several reasons why neck massage is not recommended without supervision or prior consultation: • *Neck injuries or problems*: If someone has an existing neck injury or problem, such as a herniated disc, pinched nerve, or cervical instability, neck massage may aggravate the condition or cause further damage. • *High blood pressure*: Some massage techniques can temporarily increase blood pressure. If a person already has high blood pressure or cardiovascular problems, neck massage could be counterproductive and increase the risk of complications. • *Infection or inflammation*: If there is an infection or inflammation in the neck area, massage could make it worse or spread the infection. • *Risk of injury*: The neck is a delicate part of the body, containing important structures such as the spine and nerves. Poorly performed or overly forceful massage can cause injury, pain, or discomfort.	**Objective**: Reduce tension in the muscles involved in swallowing. **Load parameters**: Perform for 5 min before and after the prescribed sessions mentioned earlier.

(continued)

Table 6.8 (continued)

Exercise	Description/diagram	Objective/load parameters/ recommendations
	It is important to remember that each person is unique and may have individual medical conditions that require special precautions. It is always advisable to consult a healthcare professional, such as a physician or physical therapist, before performing neck massage or any other treatment on the neck. They can properly assess the situation and make personalized and safe recommendations (Figs. 6.36 and 6.37). 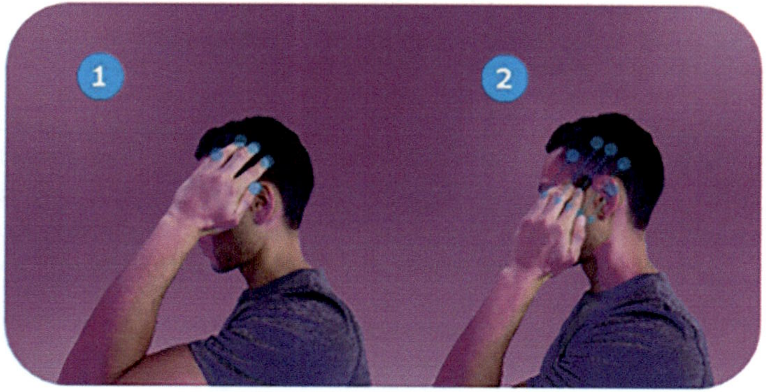 **Fig. 6.36** Bilateral massage of head and jaw muscles	

Massage the fibers of the temporal muscle in parallel, with the fingertips of the hand.

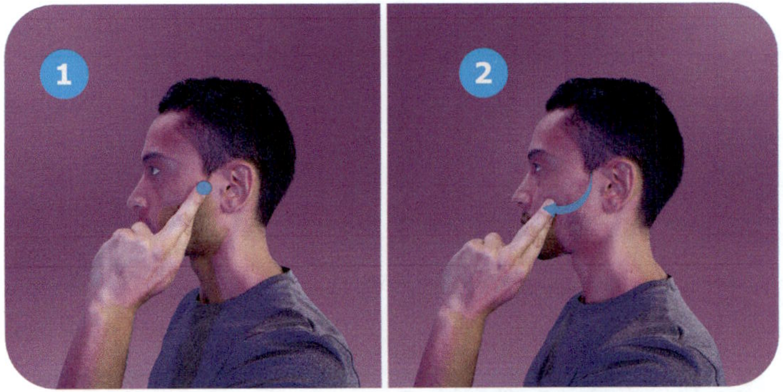

Massage the masseter muscle transversely with the fingertips of the index and middle fingers

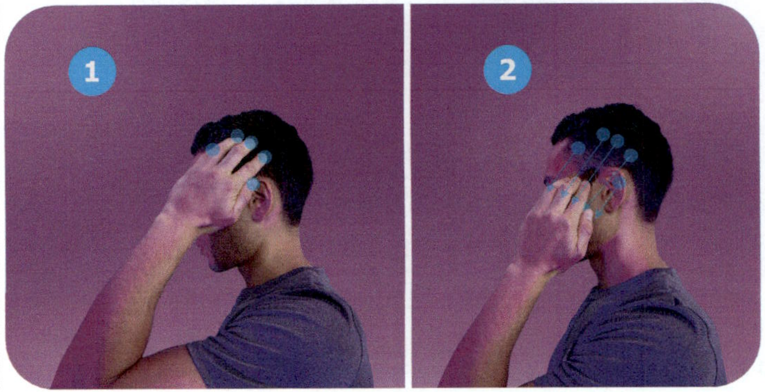

(continued)

Table 6.8 (continued)

Exercise	Description/diagram	Objective/load parameters/ recommendations
	Massage the fibers of the masseter muscle in parallel, with the fingertips of the index and middle fingers. 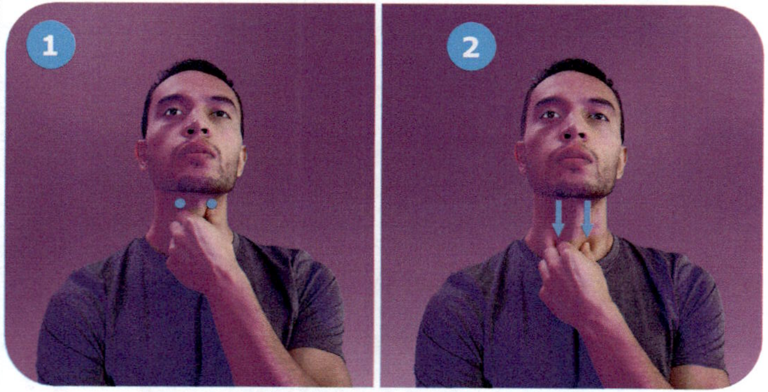 **Fig. 6.37** Laryngeal massage Massage the fibers of the sternocleidomastoid and thyrohyoid muscles in parallel with the fingertips of the index and thumb.	

Diaphragmatic breathing exercise	• Breathe slowly and deeply, in inhalation and exhalation phases, using the diaphragm. • As you inhale or take a breath, the diaphragm contracts and the chest expands in the front, back, and side. • When exhaling or blowing out air, the diaphragm relaxes and the chest shrinks all around. Imagine the navel pointing toward the ground (Fig. 6.38). 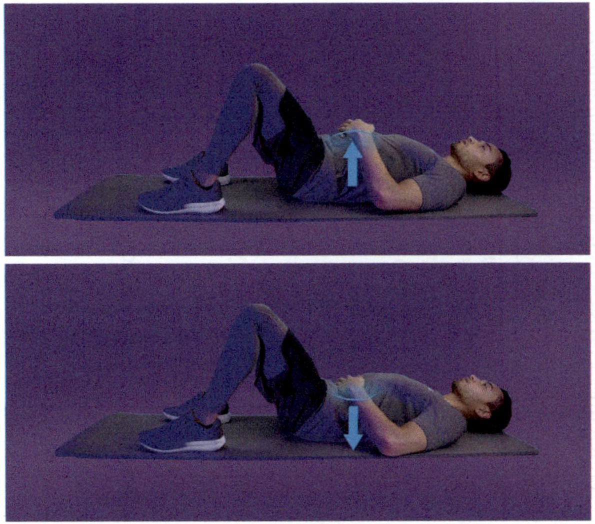 **Fig. 6.38** Diaphragmatic breathing exercise • Lie on your back with your knees bent and feet flat on the floor. • Place both hands on the abdominal area, just above the navel. • Exhale and draw the navel toward the spine (lumbar area), as if you want to pull it inside the body. • Maintain the contraction for a few seconds. • Inhale slowly and relax the muscles. • Repeat the exercise 10–15 times.	**Objective**: Strengthen respiratory muscles and improve the ability to control breathing during swallowin. **Load parameters**: • Volume: 4 sets of 8 repetitions • Frequency: 3 times per week • Density: – Between sets: 1 min. – Between repetitions: N/A **Suggestions**: • Keep your back straight and shoulders relaxed. • Focus on contracting the deep abdominal muscles, especially the transverse abdominal muscle.

Music Therapy

Music therapy is a commonly used method for the treatment of depression, prevention of isolation, and overall management of socioemotional disturbances in patients with Parkinson's disease. Currently, with the research conducted, benefits of its use in speech therapy have been found when the patient is an active participant in the intervention, that is, when they sing [53, 54].

Effects of Music Therapy

The effects of music therapy in Parkinson's disease according to Chica and Parada [53], López [54], de Oliveira and Andrade [55] are:

- Singing increases expiratory force, thereby improving voice tone.
- Singing at different pitches improves speech phonation and prosody.
- It improves vocal tone because singing involves constant changes in rhythm, pitch, and speech variation.
- Increases speech rate.
- Improves posture while speaking, which is particularly useful for Parkinson's patients who tend to have upper cross syndrome, which affects their speech and breathing processes.
- Promotes nonverbal expression, as singing encourages increased facial gestures.
- Improves both motor and non-motor symptoms of Parkinson's disease.
- Improves balance and dynamic/static postural equilibrium when music therapy is used as a rhythmic method in active therapies (such as dance).
- Improves quality of life when used in conjunction with physical therapy.

Dosage

According to the meta-analysis conducted by de Oliveira and Andrade [55], music therapy can be dosed as follows:

- Session duration: From 30 min to 2 h
- Number of sessions per week: 2–5 sessions
- Number of weeks: 4–16 weeks

When using music therapy for Parkinson's disease patients, the focus should be on improving tone, projection, and speech intelligibility [55] (Table 6.9).

Table 6.9 Suggested music therapy exercises

Exercise	Description	Objective
Dancing to music	This is an exercise in which the person with Parkinson's disease dances to the rhythm of music they enjoy, using different parts of the body and movements adapted to their abilities. It is recommended to use music with a clear and varied rhythm.	To promote mobility, balance, coordination, and a positive mood.
Group singing	The person joins a singing group where different vocal exercises are performed and singing in a choir is encouraged. It is recommended to choose songs that the person knows and enjoys.	To improve voice quality and breathing and encourage socialization and participation in group activities.
Listening to relaxing music	The person sits comfortably in a quiet place and listens to relaxing music with headphones. Deep breathing exercises and visualization may be used while listening.	To reduce stress, anxiety, and depression, and improve sleep quality.
Musical improvisation	The person plays a musical instrument or sings freely, without following any specific notes or rhythm. Various instruments such as guitar, keyboard, or percussion may be used.	To encourage creativity, spontaneity, and emotional expression, and to improve fine motor coordination and mobility.
Music therapy as a couple	The patient and their partner dance together, holding hands and moving to the rhythm of slow and gentle music.	To improve communication and emotional connection between the person with Parkinson's disease and their partner, and to promote physical contact and mutual support.

Reality Orientation Therapy

In their review of reality orientation therapy (ROT), Klimova et al.[56] present a nonpharmacological tool commonly used with Parkinson's, Alzheimer's, and/or dementia patients. ROT aims to reorient the patient temporally and spatially within their reality in order to improve self-awareness. This therapy is characterized by connecting events, characteristics, experiences, professions, among other aspects, from the person's past with their present, with the goal of relearning what has already been lived but has deteriorated or been lost due to the pathology. In addition to improving self-awareness, ROT also aims to prevent the disorientation typical of Parkinson's, Alzheimer's, and/or dementia patients and to improve their social interaction.

Effects of ROT

- Improves temporal and spatial orientation.
- Facilitates performance of activities of daily living.
- Improves mood in Parkinson's patients.
- Improves social skills and interactions.
- Facilitates verbal and nonverbal communication.
- Keeps the patient connected to their current and lived reality.

Dosage

Therapeutic exercise is essential in ROT. It is suggested that the intervention be carried out over a total period of 24 weeks, with 2 sessions of 45 min per week.

Within ROT, there are various types of therapeutic exercises that can be used in the treatment of patients with Parkinson's, Alzheimer's, and/or dementia. Some useful examples of exercises within ROT include (Table 6.10):

Table 6.10 ROT exercises

Exercise	Description
Walking in familiar places	Walking in places or on surfaces that the patient used to frequent before experiencing symptoms, such as a park, the beach, or a familiar neighborhood. The goal is to improve walking patterns and help the patient feel more comfortable and secure in their environment.
Sports and physical activities	Engaging in a sport or physical activity that the patient did or enjoyed before the disease, such as swimming, walking, dancing, or playing tennis. The exercise should be adapted to the patient's needs and abilities.
Memory exercises	Practicing memory exercises, such as recalling the words to a song the patient used to listen to in their youth, repeating lists of objects or words, and associating pictures with words. These exercises can be done individually or in a group setting.
Using familiar objects and materials	Use objects and materials related to the patient's life, such as old photographs, travel souvenirs, collectibles, books, or magazines. These items can help stimulate memory and facilitate conversations about past experiences.
Role-playing exercises	Engaging in role-playing exercises in which the patient assumes the role of a profession or character that is familiar to them or that they played in a past life, such as a chef, musician, or writer. This can help stimulate memory and creativity.
Board games and group activities	Playing board games or participating in group activities that promote social interaction and memory, such as bingo, scavenger hunts, or chess. These activities can be a fun and stimulating way to exercise memory and socialize with others.
Temporal and spatial orientation exercises	Practicing temporal and spatial orientation exercises, such as remembering important dates, giving directions to a familiar place, or drawing a map of a familiar city. These exercises can help improve memory and spatial awareness.

These exercises can help improve self-awareness and connect the current reality with the patient's memory and past experiences

Competing Interests The author have no conflicts of interest to declare that are relevant to the content of this chapter.

References

1. Loprinzi PD, Danzl MM, Ulanowski E, Paydo C. A pilot study evaluating the association between physical activity and cognition among individuals with Parkinson's disease. Disabil Health J. 2017;11:165–8. https://doi.org/10.1016/j.dhjo.2017.05.004.
2. Aho VTE, Houser MC, Pereira PAB, et al. Relationships of gut microbiota, short-chain fatty acids, inflammation, and the gut barrier in Parkinson's disease. Mol Neurodegener. 2021;16:1–14. https://doi.org/10.1186/s13024-021-00427-6.
3. Albani G, Albani S, Keshavarzian A. Editorial: role of diet, physical activity and immune system in Parkinson's disease. Front Neurol. 2020;11:1–3. https://doi.org/10.3389/fneur.2020.611349.
4. Bhalsing K, Abbas M, Tan L. Role of physical activity in Parkinson's disease. Ann Indian Acad Neurol. 2018;21:242–9. https://doi.org/10.4103/aian.AIAN.
5. Cusso ME, Donald KJ, Khoo TK. The impact of physical activity on non-motor symptoms in Parkinson's disease: a systematic review. Front Med (Lausanne). 2016;3:1–9. https://doi.org/10.3389/fmed.2016.00035.
6. Fayyaz M, Jaffery SS, Anwar F, et al. The effect of physical activity in Parkinson's disease: a mini-review. Cureus. 2018;10 https://doi.org/10.7759/cureus.2995.
7. Galimberti D, Scarpini E. Neurodegenerative diseases. 2nd ed. Springer; 2018.
8. Khalil H, Alomari MA, Khabour O, et al. The association between physical activity with cognitive function and brain derived neurotrophic factor in people with Parkinson's disease, a pilot study. J Aging Phys Act. 2017;0:1–24. https://doi.org/10.1123/japa.2016-0121.
9. Landers MR, Lopker M, Newman M, et al. A cross-sectional analysis of the characteristics of individuals with Parkinson disease who avoid activities and participation due to fear of falling. J Neurol Phys Ther. 2017;41:31–42. https://doi.org/10.1097/NPT.0000000000000162.
10. Shalash A, Roushdy T, Essam M, et al. Mental health, physical activity, and quality of life in Parkinson's disease during COVID-19 pandemic. Movement Disord. 2020;35:1097–9. https://doi.org/10.1002/mds.28134.
11. Shih CH, Moore K, Browner N, et al. Physical activity mediates the association between striatal dopamine transporter availability and cognition in Parkinson's disease. Parkinsonism Relat Disord. 2019;62:68–72. https://doi.org/10.1016/j.parkreldis.2019.01.027.
12. van Uem JMT, Cerff B, Kampmeyer M, et al. The association between objectively measured physical activity, depression, cognition, and health-related quality of life in Parkinson's disease. Parkinsonism Relat Disord. 2018;48:74–81. https://doi.org/10.1016/j.parkreldis.2017.12.023.
13. Wassenaar TM, Zimmermann K. Lipopolysaccharides in food, food supplements, and probiotics: should we be worried? Eur J Microbiol Immunol. 2018;8:63–9. https://doi.org/10.1556/1886.2018.00017.
14. Armstrong MJ, Okun MS. Diagnosis and treatment of Parkinson disease: a review. J Am Med Assoc. 2020;323:548–60. https://doi.org/10.1001/jama.2019.22360.
15. Schenkman M, Moore CG, Kohrt WM, et al. Effect of high-intensity treadmill exercise on motor symptoms in patients with De Novo Parkinson disease a phase 2 randomized clinical trial. JAMA Neurol. 2018;75:219–26. https://doi.org/10.1001/JAMANEUROL.2017.3517.
16. Pallarés JG, Morán Navarro R. Propuesta metodológica para el entrenamiento de la resistencia cardiorrespiratoria. J Sport Health Res. 2012;4:119–36.
17. Klamroth S (2018) Perturbation treadmill training in Parkinson's disease

18. Rigby BR, Davis RW, Avalos MA, et al. Acute cardiometabolic responses to three modes of treadmill exercise in older adults with Parkinson's disease. Adapted Phys Activity Quart. 2018;35:424–36. https://doi.org/10.1123/apaq.2017-0200.
19. Motek Medical BV (2023) CAREN. The world's most advanced biomechanics lab. https://www.motekmedical.com/solution/caren/#. Accessed 20 Nov 2023
20. Kirwa R. Therapy on Parkinson ' s Disease. J Regen Biol Med. 2021;3:1–5. https://doi.org/10.37191/Mapsci-2582-385X-3(6)-093.
21. Tofani M, Ranieri A, Fabbrini G, et al. Efficacy of occupational therapy interventions on quality of life in patients with Parkinson's disease: a systematic review and meta-analysis. Mov Disord Clin Pract. 2020;7:891–901. https://doi.org/10.1002/mdc3.13089.
22. Foster ER, Carson LG, Archer J, Hunter EG. Occupational therapy interventions for instrumental activities of daily living for adultswith parkinson's disease: a systematic review. Am J Occup Ther. 2021;75:1–24. https://doi.org/10.5014/ajot.2021.046581.
23. Ojeda del Pozo N, Peña Lasa J, Bengoetxea Noreña E, et al. REHACOP: programa de rehabilitación cognitiva en psicosis. Rev Neurol. 2012;54:337. https://doi.org/10.33588/rn.5406.2011514.
24. Bispo VA, Bastos JAI, Almeida CC de, et al (2021) The effects of neuromuscular electrical stimulation on strength, pain, and function in individuals with knee osteoarthritis: a systematic review with meta-analysis. Fisioterapia e Pesquisa 28:416–426. doi: https://doi.org/10.1590/1809-2950/20028528042021
25. Souza RVS, Maciel DG, Cerqueira MS. Effects of transcranial direct current stimulation associated or combined with exercise on musculoskeletal pain: systematic review. Brazil J Pain. 2021;4:167–71. https://doi.org/10.5935/2595-0118.20210029.
26. Straudi S, Buja S, Baroni A, et al. The effects of transcranial direct current stimulation (tDCS) combined with group exercise treatment in subjects with chronic low back pain: a ilot randomized control trial. Clin Rehabil. 2018;32:1348–56. https://doi.org/10.1177/0269215518777881.
27. Conceição MC, Dantas E. Control de intensidad en entrenamiento de flexibilidad. Cuerpo Cultura Movimiento. 2019;9:78–90. https://doi.org/10.15332/2422474x/5355.
28. Muñoz Daga L. Plan de intervención de fisioterapia convencional complementado con fisioterapia digital para un paciente con Enfermedad de Parkinson y Apnea Obstructiva del Sueño. A propósito de un caso. Universidad de Zaragoza; 2021.
29. Villamizar P. Fuerza prensil y riesgo de caída de los sujetos pertenecientes al programa de adulto mayor de la Universidad Santo Tomas y centros vida de la alcaldía de Bucaramanga. Universidad Santo Tomas de Bucaramanga; 2018.
30. Ángel M (2012) Terapia Ocupacional en personas con enfermedad de Parkinson: una aproximación desde distintos marcos de referencia. Tesis de grado, Universidad de Zaragoza Escuela de Ciencias de la Salud
31. Lear A (2015) Terapia Ocupacional y Enfermedad de Parkinson: una revisión basada en la evidencia. España
32. Palazón García R, Gómez del Monte C, Cantero Garlito PA, et al. Protocolo terapéutico en la enfermedad de parkinson. Rehabilitacion (Madr). 2001;35:175–8. https://doi.org/10.1016/s0048-7120(01)73164-7.
33. Radder DLM, Sturkenboom IH, van Nimwegen M, et al. Physical therapy and occupational therapy in Parkinson's disease. Int J Neurosci. 2017;127:930–43. https://doi.org/10.1080/00207454.2016.1275617.
34. Carapellotti AM, Stevenson R, Doumas M. The efficacy of dance for improving motor impairments, non-motor symptoms, and quality of life in Parkinson's disease: a systematic review and meta-analysis. PLoS One. 2020;15(8):e0236820.
35. Ismail SR, Lee SWH, Merom D, et al. Evidence of disease severity, cognitive and physical outcomes of dance interventions for persons with Parkinson's Disease: a systematic review and meta-analysis. BMC Geriatr. 2021;21 https://doi.org/10.1186/s12877-021-02446-w.
36. Ruiz MA, López RMM. Dance for people with Alzheimer's disease: a systematic review. Curr Alzheimer Res. 2019;16:919–33. https://doi.org/10.2174/1567205016666190725151614.

37. Deuel LM, Seeberger LC. Complementary therapies in Parkinson disease: a review of acupuncture, Tai Chi, Qi Gong, Yoga, and Cannabis. Neurotherapeutics. 2020;17:1434–55. https://doi.org/10.1007/s13311-020-00900-y.
38. García Arribas M (2018) Tratamiento fisioterapéutico en pacientes ancianos con daño neurológico. Demencia y Enfermedad de Parkinson. Universidad de Valladolid
39. Tung JH, Pong K, Tszlam, et al. Sarcopenia: current treatments and new regenerative therapeutic approaches. J Orthop Transl. 2020;23:38–52. https://doi.org/10.1016/j.jot.2020.04.002.
40. Fiorilli G, Quinzi F, Buonsenso A, et al. A single session of whole-body electromyostimulation increases muscle strength, endurance and prongf in early parkinson patients. Int J Environ Res Public Health. 2021;18 https://doi.org/10.3390/ijerph18105499.
41. María Sánchez A (2016) La Estimulación Complementaria Para La Rehabilitación De La Disfagia En Pacientes Con Enfermedad De Parkinson. PP. 1–39
42. Alouini S, Memic S, Couillandre A. Pelvic floor muscle training for urinary incontinence with or without biofeedback or electrostimulation in women: a systematic review. Int J Environ Res Public Health. 2022;19 https://doi.org/10.3390/ijerph19052789.
43. Centeno LF (2022) Electroestimulación neuromuscular como parte del tratamiento de la disfagia neurogénica. Revisión sistemática. Tesis de grado, Universidad de Valladolid
44. Sweeney D, Quinlan LR, Richardson M, et al. Multifaceted sensory electrical stimulation cueing for freezing of gait in Parkinson's disease. Parkinsonism Relat Disord. 2021;82:106–8. https://doi.org/10.1016/j.parkreldis.2020.11.022.
45. Berenguer M, Yévenes H. Trastornos del habla en la enfermedad de Parkinson. Revisión. Rev Cient Cienc Med. 2019;22:36–42.
46. Manor Y, Mootanah R, Freud D, et al. Video-assisted swallowing therapy for patients with Parkinson's disease. Parkinsonism Relat Disord. 2013;19:207–11. https://doi.org/10.1016/j.parkreldis.2012.10.004.
47. McDonnell MN, Rischbieth B, Schammer TT, et al. Lee Silverman Voice Treatment (LSVT)-BIG to improve motor function in people with Parkinson's disease: a systematic review and meta-analysis. Clin Rehabil. 2018;32:607–18. https://doi.org/10.1177/0269215517734385.
48. Saffarian A, Shavaki Y, Shahidi G, et al. Lee Silverman voice treatment (LSVT) mitigates voice difficulties in mild Parkinson's disease. Med J Islamic Republic Iran. 2019;33:5.
49. Zárate C (2021) Rehabilitación logopédica en la enfermedad de parkinson. Tesis, Universidad de la Laguna
50. Claus I, Muhle P, Czechowski J, et al. Expiratory muscle strength training for therapy of pharyngeal dysphagia in Parkinson's disease. Movement Disord. 2021;36:1815–24. https://doi.org/10.1002/mds.28552.
51. ASPIRE Respiratory Products (2023) EMST150
52. Park MS, Choi JY, Song YJ, et al. Systematic review of behavioral therapy to improve swallowing functions of patients with Parkinson's disease. Gastroenterol Nursing. 2019;42:65–78. https://doi.org/10.1097/SGA.0000000000000358.
53. Chica R, Parada A. Musicoterapia grupal y bienestar emocional en la enfermedad de Parkinson. Propuesta de intervención. Rev Misostenido. 2021;2:1–8.
54. López AP (2020) Papel da musicoterapia no tratamento logopédico. Tesis, Universidade da coruña
55. de Oliveira L, Andrade PGG. A aplicação da musicoterapia na doença de Parkinson: uma revisão integrativa. Rev Eletrôn Acervo Saúde. 2021;13:1–11. https://doi.org/10.25248/reas.e8625.2021.
56. Klimova B, Toman J, Kuca K. Effectiveness of the dog therapy for patients with dementia: a systematic review. BMC Psychiatry. 2019;19:1–7. https://doi.org/10.1186/s12888-019-2245-x.

Chapter 7
Nonconventional Therapeutic Exercises: Explanation, Examples, Effects, and Dosage

Initial Questions

- What is the relevance and effectiveness of integrating nonconventional active therapeutic means and methods compared to conventional approaches in the treatment of Parkinson's disease?
- What expectations can we have regarding the scientific evidence of the effectiveness of these nonconventional therapeutic methods and how can we anticipate their integration into clinical practice for the treatment of neurodegenerative pathologies?

Below is a description of a series of methods and means of nonconventional or alternative therapeutic training, as opposed to conventional approaches. The aim is to prescribe movement in a dosed manner based on scientific evidence for patients with Parkinson's and related disorders.

Cueing Exercises

This type of training focuses on a set of common visual, auditory, and/or kinesthetic stimuli that facilitate mindful and focused attention to movement in patients with motor limitations, such as the freezing of gait (FOG) phenomenon in Parkinson's disease [1]. The goal of cueing is to maintain and restore a natural pattern of movement by preventing episodes of freezing of gait, freezing of speech, or freezing of any limb movement. This is achieved by redirecting affected neural circuits to use new or less impaired circuits.

Movement difficulties in Parkinson's patients arise from instability between cortical and subcortical areas of the brain, making it difficult to perform multiple tasks simultaneously, such as walking and talking. To address this problem, cueing is used to increase activity in the upper and lower parietal lobes of the brain. This

C. A. A. Mejía, *Therapeutic Exercise for Parkinson's Disease and Related Disorders*, https://doi.org/10.1007/978-3-031-62119-2_7

technique involves providing stimuli that guide and focus attention on movement, thereby reducing cognitive load and facilitating the performance of motor tasks [1].

There are different types of cueing, including auditory, visual, and kinesthetic. Similarly, there are different ways to apply cueing through different attentional focuses (internal, external, specific neutral, and nonspecific neutral), as described below:

- **Internal focus:** These refer to signals or stimuli that direct the patient's attention to parts of his or her own body, such as the head, feet, and hands, while recalling, performing, or planning a motor action.
- **External focus:** On the other hand, external focuses are signals or stimuli that direct the patient's attention to objects or elements in the environment, such as the ceiling, floor, walls, a chair, and the weather, while recalling, performing, or planning a motor action.
- **Neutral focuses:** Neutral focuses refer to attentional cues or stimuli that are neither external nor internal, that is, they are not focused on body parts or environmental elements. These neutral focuses can be divided into two types:
  - *Specific neutral focuses:* These are signals or stimuli that explicitly direct the patient's attention to specific aspects of the motor task. For example, the focus may be on performing the maximum number of repetitions of an exercise or lifting the heaviest possible weight during a specific motor activity.
  - *Nonspecific neutral focus:* In this case, the stimuli do not focus on specific or explicit aspects of the motor task. Instead, they are aimed at general motivation or optimal performance. For example, patients may be encouraged to exert their best effort or achieve the highest possible performance without focusing on specific aspects of the task.

As science has progressed, cueing has evolved and adapted to address different motor impairments presented by patients. A clear example of cueing is the use of visual stimuli, such as wireless devices placed on the toe of the patient's shoe. These devices emit a LED light in the form of a line in front of the foot that is activated only when the opposite foot touches the ground. This light serves as a visual cue to initiate walking, motivating the patient to take steps, reducing gait freezing, and decreasing the risk of falls. In addition to visual cues, there are also auditory cues, such as metronomes, which emit sounds at regular intervals to guide step and gait frequency. These sounds provide a rhythm that helps the patient maintain a more stable and coordinated gait. On the other hand, kinesthetic stimuli involve the use of devices that emit vibrations or minimal currents to indicate to the patient when to take a step, especially during episodes of gait freezing.

It is important to follow some suggestions when choosing the type of signal or stimulus to be used:

- **Generate safe and logical stimuli that promote the desired biomechanical movement:** It is important that the stimuli are appropriate for the type of movement you are trying to improve, so that they are safe and appropriate for the patient.

- **Know the specific timing of the stimulus activation:** This stimulus activation must be synchronized with the time when the patient's movement changes or freezes. In this way, cueing will be effective and timely.
- **Choose stimuli that provide feedback to the patient about his or her performance or change:** Cueing should provide the patient with information about how they are performing the movement and whether they are improving in response to the stimulus.
- **Select stimuli that allow modification of movement frequency, amplitude, and intensity:** This adds flexibility and adaptability to the rehabilitation process by allowing adjustments to the stimuli based on the patient's changing needs.
- **Select a few stimuli at a time to avoid overwhelming the patient:** Too many stimuli can disrupt the patient's focus and reduce the effectiveness of cueing.
- **Ensure that cueing can be done anywhere, on any surface, even in the patient's home:** Accessibility and practicality of cueing are key to its effective integration into the patient's daily life and rehabilitation process.

Effects of Cueing

- Promotes the generation of motor responses.
- Facilitates concentration on movement.
- Prevents deterioration of movement patterns.
- Integrates postural control with movement.
- Improves visuomotor and visuopedic coordination.
- Prevents the freezing of movement phenomena, such as FOG, during times when overcoming obstacles, changing directions, and/or triggering circumstances are required.
- Improves gait stability through functional rehabilitation of gait amplitude and timing.
- Contributes to the improvement of spatiotemporal perception.
- Visual cueing appears to contribute to the control and regulation of stride length. It increases the flow of information in the motor networks of the occipitoparietal lobes of the brain.
- Auditory cueing contributes to correct frequency and timing of gait as well as improved coordination of the upper and lower extremities.

Dosage

A meta-analysis conducted by Ghai et al. [2] on the effects of cueing on motor performance and quality of life in people with Parkinson's disease concludes that adherence to a cueing program using rhythmic auditory stimuli significantly improves gait. The author suggests that the intervention be performed 3–5 times per week, with sessions lasting 20–45 min. Regarding the total duration of the program, a period of more than 6 weeks and not less than 2 weeks is recommended, as the retention of information acquired during the sessions is easily lost in Parkinson's disease patients [1, 2].

When teaching cueing exercises, it is essential to consider the following tips to facilitate the professional's work and improve the patient's movement:

1. Use simple and correct words or commands that allow the patient to perform the movement correctly without requiring much technical knowledge.

For example, when performing a squat:

× Wrong: Prolong the eccentric phase of the squat.
✓ Correct: Make sure to descend slowly during the squat.

2. Facilitate the performance of a movement sequence in the correct direction by first instructing the patient to perform the movement in the opposite direction.

For example, when teaching scapular retraction:

× Wrong: Retract the shoulder blades.
✓ Correct: Bring the shoulders forward as much as possible, then bring the shoulders back as much as possible without lifting them.

3. Avoid explaining a movement in detail. The patient is already trying to perform the movement, so paying attention to every detail can be overwhelming. It is best to teach the movement gradually.

Example of teaching shoulder external rotation:

× Wrong: Stand with arms fully extended, shoulders relaxed, and perform shoulder external rotation as if rotating the palms outward, making sure the shoulder rotates as well.
✓ Correct: Stand with arms extended and relaxed, rotate palms outward and forward.

4. Touch the muscle you want the patient to contract, not the area that is causing the movement problem.

For example, when teaching to activate the lower fibers of the trapezius muscle for scapular depression movement:

× Wrong: Touch the upper part of the shoulder and indicate to lower the shoulders.
✓Correct: Touch the lower trapezius fibers and indicate their contraction and shoulder depression.

Cueing Exercises

See Tables 7.1, 7.2, 7.3, 7.4, 7.5 and 7.6.

Table 7.1 Cueing sit-up exercise

Sit-up		
Objective: Facilitate muscle contraction, proprioception, and muscular hypertrophy		
Initial position		
See Fig. 7.1 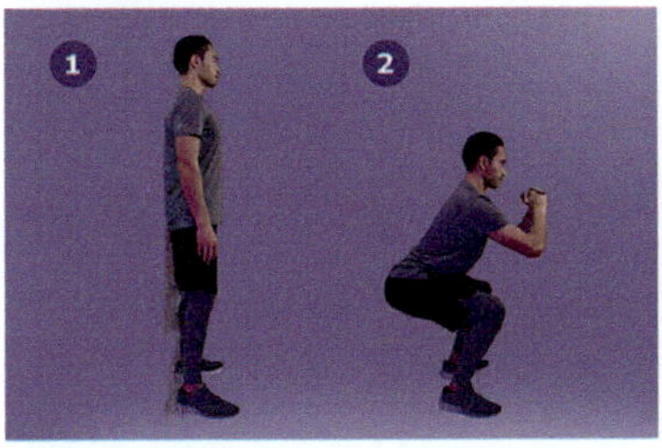 **Fig. 7.1** Lateral view sit-up exercise	See Fig. 7.2 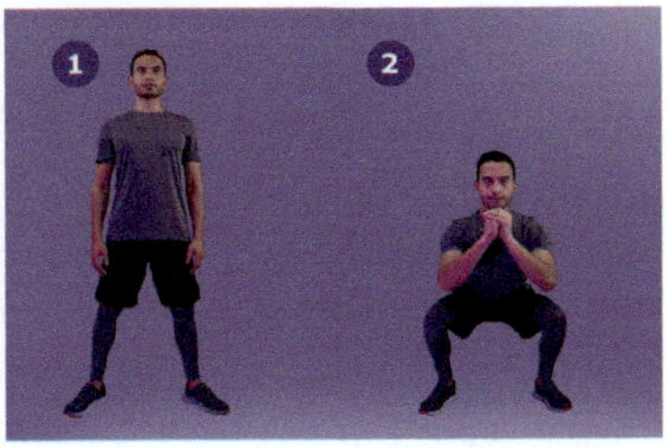 **Fig. 7.2** Frontal view sit-up exercise	
Step 1	**Step 2**	**Step 3**
• Initial position: Start standing with feet approximately shoulder-width apart and externally rotate the hips (pointing the toes outward). Maintain a straight back and relaxed shoulders. You can have your arms extended forward or crossed over the chest.	• Descent: Initiate the movement by flexing the knees and hips simultaneously, as if sitting in a chair. Aim for a knee flexion of approximately 90°. • Lower yourself slowly, keeping the heels in contact with the ground and maintaining a straight back. Make sure to engage the abdominal area and keep your gaze forward to maintain good posture.	• Ascent: Push through the heels and extend the knees and hips to return to the starting position. As you ascend, keep your back straight and avoid leaning forward. • It is essential to remember to perform the squat in a safe and proper manner. Keep the heels on the ground, prevent the knees from collapsing inward, and avoid arching the back.
Auditory cueing (instructions given to the patient)		
• Focus on strongly contracting the glutes and quadriceps before initiating the movement (this facilitates muscle activation). • Begin the knee and hip flexion without losing that contraction.	• Concentrate on the muscular contraction of the quadriceps and glutes while descending (this facilitates a longer eccentric phase of the squat, resulting in increased metabolic stress that promotes hypertrophy).	• While ascending or extending the knees and hips, strongly contract the glutes (an additional stimulus that enhances proprioception, muscle activation, and hypertrophy).
Visual cueing		
• Use a looped video demonstrating the correct execution of a squat and muscle activation during the movement (using cues to highlight points of greater muscle contraction). The video should emphasize a prolonged eccentric phase and a short concentric phase. • Instruct the patient to mimic the movement shown in the video as accurately as possible.		

(continued)

Table 7.1 (continued)

Sit-up	
Kinesthetic cueing	
• Instruct the patient to touch their hands to the quadriceps and glutes and to contract the muscles forcefully while performing the squat. This sensory stimulus facilitates proprioception, muscle activation, and muscle contraction.	
Training method: • Sensorimotor through cueing **Load control/instrument used for load control:** • Execution speed/video duration, stopwatch, metronome, etc. • Level of muscle contraction and activation/utilization of hands as kinesthetic instrument, electromyography **Load dosage for hypertrophy** [3]**:** • **Volume:** – Repetitions: 15 – Duration of eccentric phase: 5 s – Duration of concentric phase: 2 s – Sets: 3 • **Intensity:** – 40% of 1RM (repetition maximum) • **Density (rest periods between sets and repetitions, values are given as follow "load phase: Recovery phase ratio"):** – Between repetitions: Not applicable – Between sets: 1:2	
Modifications of the exercise	
Easier level: • *Option 1:* Squat on a fit-ball or a bench. Involves sitting down and standing up. • *Option 2:* Wall-sit squat with isometric contraction. Lean against the wall while performing the squat.	**Advanced level:** • *Option 1:* Single-leg squat • *Option 2:* Squat with increased external load and a longer eccentric phase. • *Option 3:* Squat with the use of occlusion bands for hypertrophy training.
Notes: Visual, auditory, and kinesthetic cueing can vary based on the creativity of the professional or the patient and the attentional focuses used to execute the movement. These attentional focuses can be internal, external, or neutral. Example: • Internal focuses: – Concentrate on contracting the glutes during the eccentric phase of the squat. – Think about how each quadriceps muscle contracts during the concentric phase of the squat. • External focuses: – Imagine pushing the floor away from you as far as possible during the concentric phase of the squat. – Focus on lowering the weight or barbell as slowly as possible. • Neutral focuses: – Specific: Instruct the patient to perform the exercise as fast or slow as possible. – Nonspecific: Highlight the patient's correct postures and successes. This methodology can be applied to any strength exercise.	

Table 7.2 Cueing isometric ball lunge exercise

Isometric ball lunge
Objective: Contribute to the improvement of static stability through isometric and isotonic contraction exercises.
Initial position
See Fig. 7.3 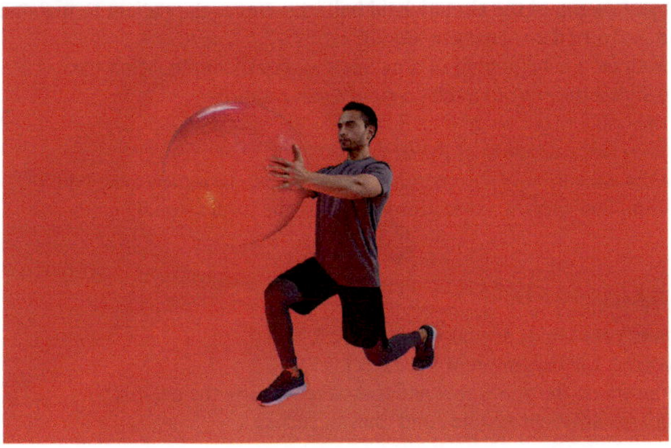 **Fig. 7.3** Initial position, isometric ball lunge exercise • Static lunge position, with arms extended and shoulders flexed at 90°, holding the ball with both hands

Step 1	**Step 2**	**Step 3**
See Fig. 7.4 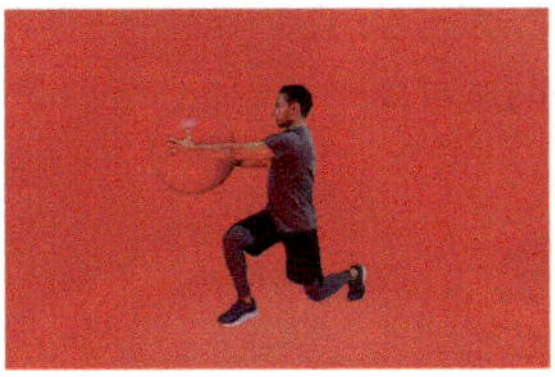 **Fig. 7.4** Right side turn, isometric ball lunge exercise Bring the ball to the right side with arms extended.	See Fig. 7.5 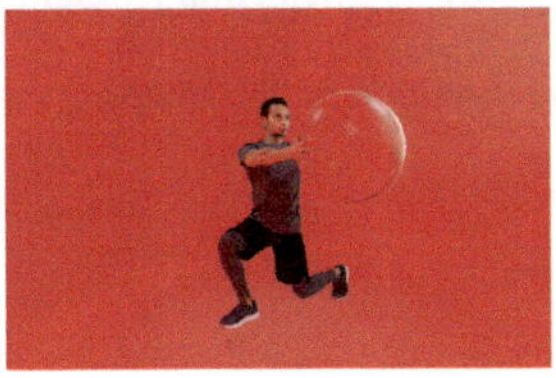 **Fig. 7.5** Left side turn, isometric ball lunge exercise Bring the ball to the left side with arms extended.	See Fig. 7.6 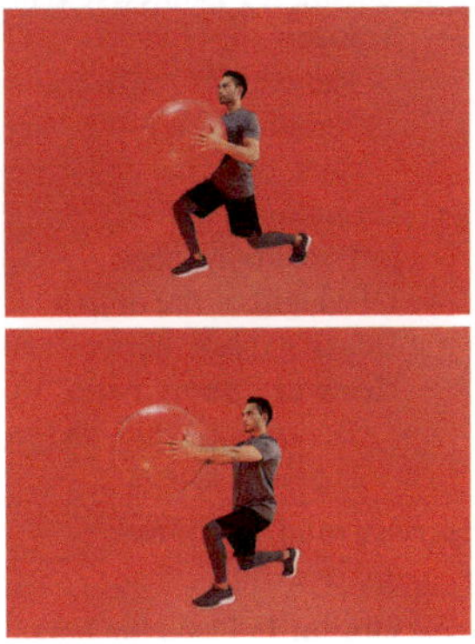 **Fig. 7.6** Front side, isometric ball lunge exercise Bring the ball back to the center and repeat the previous sequence (consider this as 1 repetition of the exercise). Alternate legs at the end of each set.

(continued)

Table 7.2 (continued)

Isometric ball lunge	
Auditory cueing (instructions given to the patient)	
• Use a metronome or verbal command to indicate the start of each trunk rotation during the lunge, controlling the number of repetitions and speed of execution.	
Visual cueing	
• Place a ball or balancing object on top of the already held ball; this forces the patient to maintain a stable scissor position and perform the movement slowly. • Use a flashlight or light to indicate the beginning of a movement. For example, blink the flashlight on a cell phone to signal the start of a left-to-right torso rotation. • Always keep your eyes on the ball. • Use videos for proper imitation and execution of the movement. • Use a laser pointer to guide the execution of the exercise. For example, to indicate the path of the ball, the speed of execution, and specific corrections given by the professional.	
Kinesthetic cueing	
• Hold the ball firmly. • Squeeze the ball as hard as you can. • Try to feel the air passing over your hands as you move the ball. • Touch specific muscles to correct the execution of the exercise. • Use electrical muscle stimulation on the zones that are contracted during the exercise. • Perform the exercise barefoot on different textures and uneven surfaces.	
Training method: • Isometric training with supplementary weights **Load control/instrument used for load control:** • Execution speed/metronome, stopwatch • Load volume/weight of the ball or object **Load dosing for isometric training with supplementary weights** [3]**:** • **Volume:** – Repetitions (only count one repetition for the complete movement of the trunk and arms from right to left): 8–12 – Sets: 6 • **Intensity:** – Execution speed – Weight of the object • **Density (rests between sets and repetitions. Values are given as follow "loading phase: Recovery phase ratio"):** – Between repetitions: Not applicable – Between sets: 1:2	
Exercise modifications	
Basic level: • **Option 1:** Place the back knee on a cushion. • **Option 2:** Perform the movement without an additional ball or weight.	**Advanced level:** • **Option 1:** Use a dumbbell or weight plate instead of the ball. • **Option 2:** Place the front foot on a Bosu ball or unstable surface.

Table 7.2 (continued)

Isometric ball lunge
Notes: Visual, auditory, and kinesthetic cues vary according to the creativity of the practitioner or patient, as well as the attentional focus used to perform the movement. These attentional focuses can be internal, external, or neutral. *Example:* • Internal focus: – Strongly and continuously contract the muscles in the legs, torso, and arms. – Imagine the slow contraction of the muscles that rotate the trunk. • External focuses: – Visualize the path of the ball with your eyes closed as you perform the movement. – Always keep your eyes on the path of the ball. • Neutral focuses: – Specific: Instruct the patient to hold the position as long as possible. – Nonspecific: Encourage the patient to do their best. This method can be applied to any isometric exercise.

Table 7.3 Gait training with cueing exercise

Gait training
Objective: Contribute to the re-adaptation and/or rehabilitation of dynamic stability during walking.
Exercise framework and explanation
In this exercise, various objects are placed on the floor and must be crossed without touching them. The goal is to get from a starting point to a final point by overcoming the obstacles. Various obstacles can be used, such as wooden blocks, cones, sport's saucers, and square wooden bars, as long as the patient's safety is ensured, and the path remains free of dangerous objects during the exercise. The difficulty of the exercise can be adjusted by varying the size, type, position, and distance between obstacles. It is important to note that, depending on the patient's stage of Parkinson's disease (see Fig. 7.2), the patient must be always accompanied by an assistant to ensure his or her safety during the exercise. Below are various illustrations showing different alternatives for the obstacle course exercise, with variations in size, type, position, and distance between obstacles (Figs. 7.7, 7.8, 7.9, and 7.10).

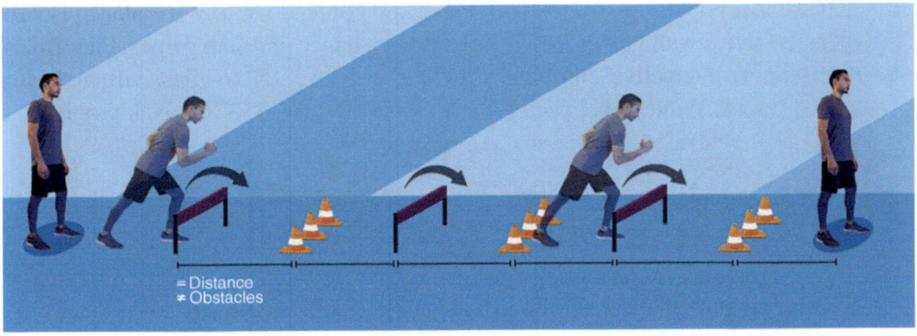

Fig. 7.7 Gait training with different obstacles and equal distances between them

(continued)

Table 7.3 (continued)

Gait training

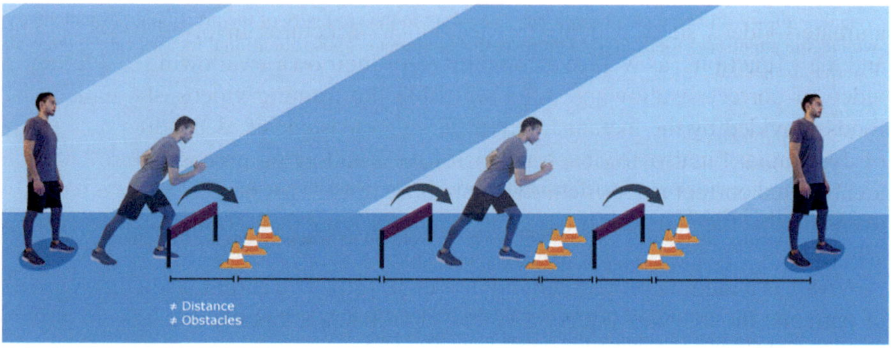

Fig. 7.8 Gait training with different obstacles and varying distances between them

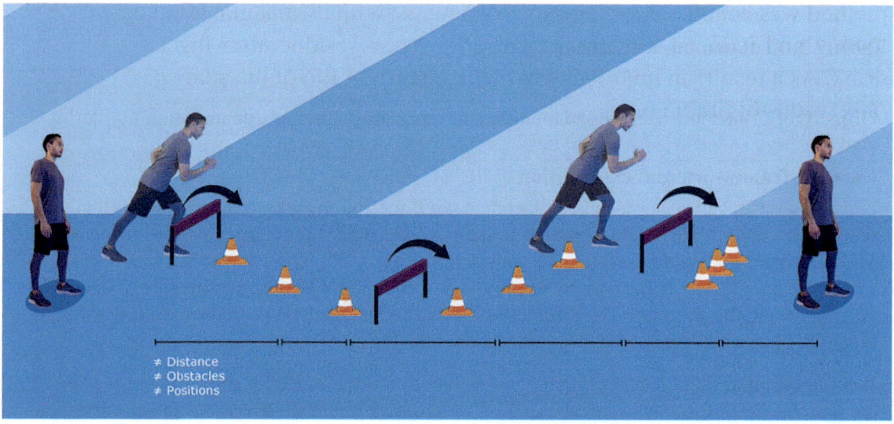

Fig. 7.9 Gait training with different obstacles, distances, and positions between them

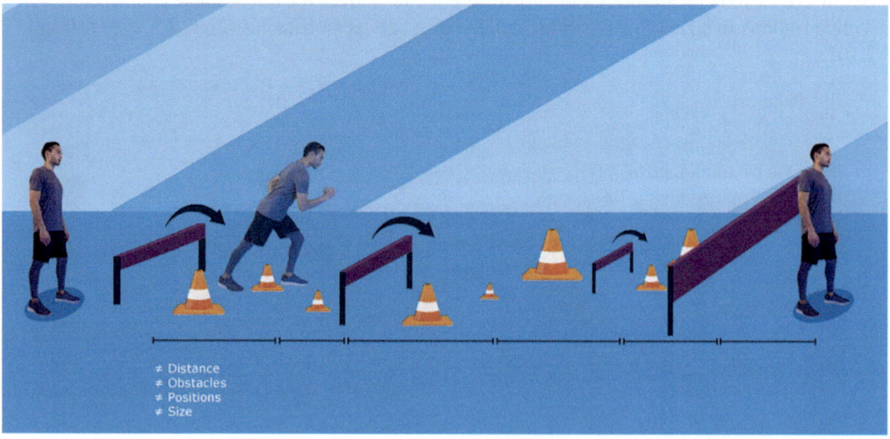

Fig. 7.10 Gait training with different obstacles, distances, sizes, and positions between them

(continued)

Table 7.3 (continued)

Gait training
Auditory cueing (instructions given to the patient)
• Walk to the rhythm of a metronome, taking a step with each beat. • Take a step with each clap. • Walk to the rhythm of a song or sound. • Walk at different speeds according to the verbal instructor's instructions (e.g., "walk slowly" for "white" or "walk faster" for "blue").
Visual cueing
• The objects placed during the walk serve as visual cues. Therefore, we can vary the textures, dimensions, and distances between obstacles. • Use colored cards to show the patient how to walk (blue: Walk forward, green: Walk sideways, red: Walk backward). • Create three obstacle courses in different directions, with the patient starting from a starting point and returning to that point after completing each obstacle as quickly as possible. • Use different colored obstacles to indicate walking speed (blue obstacles: Slow walk, green obstacles: Medium walk, red obstacles: Fast walk).
Kinesthetic cueing
• Use electrostimulation of certain muscles during walking. • Touch the lower limb or leg (by either the patient or the professional) that affects walking (e.g., during freezing of gait moments) during the exercise. • Walk barefoot on different textures and inclinations of the ground.
Load control/instrument used for load control: • Speed and coordination/stopwatch, metronome, claps, verbal commands, music, or melodies • Gait amplitude/distance between obstacles • Reaction speed/spatial distribution of obstacles, muscular electrostimulation **Load dosage** • **Volume:** – Repetitions (one repetition is the total distance traveled from the initial point to returning to it): 6 – Sets: 6 • **Intensity:** – Walking rhythm – Walking direction – Ground incline – Type of obstacle • **Density (rests between sets and repetitions. Values are given as follow "load phase: Recovery phase ratio"):** – Between repetitions: No rests – Between sets: 1:1/2

(continued)

Table 7.3 (continued)

Gait training	
Exercise modifications	
Basic level: • **Option 1:** Objects distributed at equal distances • **Option 2:** Objects of the same dimensions	**Advanced level:** • **Option 1:** Objects distributed at variable distances • **Option 2:** Objects of different dimensions
Notes: Visual, auditory, and kinesthetic cues may vary depending on the creativity of the practitioner or patient and the attentional focus used to perform the movement. These attentional focuses may be internal, external, or neutral. *Example:* • Internal focus: – Focus on a specific muscle as you walk. – Feel the ground contact with each step. • External focus: – Focus on overcoming one obstacle at a time. – Focus on the finish line. • Neutral focus: – Specific: Walk as fast as you can. – Nonspecific: Motivational message This methodology can be applied to any gait exercise.	

Table 7.4 Multidirectional jumps with cueing exercise

Multidirectional jumps

Objective: Contribute to fall prevention and gait speed through explosive strength training.

Initial position

See Fig. 7.11

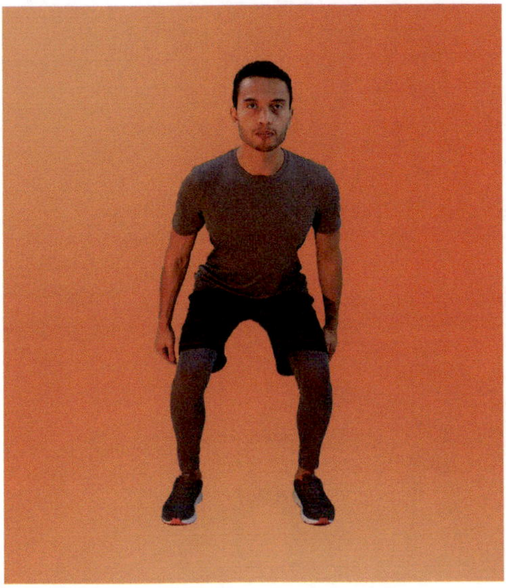

Fig. 7.11 Initial position (multidirectional jumps exercise)

- Ensure that the exercise area is safe, with at least 2 m of obstacle-free and stable ground.
- Begin with a landing position, slightly flexing knees, and hips.

Step 1

See Fig. 7.12

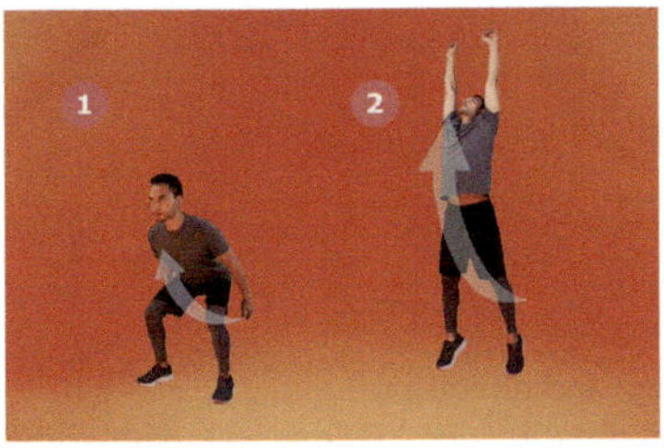

Fig. 7.12 Step 1: Vertical jump (multidirectional jumps)

- Upon the signal, perform the first vertical jump (submaximal force) with both legs, extending arms, hips, knees, and ankles.
- Land in the same manner as the initial position.

Step 2

See Fig. 7.13

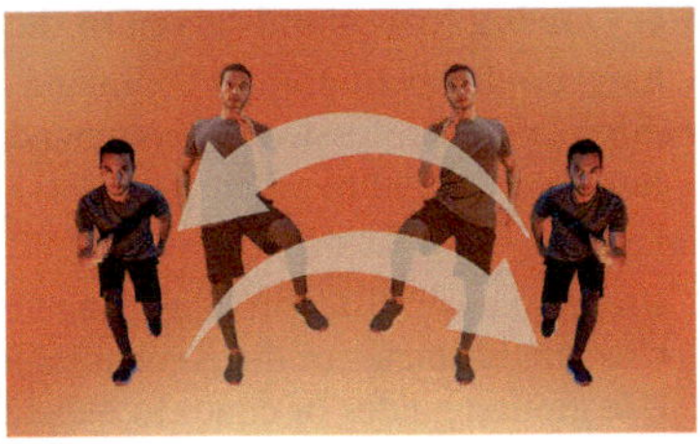

Fig. 7.13 Step 2: Lateral jump (multidirectional jumps)

- Upon the signal, perform a left lateral jump (submaximal force) on one leg.
- Then perform a right lateral jump.

(continued)

Table 7.4 (continued)

Multidirectional jumps
Step 3
See Fig. 7.14

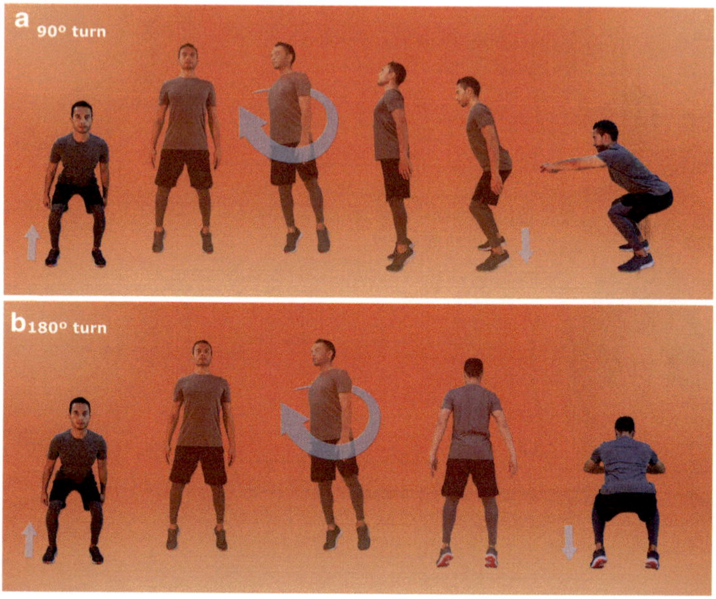

Fig. 7.14 Step 3: 90° and 180° jump (multidirectional jumps)

- Upon the signal, perform a vertical jump with a 90° or 180° twist to the right (submaximal force) with both legs and extending hips, knees, and ankles.
- Return with a vertical jump and twist to the starting position, then execute it on the opposite side.

Auditory cueing (commands given to the patient)

- Jump on the metronome's command.
- Jump on the professional's command.
- Jump to the rhythm of a melody.

Visual cueing

- Use hurdles of different heights and colors to jump over.
- Use safe obstacles of different sizes for vaulting.
- Use ground guides or cones to indicate jump distance and direction.
- Use applications or programmed slides to indicate jump direction and distance with arrows or colors.
  - For example:
    Create slides in a program such as PowerPoint that indicate jump directions with arrows and jump intensity with colors (green arrow: Low intensity; blue arrow: Medium intensity; red arrow: High intensity). The slides should be animated to alternate and be presented at specific intervals.
    Mobile applications such as "SwitchedOn" can also serve as alternatives.

(continued)

Table 7.4 (continued)

Multidirectional jumps	
Kinesthetic cueing • Jump barefoot on various firm and safe surfaces. • Jumping while the muscles of the lower limbs are stimulated with electrical impulses. • Jumping with eyes closed, where the signal to start jumping is a touch on the shoulder of the patient by the professional.	
Training method: • Plyometric **Load control/load control instrument:** • Velocity/stopwatch, frame-by-frame analysis through slow-motion videos • Range of motion/video program for biomechanical analysis, videos • Distance/meter **Load dosage:** • **Volume:** – Repetitions (number of contacts of both feet with the ground): 20–30 – Sets: 3 • **Intensity:** – Low Note: Intensity is classified as low (low speed, amplitude, and jump distance), medium (medium speed, amplitude, and jump distance), and high (high speed, amplitude, and jump distance). • **Frequency:** – Number of sessions per week: 2–3, with at least 1 day of rest between them • **Density (rest intervals between sets and repetitions. Values are given as follow "loading phase: Recovery phase ratio"):** – Between repetitions: No rest – Between sets: 1:5–1:10	
Exercise modifications	
Basic level: • **Option 1:** Jumping in a single direction and short distances • **Option 2:** Jumps in place	**Advanced level:** • **Option 1:** Jumps over greater distances, using obstacles to overcome • **Option 2:** Single-legged jumps
Notes: Visual, auditory, and kinesthetic cueing may vary based on the creativity of the professional or patient and the attentional focuses used to execute the movement. These attentional focuses can be internal, external, or neutral. *Example:* • Internal focuses: – Concentrate on the contraction of the quadriceps and glutes during the concentric phase of the jump. • External focuses: – Imagine pushing the ground as far away as possible. – Visualize jumping as far as possible before executing. • Neutral focuses: – Specific: Focus on making the landing as quiet as possible. – Nonspecific: Instruct the patient to "give their best effort in each jump". This methodology can be applied to any plyometric exercise.	

Table 7.5 The Russian march exercise demonstrated with cueing method

Russian march
Objective: Contribute to the improvement of walking speed and acceleration.
Description
See Fig. 7.15

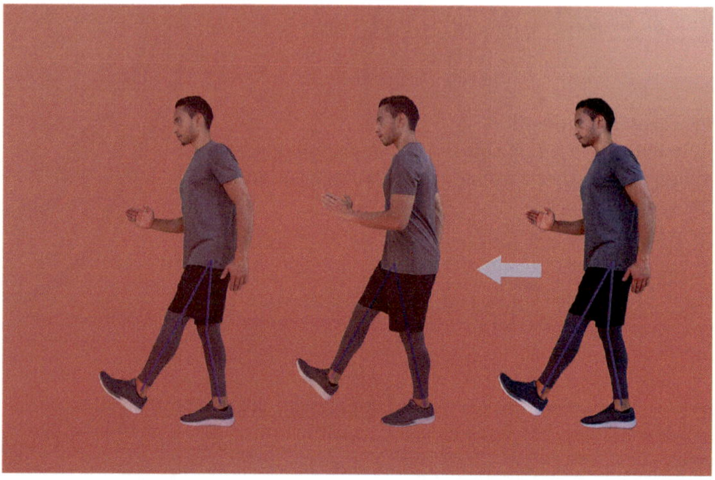

Fig. 7.15 The Russian march exercise demonstrated with cueing method

The Russian march is an exercise that can be done dynamically or statically. This exercise is like static or moving walking, the only difference being that the legs are always extended. The procedure is described step by step:

- To start the movement, flex your hips while extending one leg.
- Then contact the ground quickly, making sure that the supporting phase of the foot is with the forefoot and that the hip is slightly extended at the end of the supporting phase.
- Immediately after contacting the ground with the first leg, begin the movement with the opposite leg in the same manner, extending the leg, flexing the hip, and supporting on the forefoot.

Note:

- It is important to keep the knees extended throughout the exercise and to avoid bending them while performing the Russian march.
- In addition, the leg movement should be accompanied by a natural arm swing that follows the rhythm of the leg movement.
- It is worth noting that the Russian march can be performed while moving forward, that is, walking while performing the exercise. It can also be done statically, staying in the same place while performing the leg movement.

Auditory cueing (instructions given to the patient)

- Perform the march to the rhythm of a metronome, that is, take steps each time a beat is heard.
- Take a step every time you hear a clap.
- Walk to the rhythm of a song or sound.
- Walk at different speeds according to the professional's instructions (e.g., when saying "white," the patient should walk slowly; when saying "blue," the patient should walk faster).

(continued)

Table 7.5 (continued)

Russian march

Visual cueing

- Use colored cards to show the patient how to walk (blue: Walk forward, red: Walk backward).
- In a 100-meter obstacle-free field, use markers on the ground placed sequentially at 30, 60, and 90 meters, with the goal of increasing the speed of the Russian march as each distance is reached.

Kinesthetic cueing

- Use electrostimulation of specific muscles during the march.
- Touch the lower limb or leg (either by the patient or professional) that affects the gait (e.g., during freezing of gait moments) during the execution of the exercise.
- Perform the march barefoot on different textures and inclines of the ground.

Training method:

- Speed and agility training

Load dosage:

- **Volume:**
  - Repetitions: 1
  - Repetition duration: 25–60 s
  - Sets: 5–8.
  - Frequency:
    Sessions per week: 2 (preferably one session of maximum speed and another of agility)
- **Intensity:**
  - 80–100%
  Note: Intensity varies in speed of movement and range of motion, divided into three levels: Low (0–33%), medium (34–66%), and high (67%–100%).
- **Density (rests between sets and repetitions. Values are given as follow "load phase: Recovery phase ratio"):**
  - Between repetitions: N/A
  - Between sets: 1:12–1:20

Exercise modifications

Basic level:	Advanced level:
• **Option 1:** Static march, without any speed • **Option 2:** Moving march, slightly flexing the hips	• **Option 1:** Moving march at the highest possible speed • **Option 2:** Moving march while overcoming obstacles

Notes:

Visual, auditory, and kinesthetic cues vary according to the creativity of the practitioner or patient and the attentional focus used to perform the movement. These attentional focuses can be internal, external, or neutral.

Example:

- Internal focus:
  - Focus on specific muscles as you march.
  - Feel ground contact with each step.
- External focus:
  - Focus on touching an object with the tip of your foot.
  - Focus on the finish line.
- Neutral focus:
  - Specific: Perform the march as quickly as possible.
  - Nonspecific: Motivational message

This methodology can be applied to any speed exercise.

Table 7.6 React exercise utilizing cueing

React!
Objective: Contribute to agility and reaction speed.
Initial position
See Fig. 7.16

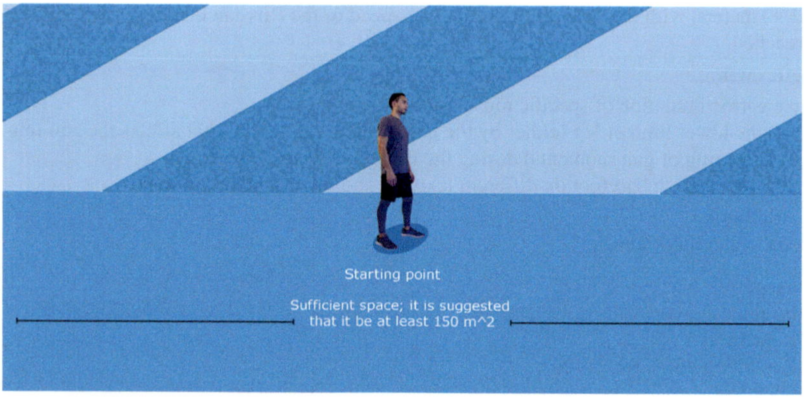

Fig. 7.16 Initial position (react exercise utilizing cueing)

- The goal of this exercise is for the patient to perform the action associated with a number from 1 to 4 as quickly as possible after receiving the instruction. It is important for the professional to give clear signals to the patient to avoid confusion and ensure safe and effective execution of the exercise.

Action # 1
See Fig. 7.17

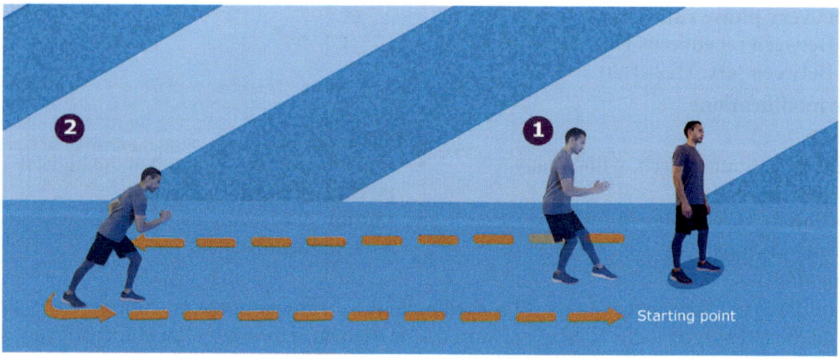

Fig. 7.17 Action # 1 (react exercise utilizing cueing)

1. Backward march.
2. Sprint forward, returning to the starting point.

(continued)

Table 7.6 (continued)

React!
Action # 2
See Fig. 7.18

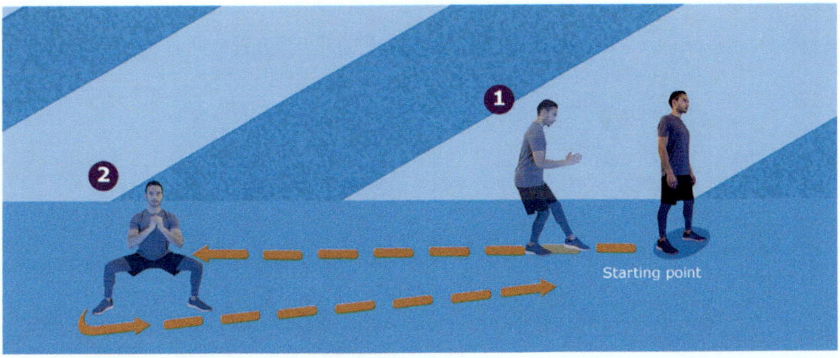

Fig. 7.18 Action # 2 (react exercise utilizing cueing)

1. Backward march.
2. Move laterally back to the starting point.
   Note: Lateral movement should be performed on both hemispheres: Left and right.

Action # 3
See Fig. 7.19

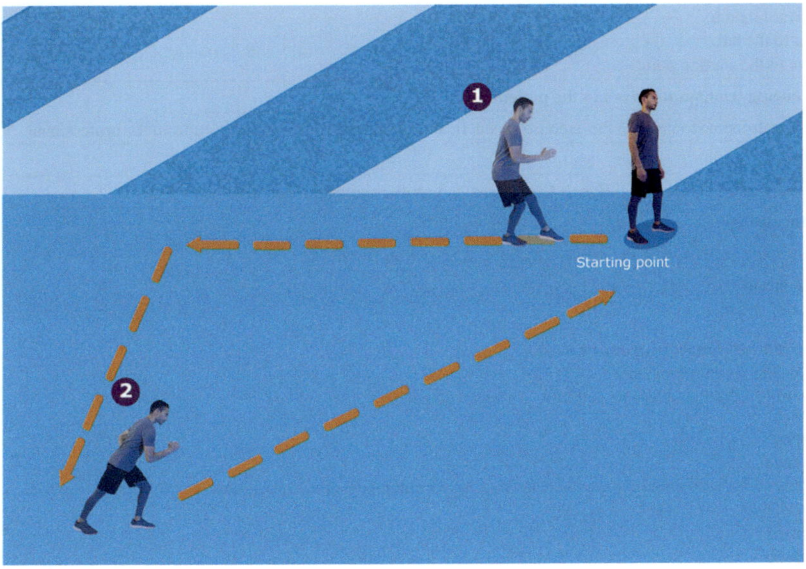

Fig. 7.19 Action # 3 (react exercise utilizing cueing)

1. Backward march.
2. Sprint to the right.
3. Return to the starting point.

(continued)

Table 7.6 (continued)

React!
Action # 4
See Fig. 7.20

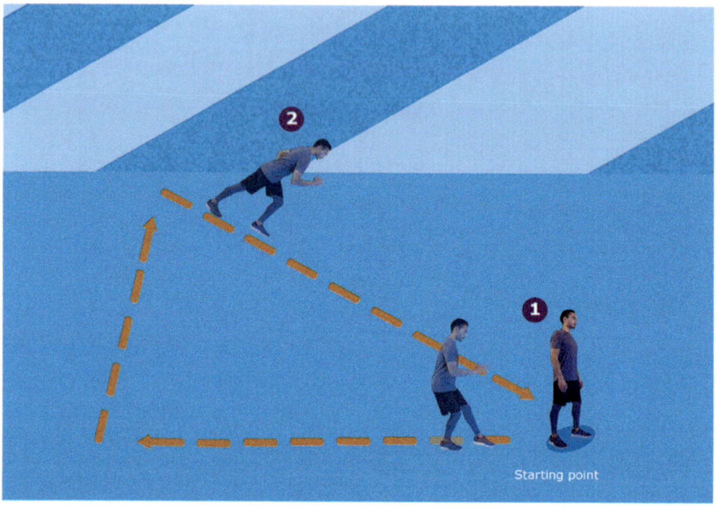

Fig. 7.20 Action # 4 (react exercise utilizing cueing)
1. Backward march.
2. Sprint to the left.
3. Return to the starting point.

Auditory cueing (commands given to the patient)

- Use a metronome to indicate the exercise speed, in addition to the verbal instructions from the professional.

Visual cueing

- Use a digital screen or visual signals to indicate the exercise number of action.

Kinesthetic cueing

- Perform the exercise with the assistance of a muscle electro stimulator.

Training method:
- Reaction speed

Load control/load control instrument used:
- Movement speed/metronome
- Reaction speed/digital screen, auditory, or visual signals

Load dosage:
- **Volume:**
  - Repetitions (one repetition equals indicating the four numbers of actions corresponding to each exercise): 3
  - Sets: 4–6
- **Intensity:**
  - 70–90%

    Note: Intensity varies in reaction speed, displacement, and range of motion, divided into three levels: Low (0–33%), medium (34–66%), and high (67–100%).
- **Density (rests between sets and repetitions. Values are given as follow "loading phase: Recovery phase ratio"):**
  - Between repetitions: 1:1
  - Between sets: 1:10–1:20

(continued)

Table 7.6 (continued)

React!	
Exercise modifications	
Basic level: • **Option 1:** Perform forward marches. • **Option 2:** Perform a static march.	**Advanced level:** • **Option 1:** Perform a march while overcoming obstacles. • **Option 2:** Perform a march while lifting the knees as high as possible.
Notes: Visual, auditory, and kinesthetic cues vary according to the creativity of the professional or patient and the attentional focuses used to execute the movement. These attentional focuses can be internal, external, or neutral. *Example:* • Internal focuses: – Concentrate on specific muscles during the exercise. – Feel the ground contact with each step. • External focuses: – Focus on the finish line. – Focus on the auditory or visual signal provided by the professional. • Neutral focuses: – Specific: Perform the exercise as quickly as possible. – Nonspecific: Motivational message This methodology can be applied to any coordination exercise.	

Qigong Exercises

Ancient practice of Chinese tradition, used as a therapy in alternative medicine. Qigong promotes health through movement, meditation, breathing techniques, and posture control. Its practice goes beyond mere physical discipline; it preserves deeply rooted tradition, culture, and customs. The term "Qigong" is best understood when broken down into "Qi," which means vital energy, and "Gong" (derived from the word Gongfu), which means work or practice. Therefore, we technically define Qigong as any practice, training, and/or cultivation that requires internal or external vital energy (qi) that is sustained over time and achieved through considerable effort or work (gong). In the context of our interest in this book (leaving aside its tradition and the culture associated with it, we focus on the scientific aspect and the evidence that supports it), Qigong is a set of exercises that holistically train the mind (cognitive aspect) and body (motor aspect) with the goal of regulating and balancing them [4].

Its practice has sufficient scientific evidence to support its use in the management of both motor and non-motor symptoms of Parkinson's disease [4].

There are several schools and/or lineages of Qigong, for information purposes:

- Medical Qigong.
- Wudang School Qigong.
- Dragon Gate Qigong.
- Yellow Emperor Qigong.

- White Snake Qigong.
- Emei Mountain Qigong.
- Yang Palace Qigong.
- Wu Family Qigong.
- Chen Family Qigong.
- Yang Family Qigong.
- Sun Family Qigong.
- Li Family Qigong.
- Guo Family Qigong.
- Zhong Yuan School Qigong.
- Polar Bear Qigong.
- White Tiger Qigong.
- Five Animals Qigong.
- Black Turtle Qigong.
- Golden Monkey Qigong.
- White Heron Qigong.

Effects of Qigong on the Control of Motor Symptoms

- Reduces muscle stiffness.
- Improves functional mobility, reducing the risk of falling.
- Increases endurance through mitochondrial oxidative pathways (aerobic).
- Increases gait speed and dynamic stability.
- Improves postural stability and balance.
- Increases confidence in performing daily motor activities.
- Reduces risk of falls and fractures.

Effects of Qigong on the Control of Non-motor Symptoms

- Reduces intestinal constipation.
- Lowers blood pressure.
- Relieves nonspecific low back pain.
- Relieves neck pain.
- Reduces pain perception.
- Reduces the number of daytime sleep episodes.
- Improves patient's social interaction.
- Facilitates verbal and nonverbal communication.
- Improves sleep quality and reduces insomnia episodes.
- Provides remarkable results in the Parkinson Disease Sleep Scale (PDSS), which evaluates sleep biomarkers in Parkinson's patients.

Dosage

According to various studies presented in the systematic review by Deuel and Seeberger [4], the effects of qigong are most pronounced and sustained after a practice period of 6–8 weeks. In terms of training volume, sessions of 45–60 min, 3–5 times a week, twice a day are suggested.

Qigong Exercises

Below are several exercises commonly practiced in Qigong. It is important to emphasize that this discipline and way of life could provide material for an entire book on Qigong, covering aspects such as its foundations, its relationship to martial arts, its breathing techniques, and numerous unique and practical concepts. Therefore, the reader is encouraged to delve deeper into this art, discipline, and lifestyle.

See Table 7.7.

Table 7.7 Warm-up techniques and fundamental postures in qigong exercises

Warm-up
Objective: Prepare the body physiologically and psychologically for subsequent exertion through stretching and dynamic mobility.
Sequence of dynamic stretches and mobility exercises for the hips, torso, shoulder girdle, and arms **Exercise modifications:** If your health does not allow it, or if you find it difficult to exercise standing up, you can always do the exercises in Figs. 7.21, 7.22, and 7.23 sitting on the floor with your legs stretched out.

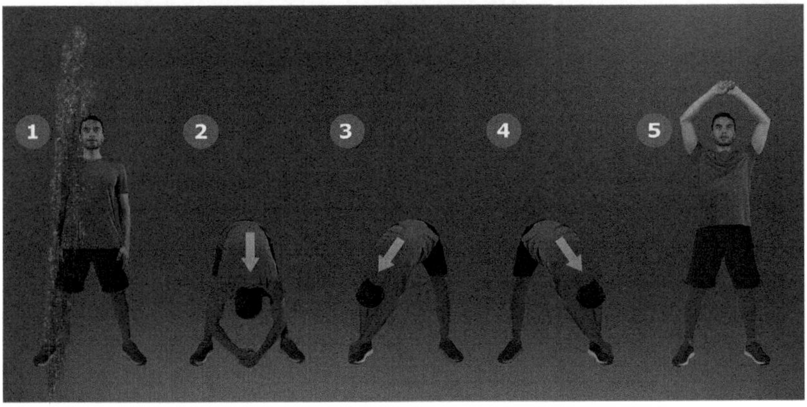

Fig. 7.21 Labei (hip flexion)

(continued)

Table 7.7 (continued)

Warm-up
• *Starting position:* The person should separate their feet and perform a hip abduction slightly wider than hip width. • Slowly and gradually flex the hips, one vertebra at a time, while directing the head and outstretched arms toward the center of the legs. • While maintaining hip flexion, perform a lateral tilt of the body to either side. First direct the head and hands to the right leg. • Then to the center of the body and finally to the left leg. • To return to the starting position, extend the hips and torso vertebra by vertebra, starting from the lumbar region and moving up to the cervical region. Next, perform a 180° shoulder flexion and extend the arms above the head. *Note:* It is important to keep the knees straight and the shoulders relaxed throughout the exercise. Continue with the Shuan Yao movement described below (Fig. 7.22).
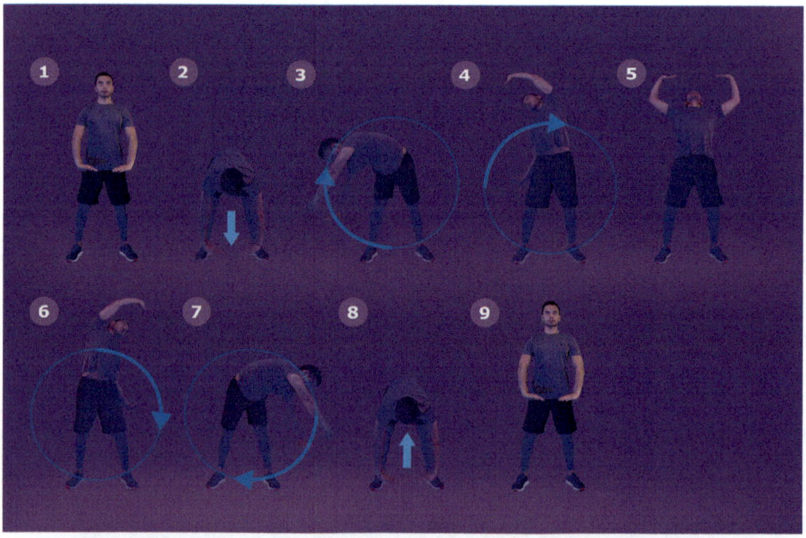 **Fig. 7.22** Shuan Yao (hip circumduction)
• In the starting position, the feet are separated with a hip abduction slightly wider than the hip width. The arms are extended in front of the body and a wrist extension is performed. • Slowly and gradually flex the hips, vertebra by vertebra, while directing the head and extended arms toward the center of the legs. • Next, perform circles with the torso and arms through movements of lateral tilt, extension, and flexion of the hips. The goal is to create circles in a clockwise or counterclockwise direction. *Note:* During hip flexion, the knees can be slightly bent, and during hip extension, the knees should also be extended. Continue with the Gong Bu La Jian movement described below (Fig. 7.23).

(continued)

Table 7.7 (continued)

Warm-up

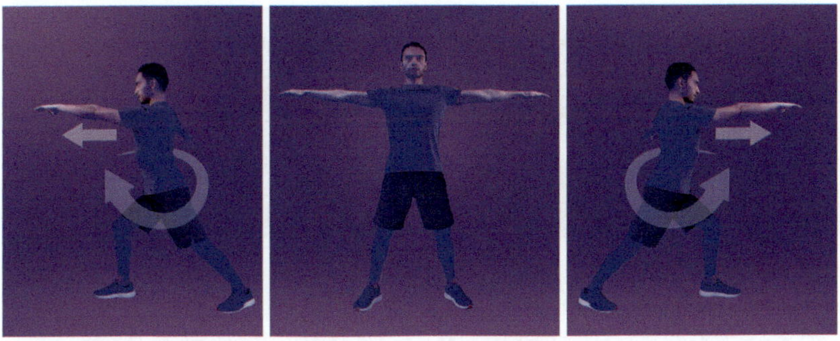

Fig. 7.23 Gong Bu La Jian (trunk rotation)

- In the starting position, the person should separate the feet and perform a hip abduction slightly wider than hip width. Additionally, extend the arms and perform a 90° shoulder horizontal abduction.
- Continue to rotate the torso and hips to the left. At the same time, flex the left knee and extend the right knee. Both feet should rotate in the direction of motion.
- During the rotation, the left arm is directed sideways in horizontal abduction, and the extended right arm is directed forward, maintaining 90° of shoulder flexion.
- Once the rotation to the left is complete, return to starting position and perform the same movement, this time to the opposite side.

Note: It is important to maintain full extension of the arms and fingers. In addition, rotate the entire body, including the feet, during the movement.

Circumduction of the neck (see Fig. 7.24):

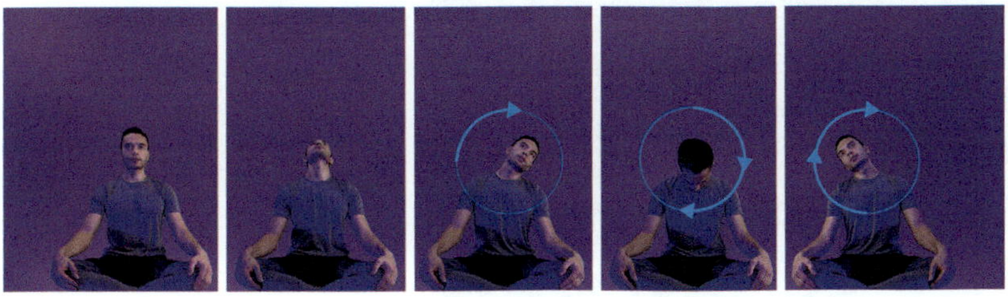

Fig. 7.24 Circumduction of the neck

Circumduction of the elbows (see Fig. 7.25):

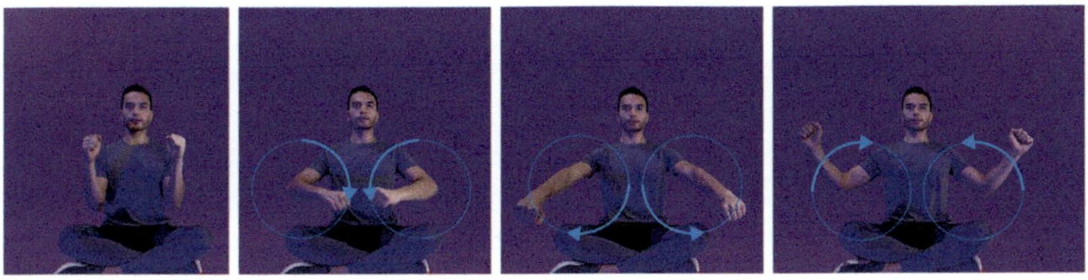

Fig. 7.25 Circumduction of the elbows

(continued)

Table 7.7 (continued)

Warm-up

Circumduction of the wrists (Fig. 7.26):

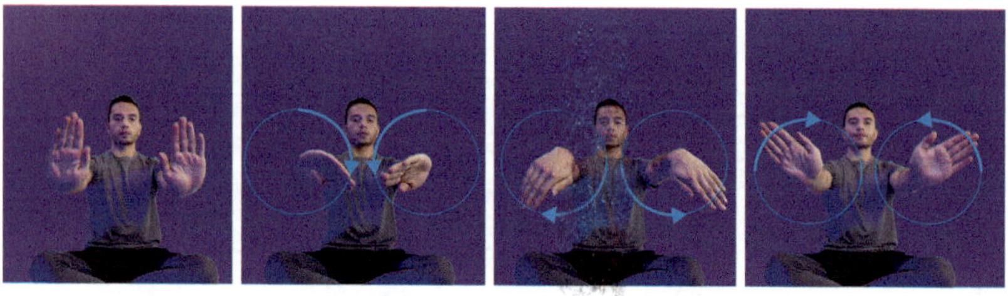

Fig. 7.26 Circumduction of the wrists

Flexion and extension of the fingers (Fig. 7.27):

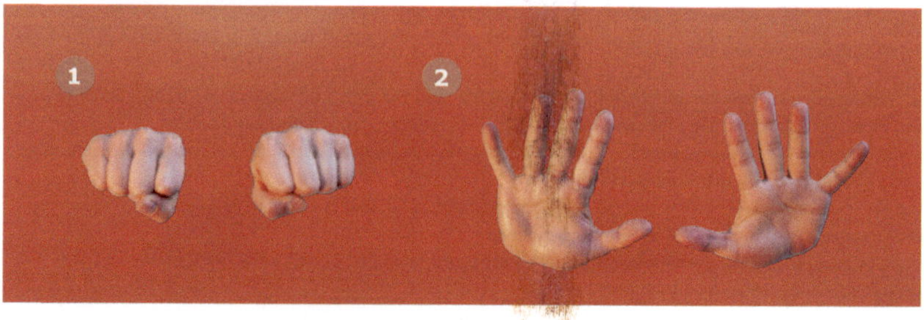

Fig. 7.27 Flexion and extension of the fingers

Circumduction of the ankles (Fig. 7.28):

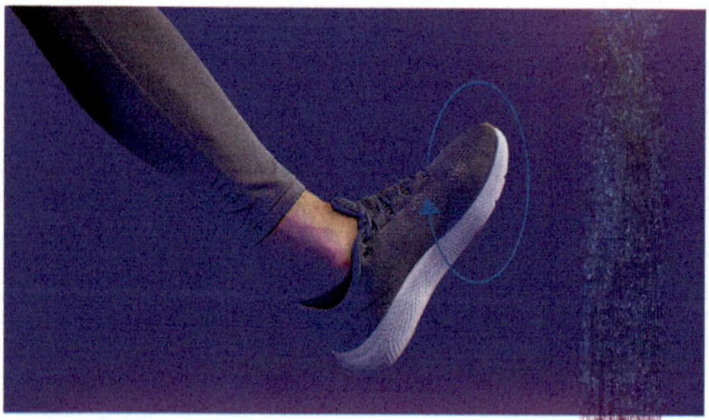

Fig. 7.28 Circumduction of the ankles

Training parameters

Training method:
- Dynamic stretching

Dosage of the load:
- **Volume:**
  - Repetitions: 15–20
  - Series: 2–3
- **Intensity:**
  - Intensity is controlled by the speed of the movement. That is, if the goal of the central phase of training is to perform fast, explosive, and wide movements, dynamic stretching should be wider and faster, but if the goal is to perform slow and not very wide movements, dynamic stretching does not require amplitude and speed.
- **Density:**
  - Does not apply since it is a continuous work.

(continued)

Table 7.7 (continued)

Warm-up

Tips

- The speed of dynamic stretching should be progressive, from slow to fast.
- Perform the exercises always being aware of the position of your body in space, how you feel your muscles, your posture, your breathing, and your balance.
- If any exercise causes you discomfort, ask your practitioner for a modification or recommendation.

Fundamental postures

Ma Bu

See Fig. 7.29

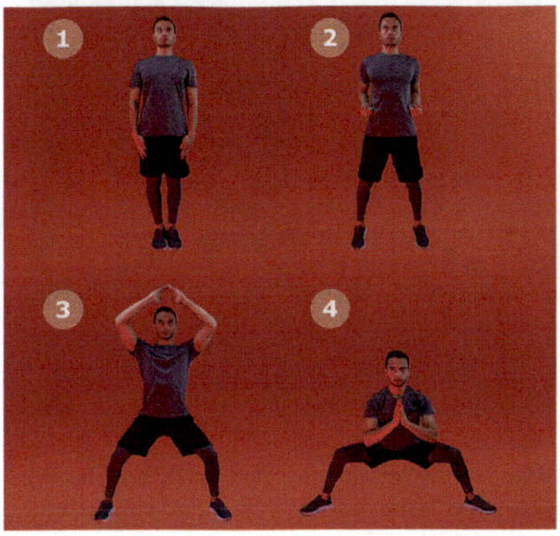

Fig. 7.29 Ma Bu

1. To begin, stand with legs together and arms next to body.
2. Next, take a sidestep to separate the feet beyond shoulder width. At the same time, make a fist with both hands and bring the elbows back, pointing both fists toward the anterosuperior iliac crests.
3. Flex shoulders to 180° and raise arms above head.
4. Again, direct the arms to the front of the chest and bring the palms together, simulating the prayer position, while squatting to assume the “"Ma Bu" position.
5. Hold the position in isometric muscle contraction and repeat the exercise on the opposite side.

Note: The gaze should be directed forward throughout the exercise. Feet should be firmly planted on the floor.

Xie Bu

See Fig. 7.30

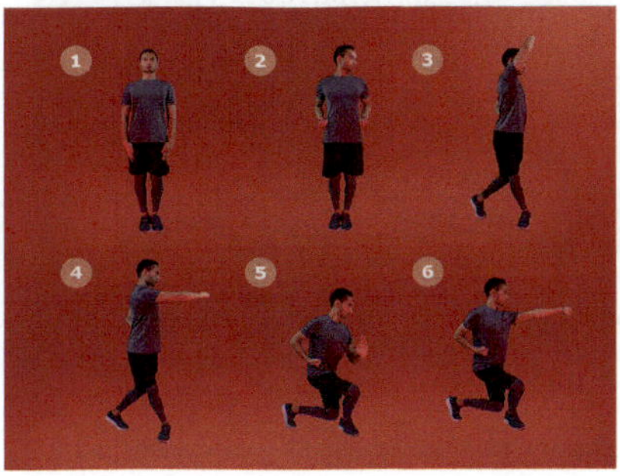

Fig. 7.30 Xie Bu

1. Begin by standing with feet together and arms out to sides.
2. Bring the elbows back and place the hands in a fist next to the anterior superior iliac crests while turning the neck to the left.
3. Step back with left foot crossing behind right foot, raise right arm above head with elbow slightly flexed and hand pointing outward in dorsal flexion.
4. Keeping the position of the legs, lower the right arm in semi-flexion at the elbow to 90° shoulder flexion.
5. Perform hip and knee flexion, shifting weight to right leg. At the same time, lower the right arm toward the right anterosuperior iliac crest, grasping the hand. The left arm is flexed and directed toward the front of the chest with the palm open.
6. Perform a left arm strike and bring the right elbow back and close to the torso.
7. Hold the position in isometric muscle contraction and repeat the exercise on the opposite side.

Gong Bu

Pu Bu

(continued)

Table 7.7 (continued)

Warm-up	
See Fig. 7.31 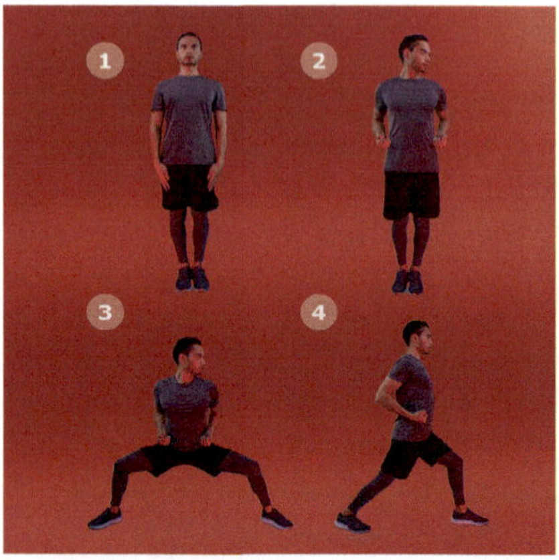 **Fig. 7.31** Gong Bu 1. Starting position: Stand with legs together and arms out to sides. 2. Bring the elbows back and place the clasped hands next to the anterosuperior iliac crests, at the same time turn the neck to face to the left. 3. Take a sidestep with the left foot and squat down, imitating the position of a rider on a horse. 4. Turn the lower limbs and trunk to the left, bending the left leg and extending the right leg. 5. Hold the position with an isometric muscle contraction and repeat the exercise on the opposite side.	See Fig. 7.32 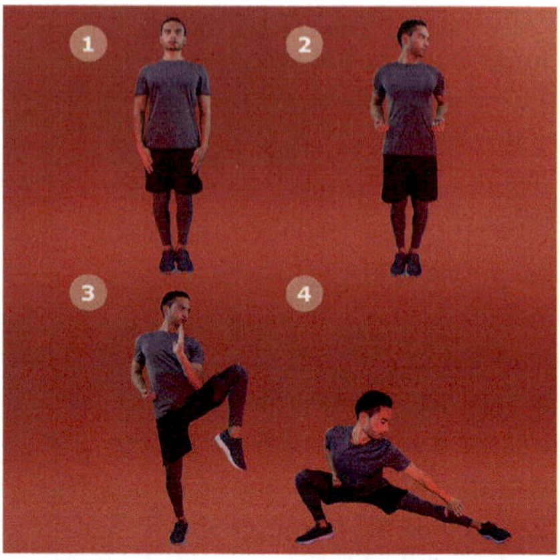 **Fig. 7.32** Pu Bu 1. Stand in starting position with both legs and arms together. 2. Bring the elbows back and place the closed hands next to the anterosuperior iliac crests while turning the neck to the left. 3. Flex the left hip by lifting the leg over the anterosuperior iliac crest and direct the left hand with the palm open toward the center of the chest. 4. Slowly lower the left leg while gradually flexing the right leg. The left leg will gradually extend sideways and slide across the floor. At the same time, extend the left arm and turn the palm inward (radial deviation), bringing it as close as possible to the left foot. *Note:* This pose requires good balance. It is recommended to be practiced gradually and on a safe surface.

Training parameters

Training method:
- Training with auxotonic contractions.

Dosage of the load:
- **Volume:**
  - Repetitions: 2 for each hemisphere (right and left)
  - Isometric time for each repetition: 30–60 s
  - Sets: 3–6
- **Intensity:**
  - The intensity of the isometric muscle contraction can be maximal, submaximal, or mild.
  - The intensity of isotonic contractions varies according to the speed at which they are performed.
- **Density:**
  - Repetitions: Not applicable
  - Sets: 1:1

(continued)

Table 7.7 (continued)

Warm-up
Tips • All the positions described have a movement phase and a static phase, we should focus mainly on the static phase, being aware of the good position and the muscles involved. • The more you practice these positions, the easier they will be to perform, so creatively and safely incorporating external loads, contraction speeds and higher intensities will significantly modify the quality and quantity of your training.

Tai Chi exercises

Tai Chi is one of the branches of Chinese martial arts based on Taoist philosophy. This martial discipline is used as an alternative medicine for the prevention and treatment of disorders and pathologies. More than 600 scientific studies, including reviews, meta-analyses, and experimental research, provide evidence of its benefits in managing both motor and non-motor symptoms of Parkinson's disease [4].

Tai Chi is divided into several schools and families, including:

- Chen
- Yang
- Wu/Hao
- Wu
- Sun
- Hebei
- Cheng Man-ch'ing
- Li style
- Fu style
- Combination style
- Qigong Tai Chi

Effects of Tai Chi on the Control of Motor Symptoms

- Increases walking speed.
- Increases the number of steps the Parkinson's patient takes during the day.
- Improves mediolateral and anteroposterior stability in both static and dynamic states.
- Helps improve the Parkinson's patient's confidence in performing daily physical activities.
- Promotes independence and self-sufficiency.
- Improves mobility.
- Increases upper and lower extremity strength, preventing falls and fractures.
- Facilitates joint range of motion (ROM), both passive and active.

Effects of Tai Chi on Non-motor Symptom Control

- Improves mood.
- Prevents fatigue and insomnia.
- Reduces sleep disturbances.
- Decreases depression and anxiety.
- Reduces blood pressure.
- Facilitates socialization.

Dosage

Most studies provide evidence that 8–14 weeks of Tai Chi training, with 60-min sessions repeated 3–4 times per week, significantly improves motor and non-motor symptoms in people with Parkinson's disease.

Tai Chi Exercises

The following are examples of Tai Chi exercises:

- Sun Salutation (Tai Chi Chuan).
- White Crane Spreading Wings (Bai He Liang Chi).
- Silk Reeling (Tai Chi Chuan).
- Golden Eagle Soaring (Jin Ying Ti Shi).
- Walking like a cat (Tai Chi Chuan).
- Snake Crawls Down (She Xin Shi).
- Silk Winding Hands (Tai Chi Chuan).
- Root Tree Posture (Zhan Zhuang).
- Waving Hands Like Clouds (Tai Chi Chuan).
- Initial Greeting (Qǐ Shì).
- Cloud Hands (Yún Shǒu).
- Parting the Wild Horse's Mane (Yě Mǎ Fēn Zōng).
- Single Whip (Dān Biān).
- Joining Hands (Tí Shǒu Shàng Shì).
- Forward foot kick (Jìn Bù Bān Lán Chuí).
- High Step on Horse (Zhǒu Dǐ Kàn Chuí).
- Covering Body Punch (Shuāng Fēng Guàn Ěr).
- Lotus Kick (Tà Lián Shì).
- Brush Knee (Yáo Bù Bān Lán Chuí).
- Heel Kick (Dēng Jiǎo).
- Spreading Wings (Yún Shǒu Huí Shēn Piē Shēn Chuí).
- Monkey Kick (Hóu Zǐ Tiào).

- Bird's Tail Grab (Bái Hè Liàng Chì).
- Rider's posture (Dān Biān).
- Final Salute (Shōu Shì).

Virtual Reality Training

Virtual reality (VR) training is based on three key therapeutic principles: interaction, immersion, and imagination. Interaction refers to the patient's ability to interact with virtual elements displayed on the screen, allowing them to make decisions and take actions to overcome challenges presented in the training program. Immersion refers to VR's ability to create an experience that feels real, as if the patient were in the virtual environment. Finally, imagination refers to the patient's ability to visualize and reproduce situations and movements that may be challenging in real life.

Thanks to the use of VR, patients with Parkinson's disease can experience, simulate, and visualize everyday situations that may be difficult for them to carry out in real life. In this way, VR becomes a valuable tool for these patients [5].

VR training can be divided into three main categories:

1. *Nonimmersive VR:* Also known as a window system, where the patient observes virtual reality through a screen. Interaction in this type of VR is through devices such as keyboards, microphones, or joysticks. Examples of this type of training include Wii Fit.
2. *Semi-immersive VR:* Also known as augmented or projection-based virtual reality, it aims to bring VR partially into the real world, such as using applications to assess a patient's posture or biomechanical analysis of gait, among other applications.
3. *Immersive VR:* Uses accessories such as VR goggles or 360° headsets, along with gloves or special suits, to fully immerse the patient in a virtual reality that is different from the real world. Examples of this type of VR include Rift, Sony PlayStation VR, Virtuix Omni, HTC Vive, and Oculus Cardboard. Immersive VR enhances the patient's perception and allows them to experience a variety of situations in a safe and controlled environment, making it a highly effective therapeutic tool for Parkinson's patients.

Effects of Virtual Reality Training

Immersion in the world of VR benefits people with Parkinson's disease in the recreation of situations and exercises that prevent and/or reduce [5, 6]:

- Gait problems.
- The risk of falls, increasing both dynamic and static stability.
- Gait rehabilitation time in patients with mild and advanced Parkinson's.

- Space-time gait disturbances.
- Patient dependence, improving daily life activities.
- Hyposensitivity of the senses, such as vision, hearing, and kinesthetic sense.
- Demotivation (as video games or exercises are highly interactive).
- Sedentary behavior.
- High economic costs for the care of Parkinson's patients.
- Deterioration of motor skills, facilitating the transfer of exercises performed in VR to their application in daily real life.
- Stagnation of a therapeutic process or intervention, as it improves sensory feedback of performance, necessary for patient rehabilitation.
- Loss of motor coordination, integrating motor training with cognitive skills.
- Cognitive decline, improving learning capacity. This is because VR activates mirror neurons in the cerebral cortex.

Dosage

According to studies, the typical duration of an effective VR intervention is usually 6–14 weeks, with sessions occurring 2–3 times per week, with each session lasting 30–45 min [7].

According to Ruiz [7], to ensure the effectiveness of a VR exercise program in patient treatment, it is critical that it meets three essential requirements:

1. *Interactive simulation:* VR should allow the patient to actively interact, make decisions, and solve problems. This ensures a realistic and meaningful experience for the patient.
2. *Implicit interaction:* VR should have sensors that allow interaction between the patient's real world and the virtual world. Devices such as goggles, suits, microphones, and similar tools play an important role in this interaction.
3. *Sensory immersion:* VR should be able to stimulate the patient's senses and create an immersive experience. This leads to a greater sense of reality and increases the patient's motivation in the exercise program.

Gait Training with Obstacles

Gait training with obstacles is characterized by the placement of various objects of varying heights, widths, and distances between them. The individual must navigate these obstacles to the best of their ability and overcome them while walking. This training is often used with Parkinson's patients and serves as a guide or track to facilitate continuous and smooth walking under these stimuli. This is particularly important as Parkinson's patients often experience gait freezing, a condition where they struggle to maintain a continuous walking pattern.

For Parkinson's patients who have also suffered a stroke, obstacle course walking serves as a stimulus to reduce the risk of falls or gait abnormalities [8–10].

Effects of Gait Training with Obstacles

- Prevents gait freezing by providing a stimulus to maintain a steady gait pattern.
- Improves gait stability, reducing the risk of falls.
- Improves proprioception, increasing the patient's awareness of temporal and spatial balance during gait biomechanics.
- Increases walking speed.

Dosage

The protocol proposed by Alcock et al. [8] to assess and train obstacle crossing during walking consists of some steps.

- First, the patient is positioned in front of the obstacles with eyes closed to prevent preplanning how to negotiate them.
- Next, the blindfold is removed, and a 7-m walk is initiated over obstacles that should be easily visible and preferably soft, non-pointed, or hazardous.
  Note: It is important to note that a professional or companion should always be present during the intervention to avoid the risk of falling.

When training the patient, it is advisable to follow a principle of progression. This involves starting with low and short obstacles and progressing to higher and longer obstacles. To challenge the patient's proprioception and balance, higher and shorter obstacles are recommended, requiring a longer stride to negotiate, thus extending the foot's support phase. Varying the dimensions of the obstacles in terms of height, width, and depth is also crucial as it closely simulates real-life situations that patients may encounter daily, thus reducing the risk of falls. Therefore, incorporating such variability into training is suggested to improve the patient's ability to navigate different situations and obstacles in their everyday environment.

Examples Protocols

Proposal by Jeong and Koo [9]

A possible intervention for gait training with obstacles is proposed by Jeong and Koo [9] using a treadmill. During the session, obstacles of different dimensions (1–8 cm in height and 2–4 cm in width) are placed, considering the patient's motor capacity to individualize and ensure safety during the stimulus. The professional positions the obstacles while the patient walks on the treadmill and overcomes them. The intensity of the training is adjusted based on the measurements of the obstacles, increasing both their height and width to increase the level of difficulty. The frequency of obstacle placement also affects the intensity of the intervention. In addition, the speed of the treadmill can be adjusted gradually and safely for the patient.

The intervention consisted of 1 month of training with five sessions per week, each lasting 1 h. The first half of the session was dedicated to obstacle avoidance on the treadmill, while the second half focused on lower limb strength training and concluded with joint mobility and flexibility exercises. It's important to emphasize that the obstacles must always ensure the patient's safety, and constant supervision by a professional or trained individual is required.

Proposal by Maeda et al. [10]

Maeda et al. [10] proposed a specific intervention protocol for older adults, including Parkinson's disease patients, consisting of 12 weeks of training with three sessions per week. During this intervention, a wooden obstacle measuring 60 cm in length, 2 cm in width, and 2 cm in height is used. The obstacle is mounted on an adjustable metal base that allows the height to be adjusted to 15% of the patient's height. For example, if the patient is 170 cm tall, the height of the obstacle would be 25.5 cm.

To perform the exercise, the patient should stand 10 cm away from the obstacle, either to the side or to the front. He/she should then step over the obstacle first with the dominant foot and then with the other foot in a stepping motion. It is recommended that this task be performed quickly, always within the safe and biomechanical limits specific to the patient.

It is essential that the patient is constantly supervised by a trained professional throughout the procedure to ensure safety. The presence of the professional makes it possible to adjust and adapt the task according to the patient's individual needs and abilities, avoiding unnecessary risks and ensuring adequate progress during the sessions. This obstacle-crossing intervention protocol aims to improve the Parkinson's patient's mobility, balance, and coordination, providing an opportunity to practice and improve specific motor skills related to overcoming obstacles.

Exergames Therapy

The term "exergames" is derived from the combination of two words: "exercise" and "gaming." It is characterized by the use of video games as a tool for physical activity or exercise for sports, recreational and/or therapeutic purposes. Exergame platforms use motion and pressure sensors that interact with the player's body movements [11, 12]. Among the most popular platforms and brands are Nintendo Wii, Wii Balance Board, Xbox Kinect, active wall games, active floor games, dance and step games, Play Bikes, treadmill games, interactive climbing, PlayStation Move, Moto tiles, virtual reality games, BioRescue, Windows Kinect, BTS Nirvana VR, and 3D VR Kayak program.

Effects of Exergames Therapy

- Motivates patients by providing fun.
- Increases patient adherence to physical activity and/or exercise.

- Increases energy expenditure. This depends on the type of video game and platform.
- Improves muscle tone and mass.
- Improves static and dynamic balance.
- Increases joint mobility.
- Helps improve cognitive executive functions.
- Prevents the risk of falling.
- Reduces fear of falling.
- Improves gait pattern.

Dosage

According to the review conducted by Piech and Czernicki [12], the most prominent interventions in their study had beneficial effects within the following parameters:

- Total intervention duration: 5–24 weeks.
- Weekly frequency: 2–3 sessions.
- Length of each session: 20–60 min.

See Table 7.8.

Table 7.8 Examples of exergames

Examples of exergames therapy	Load parameters	Platform
Beat saber	Duration of 30–45 min, 3–4 times per week. Increase the game's difficulty and movement speed over time.	Oculus quest 2, PlayStation VR
BoxVR	Duration of 20–30 min, 3–4 times per week. Increase the training intensity over time by adjusting speed, movement complexity, and the number of strikes performed.	Oculus quest 2, PlayStation VR
Dance revolution	Duration of 30–45 min, 3–4 times per week. Increase the speed and complexity of dance steps over time.	Computer or console platforms as PlayStation or Xbox
FitXR	Duration of 20–30 min, 3–4 times per week. Increase the training difficulty over time by adjusting speed, movement complexity, and the number of repetitions performed.	Oculus quest 2
Racket: Nx	Duration of 20–30 min, 3–4 times per week. Increase the training difficulty over time by adjusting ball speed, field size, and the number of repetitions performed.	Oculus quest 2
Superhot VR	Duration of 20–30 min, 3–4 times per week. Increase the game's difficulty and movement speed over time.	Oculus quest 2, PlayStation VR

Other Therapeutic Exercises

Spanakis et al. [13] in their review, share a series of active interventions through therapeutic exercise (see Table 7.9).

Table 7.9 Therapeutic exercises and their objectives for managing motor and non-motor symptoms of Parkinson's disease

Type of therapeutic exercise	Explanation	Objectives
Robot-assisted training for gait or limb mobility	Gait impairment can indicate the presence of a neurodegenerative disease, such as Parkinson's. In response to this, new technologies have been developed to assist patients with walking difficulties due to accidents or illnesses. In the current market, there is a wide variety of robots and exoskeletons that improve gait and enable rehabilitation or the achievement of the highest level of functionality in the walking pattern. Some popular examples of these technologies include the G-EO system, LOKOMAT, bionic legs, eLEGS, ReWalk, and REX Bionics (Fig. 7.33). These devices are generally classified as static (for training in one location and not easily portable) and dynamic (for training anywhere and portable). Additionally, each robot or device is used based on the patient's level of motor disability, considering functional walking scales [14–16]. Robot-assisted training is also used in rehabilitation as therapeutic exercise for the upper limbs after injuries or associated diseases such as muscle atrophy, paralysis, hemiplegia, neurodegenerative syndromes, or neurodevelopmental disorders [17].	To improve the motor function of both lower and upper limbs.

(continued)

Table 7.9 (continued)

Type of therapeutic exercise	Explanation	Objectives
	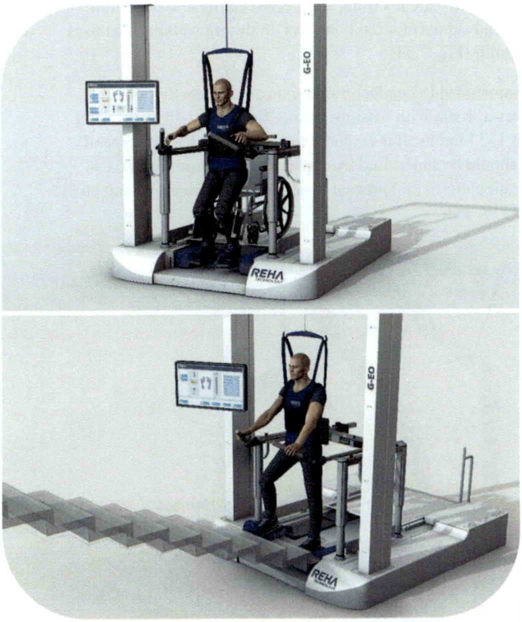 **Fig. 7.33** Figure of the G-EO systems by REHA technology. Pathological gait assistance tool, with the option of simulating different surfaces and slopes. Taken from Reha technology [photograph], 2023. https://www.rehatechnology.com/en/g-eol/ (the link provided will take you to the official page used as the source for the figure below, which provides information about the G-EO systems and other related features, including its usage and manual)	

(continued)

Table 7.9 (continued)

Type of therapeutic exercise	Explanation	Objectives
Weight-supported treadmill training	This type of training is distinguished by using a harness-like support that encircles the patient's trunk and pelvis, acting as a regulator, stabilizer, and support for the body weight during walking exercises on a treadmill (Fig. 7.34). It is recommended to conduct training on an antigravity treadmill three times a week, with sessions lasting from 20 to 45 min, over a period of 1–3 months. It is essential to emphasize that this type of training should be supervised by a qualified professional who can observe gait patterns and prevent knee collapse during walking on the treadmill [18, 19]. 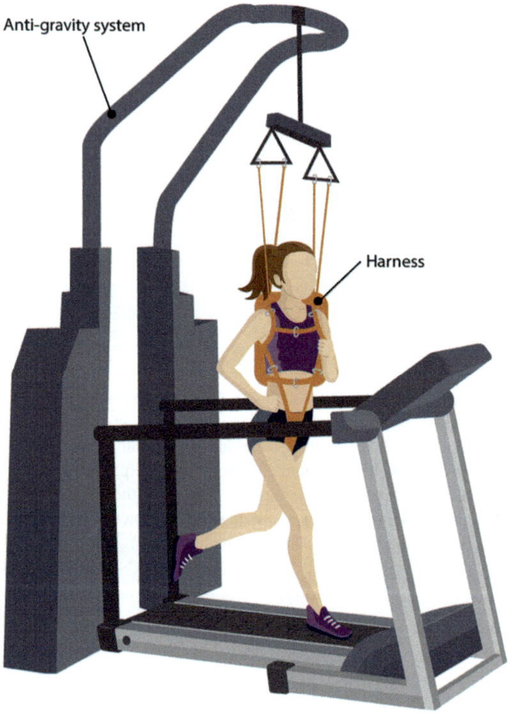 **Fig. 7.34** Illustration of an anti-gravity system designed to support body weight, with an integrated treadmill (self-created illustration) This therapeutic antigravity system is designed to enhance muscular strength and joint range of motion, with various goals, including contributing to the improvement of gait patterns.	To assist in the rehabilitation or readaptation of walking.

(continued)

Table 7.9 (continued)

Type of therapeutic exercise	Explanation	Objectives
Argentine tango	It has been found that patients with Parkinson's disease who participate in tango sessions experience an increase in their physical and social activity. Additionally, there has been an observed improvement in cognition and skill retention after 10–12 weeks of practice. An important aspect is that this intervention could potentially help slow down the motor symptoms and signs of the disease. It is recommended to engage in 1 h tango sessions, 2–4 times a week, for at least 12 months [20].	To improve motor function and emotional well-being.
Animal-assisted therapy	For many years, the importance of domestic animals (such as horses, dogs, cats, fish, and canaries) in the therapeutic process for patients, both adults and children, suffering from various conditions like autism, depression, Down syndrome, anxiety, hyperactivity, stress, apathy, eating disorders, obesity, cardiovascular diseases, fibromyalgia, neurodegenerative diseases, among others, has been recognized. The use of these animals in therapy has shown excellent results, as they fulfill the natural human need for affection and attention [21]. Animal-assisted therapy has multiple benefits for patients with Parkinson's disease, including: • Improvement of short-term memory, bringing back memories from the past or recreating previously experienced situations • Reduction of apathy • Improvement in nonverbal and verbal communication • Reduction in pharmacotherapy • Reduction of stress and agitation • Enhancement of the quality of life • Increase in social interaction • Reduction of blood pressure • Improvement in cardiovascular health Quintavalla et al. [22] propose an intervention protocol for animal-assisted therapy, where domesticated dogs were used over a total period of 12 weeks, with two 30 min sessions per week. This protocol aims to reduce stress and anxiety, improve balance and mobility, as well as promote social interaction.	To reduce stress and anxiety, improving balance and mobility, as well as promoting social interaction.

Summary

- Parkinson's disease, also known as "Shaking Palsy," is a neurodegenerative disorder that affects the central nervous system.
- It is a pathology of multifactorial etiology.
- It is characterized by the loss of dopaminergic neuronal activity and an increase in cholinergic activity.
- Mild stages of Parkinson's develop over a period of 5–6 years, while the more severe stages, with the characteristic symptoms of the disease, begin to appear 5 years after the onset of the disease.

- Risk factors include age (older age increases risk), male sex, exposure to pesticides (especially among farmers), rural living, traumatic brain injury, hepatitis C, daily consumption of dairy products, and family or personal history of melanoma.
- Protective factors include coffee consumption, high blood urea levels, daily exercise, a Mediterranean diet, and the use of nonsteroidal anti-inflammatory drugs.
- Motor symptoms include muscle and joint rigidity, resting muscle tremor (sudden onset and unilateral), bradykinesia, postural changes, urinary and anal dysfunction, digestive dysfunction, altered gait pattern, inability to walk, very small handwriting, limited or absent facial expression, hyper kyphosis, or hunched posture, hypotonia and muscle weakness in the oropharyngeal, esophageal, gastric, and facial muscles, erectile dysfunction, and decreased pelvic floor muscle tone.
- Non-motor symptoms include loss of sense of smell, sleep and mood disturbances, low blood pressure, chronic fatigue, bladder dysfunction, neuropsychiatric disorders such as depression, anxiety, apathy, and psychosis, impulsive behavior, generalized sensory impairment, constipation, nephrotic disorders, deficits in executive cognitive functions (structuring, creating, planning, evaluating, and testing), and dementia.
- The diagnosis of Parkinson's disease should be multidisciplinary because its cause is multifactorial and there is no single biomarker that indicates the etiology of this disease.
- Early diagnosis of Parkinson's disease is not enough. Both motor and non-motor symptoms that develop gradually over time must be evaluated.
- Two commonly used tests to diagnose Parkinson's disease are the Unified Parkinson's Disease Rating Scale (UPDRS) and the Montreal Cognitive Assessment (MOCA). It is recommended that these tests include assessment of both motor and non-motor symptoms of the disease.
- Non-pharmacological treatments, such as clinical exercise prescription, physical therapy, occupational therapy, and speech therapy, aim to prevent, treat, and improve both motor and non-motor symptoms of the disease.
- When prescribing exercise, it is necessary to consider the pharmacologic interaction of the medications a Parkinson's disease patient is taking.
- Include dynamic and static stability training as a primary component to reduce the risk of falls.

Summary Table of Proposed Methods

See Table 7.10.

Table 7.10 Summary of all proposed methods

Methods	Objective	Types/techniques	Effects	Dosage
Cueing	To facilitate mindful and focused attention to movement in patients with motor limitations using multisensory stimuli.	• Visual cueing • Auditory cueing • Kinesthetic cueing	• Promotes the generation of motor responses. • Helps maintain focus on movement. • Prevents deterioration of movement patterns. • Aligns and integrates postural control with movement. • Improves visuomotor and visuopedic coordination. • Prevents movement freezes, such as FOG, during obstacle overcomes, direction changes, and triggering circumstances. • Improves gait stability through functional rehabilitation of gait amplitude and timing. • Contributes to improved spatiotemporal perception. • Visual cueing appears to contribute to the control and regulation of stride length by increasing information flow in the occipitoparietal cerebral motor networks. • Auditory cueing helps maintain correct frequency and timing of gait and improves upper and lower extremity coordination.	• Recommended total intervention time: 2–6 weeks • Number of sessions per week: 3–5 • Session length: 20–45 min
Qigong	To balance multiple bodily functions through movement, meditation, breathing techniques, and postural correction.	There are various schools of qigong associated with different doctrines such as Buddhist, Confucian, and Taoist, which influence the style of practice and the movements performed. Some of them include: • Medical qigong • Wudang school qigong • Dragon gate qigong • Yellow Emperor's qigong • White Snake qigong • Emei Mountain qigong • Yang palace qigong • Wu family qigong • Chen Family qigong • Yang family qigong • Sun family qigong • Li family qigong • Guo family qigong • Zhong yuan school qigong • Polar bear qigong • White Tiger qigong • Five animals qigong • Black turtle qigong • Golden monkey qigong • White crane qigong	• Reduces muscle stiffness. • Improves functional mobility, reducing the risk of falls. • Enhances aerobic endurance through mitochondrial oxidative pathways. • Increases walking speed and dynamic stability. • Improves postural stability and balance. • Boosts confidence in performing daily motor activities. • Reduces the risk of falls and fractures. • Alleviates intestinal constipation. • Lowers blood pressure. • Reduces nonspecific lower back pain. • Reduces neck pain. • Decreases the perception of pain. • Reduces the number of daytime drowsiness episodes. • Enhances the patient's social interaction. • Facilitates verbal and nonverbal communication. • Improves sleep quality and reduces insomnia episodes. • Achieves outstanding results in the "Parkinson disease sleep scale" (PDSS) test, evaluating sleep biomarkers in Parkinson's patients.	• Recommended total intervention duration: 6–8 weeks • Sessions per week: 3–5 • Sessions per day: 1–2 • Session duration: 45–60 min

(continued)

Table 7.10 (continued)

Methods	Objective	Types/techniques	Effects	Dosage
Tai Chí	To reduce pathological stress through meditation, motor imagery, and movement.	Tai chi is classified according to various schools and/or families, including: • Chen • Yang • Wu/Hao • Wu • Sun • Hebei • Cheng man-ch'ing • Li-style • Fu-style • Combination-style • Qigong tai chi	• Increases walking speed. • Increases the number of steps the patient takes during the day. • Improves mediolateral and anteroposterior stability, both statically and dynamically. • Helps improve the confidence of Parkinson's patients in performing daily physical activities. • Promotes independence and self-sufficiency. • Enhances agility. • Increases the strength of the upper and lower limbs, preventing falls and fractures. • Facilitates joint range of motion (ROM), both passive and active mobility. • Improves mood. • Prevents drowsiness and insomnia. • Reduces sleep disorders. • Reduces depression and anxiety. • Lowers blood pressure. • Facilitates socialization.	• Recommended total intervention duration: 8–14 weeks • Sessions per week frequency: 3–4 • Session duration: 60 min
Occupational therapy	To reduce and prevent dependency and disability in activities of daily living through techniques, means and methods specific to occupational therapy.	Occupational therapy itself is a distinct field that employs various intervention techniques, such as active and/or passive manual and instrumental therapies.	• Occupational therapy, along with physical therapy and speech therapy, significantly increases the independence of Parkinson's patients. • Occupational therapy, combined with brain stimulation and virtual reality, has been shown to be effective in promoting patient independence. • Improves joint mobility. • Contributes to static and dynamic postural balance control. • Reduces the risk of falls. • Improves cognitive abilities. • Increases focused attention. • Improves memory. • Promotes physical activity. • Improves endurance through mitochondrial oxidative pathways, flexibility and gait. • Contributes to necessary rehabilitation to maintain or improve fine motor skills, such as writing. • Improves emotional Well-being. • Facilitates medication adherence. • Promotes social participation when occupational therapy activities, methods, and resources are used in heterogeneous groups (considering cognitive and motor disabilities).	**REHACOP (cognitive rehabilitation program of psychosis):** • Recommended total duration of intervention: 12–20 weeks • Weekly session frequency: 3 sessions • Session duration: 90 min **Sensory stimulation using cues combined with electrotherapy and proprioception exercises:** • Recommended total intervention time: 4 weeks • Weekly session frequency: 3 sessions • Session duration: 60 min **Transcranial direct current stimulation (tDCS) in conjunction with occupational therapy:** • Recommended total intervention time: 8 sessions • Session duration: 60 min of occupational therapy and 20 min of tDCS **Hand and forearm muscle strengthening and writing exercises:** • Recommended total intervention time: Throughout the development or progression of the condition

				• Weekly session frequency: 4 sessions • Session duration: 30 min **Physical and occupational therapy:** • Recommended total duration of intervention: 12 weeks • Weekly session frequency: 3 sessions • Session length: 90–120 min **Dance:** • Recommended total intervention time: 6–12 months • Weekly session frequency: 1–3 sessions • Session length: 60–90 min **Virtual reality training:** • Recommended total intervention time: 2 months • Weekly session frequency: 3 sessions • Session length: 60 min • Rest between reps and sets: 3 min **Virtual training sessions:** • Recommended total duration of intervention: 6 months • Weekly session frequency: 3 sessions • Session length: 40–60 min **Hatha yoga:** • Recommended total intervention time: 12 weeks • Weekly session frequency: 2 sessions • Group session length: 60 min **Physical exercises through applications or software:** • Recommended total intervention time: 8 weeks • Weekly session frequency: 3 sessions • Session duration: 30–60 min **Muscle strengthening using free weights combined with exercises that activate mitochondrial oxidative pathways (aerobic):** • Recommended total duration of intervention: 12 weeks • Weekly session frequency: 2–3 sessions • Session duration: 60–90 min

(continued)

Table 7.10 (continued)

Methods	Objective	Types/techniques	Effects	Dosage
Speech and language therapy	Contributing to the improvement, prevention, and recovery of dysarthria (speech disorders) through specific exercises.	• Lee Silverman voice treatment (LSVT) • Breathing reeducation • Video-assisted swallowing therapy (VAST) • Music therapy	• Improved vocal volume and intensity. • Facilitates voice inflection and tone changes. • Enhances articulation and phonation. • Contributes to improved facial expression communication. • Supports respiratory and swallowing therapy. • Facilitates strong and high-quality coughing by strengthening respiratory muscles and increasing expiratory pressure. • Reduces momentary shortness of breath (dyspnea). • Improves and makes food and beverage swallowing safer, avoiding dysphagia. • Reduces the amount of pharyngeal residue after consuming food or drinks. • Increases expiratory strength. • Increases speech rate. • Improves posture while speaking. • Enhances nonverbal expression. • Improves motor and non-motor symptoms of Parkinson's. • Enhances overall quality of life.	**Lee Silverman voice treatment (LSVT):** • Recommended total intervention: 4 weeks • Sessions per week: 4 • Session duration: 60 min **LSVT-BIG (BIG refers to large movements used in the method):** • Recommended total intervention: 4 weeks • Sessions per week: 4 • Session duration: 60 min **Breathing reeducation:** **EMST device:** *Week 1:* • Volume: 5 sets, 5 repetitions, 5 times a day for a total of 25 minimal exhalations per day • Rest between repetitions: Rest for a minimum of 15–20 s. Do not skip the rest between repetitions; your muscles need to recover for the next maximum exhalation • Rest between sets: Rest for a minimum of 1 min • Frequency: 5 times a week • Intensity: 75% of maximum expiratory force and/or pressure *Week 2:* • Intensity: 75–100% of maximum expiratory force and/or pressure *Week 3:* • Intensity: 100–125% of maximum expiratory force and/or pressure *Week 4:* • Intensity: 125% of maximum expiratory force and/or pressure *Week 5:* • Intensity: 125%–150% of maximum expiratory force and/or pressure

				After week 5, you can continue a maintenance treatment of expiratory strength, adjusting it to the parameters from week number 5 and modifying it from there. As advice, you should reduce the training frequency to 3 times a week. **Forced expiration with open glottis technique:** • Volume: 3 sets of 3 repetitions • Frequency: 3–4 times a week • Rest between sets: 1 min • Rest between repetitions: 10 s **Directed cough:** • Volume: 3 sets of 5 repetitions • Frequency: 3 times a week • Rest between sets: 1 min • Rest between repetitions: 5–10 s **Global chest cage mobilization:** • Volume: 4 sets of 10 repetitions • Frequency: 2–3 times a week • Rest between sets: 1–2 min • Rest between repetitions: 15 s **Video-assisted swallowing therapy (VAST):** • Recommended total intervention: 2 weeks • Sessions per week: 5 • Session duration: 30 min **Music therapy:** • Recommended total intervention: 4–16 weeks • Sessions per week: 2–5 • Session duration: 30–120 min
Physical activity	To promote the control and treatment of motor and non-motor symptoms and signs of Parkinson's disease.	• High-intensity treadmill training • Perturbed treadmill training • Aquatic or suspension training on a treadmill	• Neuroprotective effects • Reduction of cerebral atrophy • Increased dopamine secretion • Elevated levels of neurotrophins • Improved vascularization • Reduction of proinflammatory bacterial lipopolysaccharides content • Increased production of short-chain fatty acids by bacteria • Elevated peripheral levels of BDNF • Reduction and/or delay in Parkinson's neuropathology • Modulation and availability of dopamine transporter proteins	**High-intensity treadmill training:** • Total intervention: 26 weeks • Intensity: The goal is to reach 80–85% of maximum heart rate (MHR) during exercise. Intensity increases gradually from week 1 to week 8 to achieve the target percentage of MHR. It is recommended to have supervision by first aid-trained professionals during the first 2 weeks. This heart rate can be achieved by adjusting treadmill speed and/or incline.

(continued)

Table 7.10 (continued)

Methods	Objective	Types/techniques	Effects	Dosage
			• Reduction of neurotoxicity in bilateral dopaminergic pathways connecting the substantia nigra and prosencephalon, facilitating neuroplasticity and increasing BDNF levels • Enhanced spatial cognition and executive cognitive functions • Prevention of dementia and cognitive disability in Parkinson's patients • Improved sleep quality, and, consequently, mood • Enhanced gait ability • Prevention of osteoporosis and cardiovascular diseases • Reduced perception and sensation of pain • Lower levels of pharmacotherapy and medication prescription • Decreased mortality due to falls and balance loss • Prevention of fear of future falls	• Volume: – Session phases: Warm-up: 5–10 min Main: 30 min at the target MHR percentage Cooldown: 5–10 min – Frequency: 4 days a week • Biological monitoring elements: Heart rate monitor **Perturbed treadmill training:** *Recommended intervention:* • Initial phase: 5 min of warm-up and familiarization without perturbing the incline. Start perturbed training 1 min before finishing the warm-up. • Main phase: 3 sets of 5 min with 3 min standing breaks on the treadmill between sets • Intensity: 70% of comfortable walking pace, determined by a previous test (10 m walk test) • Session duration: 26 min Note: If possible, train without holding onto the treadmill's handrails. **Aquatic or suspension treadmill training:** • Recommended total intervention: 10 sessions in 6 weeks with rest intervals • Initial phase: 5 min of warm-up and familiarization • Main phase: 30 min • Intensity: – Initial phase: 1 mile per h (mph) for 5 min – Main phase: Increase speed by 0.5 mph every 5 min, up to 4 mph, or until fatigue or a professional's decision • Other intensity aspects: – Treadmill incline remains constant – In suspension: 50% body weight load on the treadmill • Session duration: 35–40 min

Muscular electrical stimulation (MES)	To help prevent muscular atrophy, loss of muscle mass and lack of muscular strength by activating muscle fibers and increasing capillarization.	• Passive muscular electrical stimulation • Active muscular electrical stimulation	• Reduction of tremors and dyskinesia • Improved postural control, balance, and muscle stiffness • Pain reduction • Improved swallowing by activating muscle fibers involved in the swallowing process, reducing dysphagia through MES • Prevention of muscle atrophy • Muscle potentiation and hence a reduction in the risk of falls • Improved proprioception • Muscle tone control	**Passive muscular electrical stimulation for muscle strength enhancement:** *Recommended intervention:* • Total duration: 8–12 weeks • Session duration: 20–30 min • Frequency: 50–75 Hz • Pulse duration: 200–400 μs • Intensity: The highest tolerated without causing any harm to the patient. According to Bispo et al. [23] review, an intensity between 60–100 mA is suggested. • Electrode size: It is recommended that they cover a larger area than standard electrodes to avoid increased discomfort in the conduction area. The size depends on the area being treated and the desired stimulation intensity. **Muscular electrical stimulation for the treatment of neurogenic dysphagia:** *Recommended intervention:* • Number of sessions: 15–20 • Days per week for intervention: 3–5 days • Recommended device according to Centeno [24] commonly used in studies: "VitalStim-Therapy" • Possible electrode placement areas: Suprahyoid muscles, hyoid bone, thyroid notch, over the thyroid, and lower thyroid area. Electrodes and channels are placed depending on the area. • Session duration: 20–30 min **Active whole-body muscular electrical stimulation:** *Recommended intervention:* • Conduct an initial familiarization session for exercise technique and adaptation to devices and electrical stimuli. • It is suggested to test these stimuli with the patient beforehand to determine their tolerance limit and not exceed it during the sessions.

(continued)

Table 7.10 (continued)

Methods	Objective	Types/techniques	Effects	Dosage
Virtual reality (VR) training	To feel, to reproduce and to visualize innumerable situations of the everyday life with the purpose to facilitate them.	• Nonimmersive VR • Semi-immersive VR • Immersive VR	• Reduce the risk of falls. • Improvement of dynamic and static stability. • Reducing gait rehabilitation time in patients with mild and advanced Parkinson's disease. • Help improve spatiotemporal gait changes. • Reduction of sensory hyposensitivity, such as visual, auditory, and kinesthetic senses. • Reducing the high cost of care for Parkinson's patients. • Facilitating the motor transfer of VR exercises to real-life applications. • Improving the sensory feedback of performance necessary for patient rehabilitation. • Integrating motor training with cognitive skills. • Activation of mirror neurons in the cerebral cortex.	• Initial phase: 5 min with multijoint exercises or exercises specific to the area • Central phase: 3 min per exercise, consisting of 4 s of isometric contraction followed by 4 s of passive rest • Intensity: • Varies according to the type of exercise, workload, contraction speed, loads, and other dosage aspects. • For the electrical stimulation protocol, rectangular waves at a frequency of 75–85 Hz are suggested, with pulse times of 350 μs, alternately performing 4 s of stimulation followed by 4 s of rest. • Session duration: 20 min from electrode placement to removal **Recommended intervention:** • Total intervention duration: 6–14 weeks • Sessions per week: 2–3 • Session duration: 30–45 min
Gait training with obstacles	To help improve gait and reduce the risk of falls.	• Walking while overcoming obstacles on flat terrain • Walking while overcoming obstacles on a treadmill • Walking while repetitively overcoming an obstacle	• Prevents gait freezing and serves as a stimulus for the continuity of walking. • Enhances gait stability, reducing the risk of falls. • Improves proprioception, making the patient aware of their temporal and spatial balance during gait biomechanics. • Increases gait speed.	**Walking while overcoming obstacles on a 7-m flat terrain:** *Recommended intervention:* • Initially, the patient stands with their eyes closed in front of the obstacles so that they do not pre-plan how to overcome them. • Upon a visual, auditory, or kinesthetic cue, the blindfold is removed, and the patient starts walking 7 m while overcoming the obstacles, which should be easily visible and preferably soft, not pointed or posing an obvious danger to the patient (foam figures of different dimensions are suggested). • Total intervention duration: 6 weeks • Sessions per week: 2 • Session duration: 60 min • Intensity: Varies based on obstacle measurements (higher and wider obstacles increase intensity), frequency of obstacle placement, and walking speed.

				Walking while overcoming obstacles on a treadmill: *Recommended intervention:* • During training, the professional or assistant places obstacles while the patient walks on a treadmill. • Obstacle dimensions range from 1 cm to 8 cm in height and 2–4 cm in width; taller and wider obstacles are unnecessary. • Total intervention duration: 4 weeks • Sessions per week: 5 • Session duration: 30 min • Intensity: • Varies based on obstacle measurements (higher and wider obstacles increase intensity). • The frequency of obstacle placement on the treadmill is another intensity parameter. • Gradually and safely increasing treadmill speed can also be used to adjust intensity. **Marching in place while overcoming obstacles:** *Recommended intervention:* • Overcoming a wooden hurdle (to make a hurdle you could use a wooden stick measuring 60 cm in length, 2 cm in width, and 2 cm in height) supported by a metal base that allows adjusting the height of the stick (height corresponding to 15% of the patient's height, e.g., if the patient is 170 cm tall, the obstacle's height will be 25.5 cm above the ground). • Position the person 10 cm from the hurdle (either laterally, frontally, or alternately) to initially pass it with the dominant foot and then with the other foot. • It is suggested to perform this exercise as quickly as possible while staying within the patient's safe limits and biomechanical coherence. • Total intervention duration: 12 weeks • Sessions per week: 3 • Session duration: 20 min

(continued)

Table 7.10 (continued)

Methods	Objective	Types/techniques	Effects	Dosage
Exergames therapy	• To help improve the conditioning and coordination abilities • To serve as an adjunct tool in therapeutic processes	Exergames therapy sessions depend on the platform, its accessories, the type of games, the patient's initial conditioning and coordination skills, and cognitive abilities.	• They are motivating for the patient due to the fun they offer. • Increases the patient's adherence to physical activity and/or exercise. • Increases energy expenditure. This depends on the type of video game and platform. • Improves muscle tone and mass. • Enhances static and dynamic balance. • Increases joint mobility. • Contributes to cognitive executive functions. • Prevents the risk of falls. • Reduces the fear of falling. • Improves gait patterns.	• Number of exercises: 3 (frontal obstacle crossing, lateral obstacle crossing, and alternating obstacle crossing, which combines both frontal and lateral crossings) • Repetitions: 20 • Micro breaks: 40 s • Sets: 3 • Intensity: Varies based on the type of obstacle, its height, the speed of obstacle crossing, and other parameters that can be tailored by each professional's creativity. **Recommended intervention:** • Use gaming platforms equipped with motion and pressure sensors that interact with the patient's body movements. • Some well-known platforms and brands include Nintendo Wii, Wii balance board, Xbox Kinect, active wall games, active floor games, dance and step games, games bikes, treadmill games, interactive climbing, PlayStation move, moto tiles, virtual reality games, BioRescue, windows Kinect, BTS nirvana VR, and 3D VR kayak program. • Total duration of intervention: 5–24 weeks • Sessions per week: 2–3 • Session duration: 20–60 min
Reality reorientation therapy	To reorient individuals temporally and spatially • To improve social interaction	The duration of reality reorientation therapy varies depending on the protocol or types of exercises used.	• Enhances temporal and spatial orientation. • Facilitates performance in activities of daily living. • Improves mood. • Enhances social skills and interactions. • Facilitates verbal and nonverbal communication. • Keeps the patient connected to their current reality.	**Recommended intervention:** • Exercises aimed at improving spatial and/or temporal perception and awareness. • Total duration of intervention: 24 weeks • Sessions per week: 1 • Session duration: 45 min

Competing Interests The author have no conflicts of interest to declare that are relevant to the content of this chapter.

References

1. Ginis P, Nackaerts E, Nieuwboer A, Heremans E. Cueing for people with Parkinson's disease with freezing of gait: a narrative review of the state-of-the-art and novel perspectives. Ann Phys Rehabil Med. 2018;61:407–13. https://doi.org/10.1016/j.rehab.2017.08.002.
2. Ghai S, Ghai I, Schmitz G, Effenberg AO. Effect of rhythmic auditory cueing on parkinsonian gait: a systematic review and meta-analysis. Sci Rep. 2018;8:1–19. https://doi.org/10.1038/s41598-017-16232-5.
3. Weineck J. Entrenamiento total. 2005.
4. Deuel LM, Seeberger LC. Complementary therapies in Parkinson disease: a review of acupuncture, tai chi, qi gong, yoga, and cannabis. Neurotherapeutics. 2020;17:1434–55. https://doi.org/10.1007/s13311-020-00900-y.
5. Lina C, Guoen C, Huidan W, et al. The effect of virtual reality on the ability to perform activities of daily living, balance during gait, and motor function in Parkinson disease patients: a systematic review and meta-analysis. Am J Phys Med Rehabil. 2020;99:917–24. https://doi.org/10.1097/PHM.0000000000001447.
6. Vargas M, Vargas L. Realidad virtual aplicada como estrategia de intervención en la función motora de pacientes con Parkinson. Repositorio ECR. 2019:1–44. https://repositorio.ecr.edu.co/server/api/core/bitstreams/ab345027-1901-4f84-8de7-eaab0a187d6d/content.
7. Ruiz L. La Realidad Virtual y su aplicación en la rehabilitación de la Enfermedad de Parkinson. Tesis de grado: Universidad Miguel Hernández; 2018.
8. Alcock L, Galna B, Hausdorff JM, et al. Gait & posture special issue: gait adaptations in response to obstacle type in fallers with Parkinson's disease. Gait Posture. 2018;61:368–74. https://doi.org/10.1016/j.gaitpost.2018.01.030.
9. Jeong YG, Koo JW. The effects of treadmill walking combined with obstacle-crossing on walking ability in ambulatory patients after stroke: a pilot randomized controlled trial. Top Stroke Rehabil. 2016;23:406–12. https://doi.org/10.1080/10749357.2016.1168592.
10. Maeda Y, Sudo D, Shimotori D. Different effects of 12-week speed or accuracy training on obstacle-crossing foot motion in healthy elderly. Int J Environ Res Public Health. 2022;19 https://doi.org/10.3390/ijerph19084596.
11. Muñoz JE, Villada JF, Giraldo Trujillo JC. Exergames: una herramienta tecnológica para la actividad física. Rev Méd Risaralda. 2013;19:126–30.
12. Piech J, Czernicki K. Virtual reality rehabilitation and exergames-physical and psychological impact on fall prevention among the elderly-a literature review. Appl Sci (Switzerland). 2021;11(9):4098. https://doi.org/10.3390/app11094098.
13. Spanakis M, Xylouri I, Patelarou E, Patelarou A. A literature review of high-tech physiotherapy interventions in the elderly with neurological disorders. Int J Environ Res Public Health. 2022;19(5):9233. https://doi.org/10.3390/ijerph19159233.
14. Bergmann J, Krewer C, Bauer P, et al. Virtual reality to augment robot-assisted gait training in non-ambulatory patients with a subacute stroke: a pilot randomized controlled trial. Eur J Phys Rehabil Med. 2018;54:397–407. https://doi.org/10.23736/S1973-9087.17.04735-9.
15. Campos-Fajardo S, Campos J, Morros GE, et al. Cambios en la marcha asociados con demencia por cuerpos de Lewy: una revisión narrativa de la literatura. Acta Neurol Colombiana. 2022;38:51–9. https://doi.org/10.22379/24224022400.
16. Morone G, Paolucci S, Cherubini A, et al. Robot-assisted gait training for stroke patients: current state of the art and perspectives of robotics. Neuropsychiatr Dis Treat. 2017;13:1303–11. https://doi.org/10.2147/NDT.S114102.

17. Gueye T, Dedkova M, Rogalewicz V, et al. Early post-stroke rehabilitation for upper limb motor function using virtual reality and exoskeleton: equally efficient in older patients. Neurol Neurochir Pol. 2021;55:91–6. https://doi.org/10.5603/PJNNS.A2020.0096.
18. Anggelis E, Powell ES, Westgate PM, et al. Impact of motor therapy with dynamic bodyweight support on functional Independence measures in traumatic brain injury: an exploratory study. NeuroRehabilitation. 2019;45:519–24. https://doi.org/10.3233/NRE-192898.
19. Aras B, Yaşar E, Kesikburun S, et al. Comparison of the effectiveness of partial body weight-supported treadmill exercises, robotic-assisted treadmill exercises, and anti-gravity treadmill exercises in spastic cerebral palsy. Turk J Phys Med Rehabil. 2019;65:361–70. https://doi.org/10.5606/TFTRD.2019.3078.
20. McKee KE, Hackey ME. The effects of adapted tango on spatial cognition and disease severity in Parkinson's disease. J Mot Behav. 2014;45:1–17. https://doi.org/10.1080/00222895.2013.834288.The.
21. Parra EV, Garre JMH, Pérez PE. Benefits of dog-assisted therapy in patients with dementia residing in aged care centers in Spain. Int J Environ Res Public Health. 2021;18:1–12. https://doi.org/10.3390/ijerph18041471.
22. Quintavalla F, Cao S, Spinelli D, et al. Effects of dog-assisted therapies on cognitive mnemonic capabilities in people affected by alzheimer's disease. Animals. 2021;11:1–12. https://doi.org/10.3390/ani11051366.
23. Bispo VA, Bastos JAI, de Almeida CC, et al. The effects of neuromuscular electrical stimulation on strength, pain, and function in individuals with knee osteoarthritis: a systematic review with meta-analysis. Fisioterapia Pesquisa. 2021;28:416–26. https://doi.org/10.1590/1809-2950/20028528042021.
24. Centeno LF. Electroestimulación neuromuscular como parte del tratamiento de la disfagia. Tesis de grado: Universidad de Valladolid; 2022.

Chapter 8
Mastering the Science of Training Program Development

Initial Questions

- How can I optimize the prescription of therapeutic exercise for patients with motor and non-motor conditions who experience constant or sudden changes in their pathological states?
- What are the basic principles of the ATR model (accumulation, transformation, and realization) and how can they be applied in the development of an effective training plan?
- What is the importance of block periodization, training directions, and planning structure in the context of therapeutic exercise, especially when treating patients with Parkinson's disease?

Training Plan Proposal Based on the ATR Model (Accumulation, Transformation, and Realization)

We propose a training plan based on the ATR model with the aim of prescribing exercise for Parkinson's patients. Both the model and its content are explained below.

ATR Model

The origin of the model began with coach Bondarchuk, who developed a periodization that includes three types of mesocycles: ordinary, competition, and restoration. Each mesocycle has a duration of 4 weeks for the first two and 2 weeks for the third.

Supplementary Information The online version contains supplementary material available at https://doi.org/10.1007/978-3-031-62119-2_8.

C. A. Mejía, *Therapeutic Exercise for Parkinson's Disease and Related Disorders*, https://doi.org/10.1007/978-3-031-62119-2_8

The peculiarity of his training program is the alternation and repetition of a set of exercises in each mesocycle block.

In the 1980s, Issurin and Kaverin, based on Bondarchuk's theory, established three types of mesocycle blocks: accumulation, transformation, and realization (ATR, see Table 8.1). The duration of each mesocycle is adjusted to the corresponding physiological and biomechanical requirements. This training approach allows for an average reduction of between 5% and 10% in annual training volumes and lasting improvements in key components of physical fitness. The application of the ATR model is typically seen in the sports arena, significantly enhancing performance, as was the case in the 1988 Seoul Olympics and the 1989 and 1990 World Championships [1, 2].

Professionals in sports training adopted the idea of training blocks as a cycle of specialized loads, with a maximum of two objectives per block and a high concentration over a short period of time. This means that training loads cannot be used for different objectives simultaneously and must be developed consecutively. Sports performance requires the mastery of certain skills that can only be developed in training blocks. This idea also applies to clinical exercise prescription, as the available time for health-care professionals is limited, and they often see many patients in a day. Furthermore, the development of a process or objective that includes morphological, organic, and biomechanical changes requires a sufficiently long and specific period, changes achieved in training blocks (mesocycles) [1, 2].

In the context of therapeutic exercise applied to pathologies, block periodization of training can be an effective strategy for the consecutive development of target capabilities in successive mesocycle blocks. Their strategy is based on the residual effects of training, meaning that the effects of highly concentrated training stimuli overlap and persist for an extended period. Compared to the traditional theory of training periodization, block periodization has several benefits applicable to clinical practice. For instance, it reduces the total time volume in a therapeutic session and allows for more effective monitoring since it focuses on the consecutive development of specific capacities and can be easily adapted to the patient's needs.

Block periodization is especially effective and practical in therapeutic exercise applied to patients with Parkinson's disease. By creating a planned and structured exercise program in blocks, a gradual and safe progression in intensity and training volume can be established, which can be beneficial for patients. Moreover, block periodization can help patients with Parkinson's achieve their peak performance at specific times, which is particularly important for those who need to reach an optimal therapeutic level at specific stages of the disease.

Principles of Block Periodization with the ATR Model

- *Concentration of training loads*: Training loads should be highly concentrated to produce sufficient stimulus and achieve significant gains in a motor skill, coordination, technique, or therapeutic goal as planned.

Table 8.1 Characteristics of the ATR model for block planning

Attributes	Type of mesocycle Accumulation	Transformation	Realization
Objective	To accumulate a solid foundation of motor, coordinative, and/or technical skills, as well as the necessary physiological and biomechanical adaptations required to achieve the ultimate objective.	To transform the adaptations obtained during the accumulation phase into specific improvements for the ultimate objective. This is achieved through more specific training loads, with a greater emphasis on the specific skill, objective, or movement that needs improvement.	To attain the highest possible performance in the ultimate objective raised. This is achieved through a highly specific and personalized training approach, focused on the individual needs of the patient.
Therapeutic applicability	This block can be used to prepare the patient for more advanced exercises, enhance specific movement techniques, increase muscular endurance and strength, and reduce the risk of injuries, pathological symptoms, and signs.	This block can be employed to make specific adjustments and adaptations to the treatment or exercise plan based on the patient's progress or limitations.	This block can be utilized to assist the patient in achieving a specific performance goal, improving functional capacity, or attaining a significant therapeutic objective.
Motor and technical targeted abilities	– Basic physical abilities – Phase 1 and 2 of endurance training – Maximum strength – Maximum speed – Basic coordination abilities – Basic tactical skills – Basic flexibility	– Specific physical abilities – Phase 2 and 3 of endurance training – Endurance strength – Explosive strength – Specific flexibility – Speed endurance – Technique under physiological and psychological fatigue – Specific coordination abilities	– Comprehensive physical and coordination abilities – Strength, speed, coordination, flexibility, mobility, and specific technique according to the set objectives
Volume/intensity	High volume/low intensity	Reduce volume/increased intensity	Low to medium volume/high intensity
Density	Sufficient recovery to enable morphological modification	– Incomplete recovery – Accumulated fatigue	Total recovery
Control of training	Control of foundational skills and capacities	Control of specialized skills and capacities	Control of specific goals and accomplishments
Residual effects	30 days	Between 15 and 20 days	Unspecific, but <15 days

- *Consecutive development*: When the number of specific motor skills, coordination, techniques, or therapeutic goals exceeds the capacity to be developed simultaneously during a planned period, it is necessary to focus on the consecutive development of each of them.
- *Specialization of mesocycle blocks*: Mesocycle blocks, typically lasting 1 month, should be specialized, and organized to produce one of these three different effects: accumulation, transformation, and realization.

Directions of Training

Directions of training are fundamental aspects that help determine a patient's preparation for rehabilitation or recovery. These directions not only indicate the CONTENT of the training the patient should receive, but also relate to two basic categories of training: LOAD and METHOD.

- CONTENT, also known as the preparation component, refers to the specific exercises or activities included in a training session or rehabilitation program. The content may vary depending on the patient's goals and needs, as well as their current physical condition. As a guide, the preparation component or content includes all the exercises suggested in this book (cueing, qigong, tai chi, occupational therapy, etc.).
- LOAD refers to the amount and type of exercise the patient will perform. It is important to determine the appropriate load for the patient based on their current physical condition to prevent injury or complications. For example, a patient who has suffered a leg injury may initially require a lighter exercise load to allow the injury to heal properly. The intensity perception table (see Table 8.2) is used as a guide for load dosing in the proposed ATR planning model. This table establishes the units (ranging from 1 to 4) of intensity perception for the microcycle (usually 1 week) being worked on. Note that the unit set for each microcycle, or week should not exceed 4 or be <1.
- The METHOD/TECHNIQUE refers to how the training is performed. It is important to choose a method that is appropriate for the patient, based on their current needs and abilities. For example, a patient with balance problems may require a specific training method that focuses on improving balance and coordination, such as one-leg balance training with eyes closed. As a guide, the method and/or technique includes all subcategories of the content or preparation components.

Table 8.2 Intensity perception table for training planning according to the ATR model

Intensity perception chart		
Qualitative value of work	Unit	% of intensity
Rest	1	25
Low	2	50
Medium	3	75
High	4	100

Directions of training are a fundamental part of determining the content, load, and method of training a patient should receive based on the TRAINING EFFECTS (discussed later), the pathological stage, and the motor and non-motor signs and symptoms of the condition. The goal is to achieve successful rehabilitation, recovery, or readaptation.

Training Effects

These are the changes in a person's biological state that occur as a result of training. For example, a swimmer who trains consistently may improve cardiovascular endurance, swimming technique, and back and shoulder strength. These training effects are critical in determining the direction of training based on established therapeutic goals. They are used to plan and analyze training goals and the potential outcomes that can be achieved once they are met. These training effects are divided into several categories based on morphological and physiological changes:

- *Funnel effect*: This refers to the reduction of areas accessible to training stimuli as the patient improves and develops their skills. In other words, as a person improves in a particular skill, it becomes increasingly difficult to improve in that skill, and it becomes necessary to focus on other areas in order to continue to improve overall. For example, a novice runner can greatly improve their race time by simply running more miles, but as they improve, they need to focus on other aspects such as running technique or speed endurance to continue to make progress.
- *Acute effect*: This refers to the immediate changes that occur in the body during exercise. For example, during exercise, our heart rate and breathing rate increase, and we sweat to regulate our body temperature.
- *Immediate effect*: These are the changes that occur after a single exercise session. For example, after a weightlifting session, our muscles may feel tired and sore from the physical exertion.
- *Cumulative effect*: This refers to the changes that occur because of multiple training sessions. For example, after several weeks of consistent training, a runner may notice a significant improvement in race time and overall endurance.
- *Delayed effect*: These are the changes that occur after a specific training program. For example, a 6-week training program may produce significant improvements in athletic performance during and after the program.
- *Residual effect*: This refers to the body's ability to maintain the changes produced by training after a period of time without training. For example, an athlete who stops training for several weeks may retain certain training benefits, such as muscle strength, although he or she may lose some cardiovascular endurance. There are certain types of residual training effects, as outlined by Vladimir Issurin [2], which are categorized based on their effects over time (Fig. 8.1):

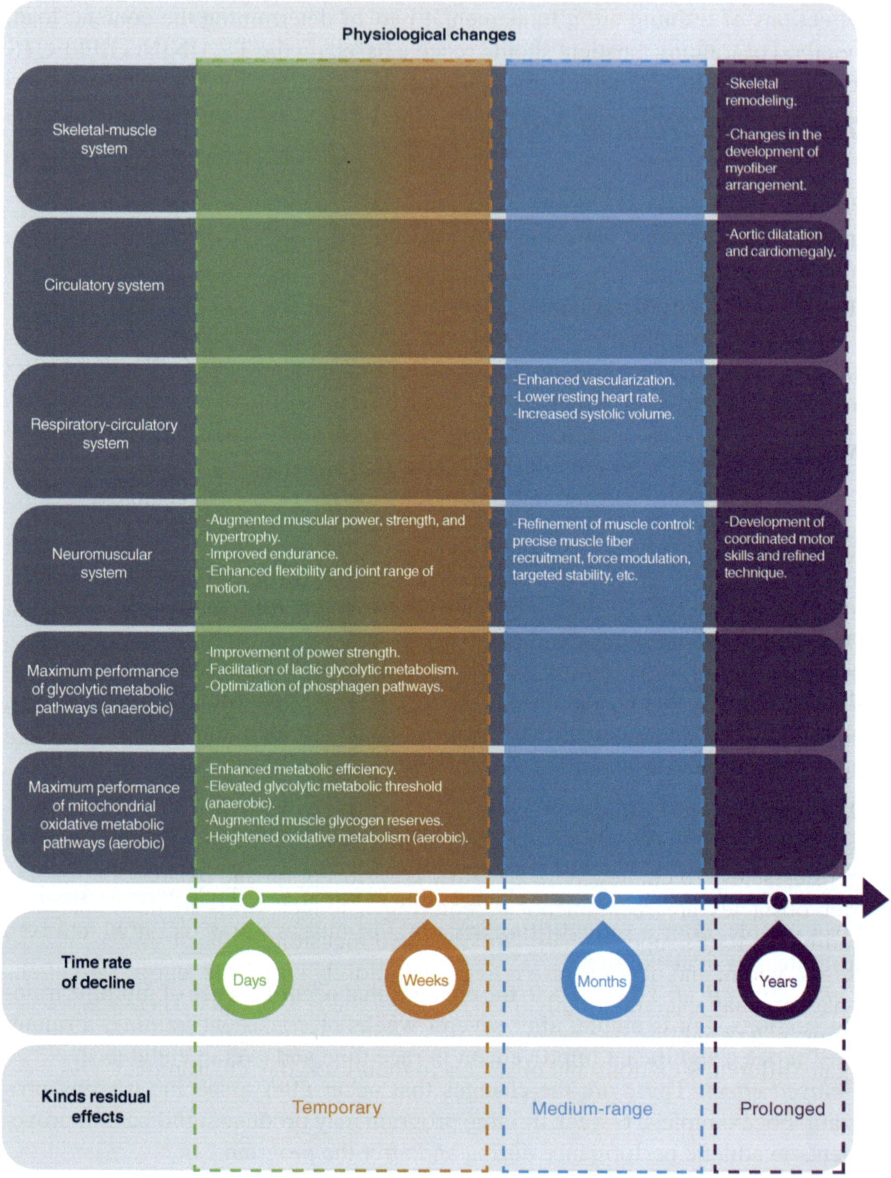

Fig. 8.1 Types of residual training effects categorized by time or rate of decay, modified from Vladimir Issurin [2]

Training Levels for Each ATR Cycle

Therapeutic training levels are useful in planning ATR block cycles to achieve specific goals based on the patient's pathological stage, coordination and physical abilities, cognitive abilities, and other biopsychosocial aspects. In this way, the prescription of therapeutic training can be tailored to the individual needs and goals of each patient in order to maximize the effectiveness of treatment and achieve optimal recovery. The following are the levels of therapeutic exercise:

1. *Basic or initial rehabilitation level*: This level is designed for patients who are beginning a rehabilitation, recovery, and/or readjustment program and do not have the experience or physical condition to perform therapeutic exercises. Exercises are simple, low-intensity, high-volume, designed to prevent injury and adapt to the patient's specific needs.
2. *Intermediate or advanced level of rehabilitation*: At this level, the patient has a solid foundation in the rehabilitation, recovery, and/or readjustment program and is ready to begin improving performance. Exercises are more intense, specific, and moderate in volume, and advanced rehabilitation, recovery, and/or readaptation tools may be used to help the patient achieve their goals.
3. *Advanced or maintenance level*: At this level, the patient has regained much of their functionality and is looking to maintain therapeutic gains. Exercises are more complex and specific, and goal tracking is added to keep the patient motivated and engaged.
4. *Follow-up level*: This level is reserved for patients who have completed their rehabilitation, recovery, and/or readjustment program and require regular follow-up to maintain their health status.

Levels of Temporal Organization in Training Planning

- *Macrocycle*: This is the highest level of temporal organization in training planning and typically ranges from several months to a year or more. The macrocycle is subdivided into several mesocycles.
- *Mesocycle*: This is the intermediate level of temporal organization in training planning and typically lasts from several weeks to several months. The mesocycle is divided into multiple microcycles.
- *Microcycle*: This is the lowest level of temporal organization in training planning and typically lasts from a few days to a week. The microcycle is the basic unit of training planning and is used to design daily or weekly training programs. Microcycles differ in their purpose, load level, design specifics, and duration. Therefore, there are different types of microcycles (see Fig. 8.2) [2].

Planning Structure

The planning structure is a visual representation of the relationship between all the above concepts to properly prescribe exercise for Parkinson's patients:

Figure 8.3 illustrates the structure of training planning hierarchically, starting from the smallest unit called a microcycle, which is associated with a specific goal or type of microcycle (adaptation, load, impact, activation, control of objectives,

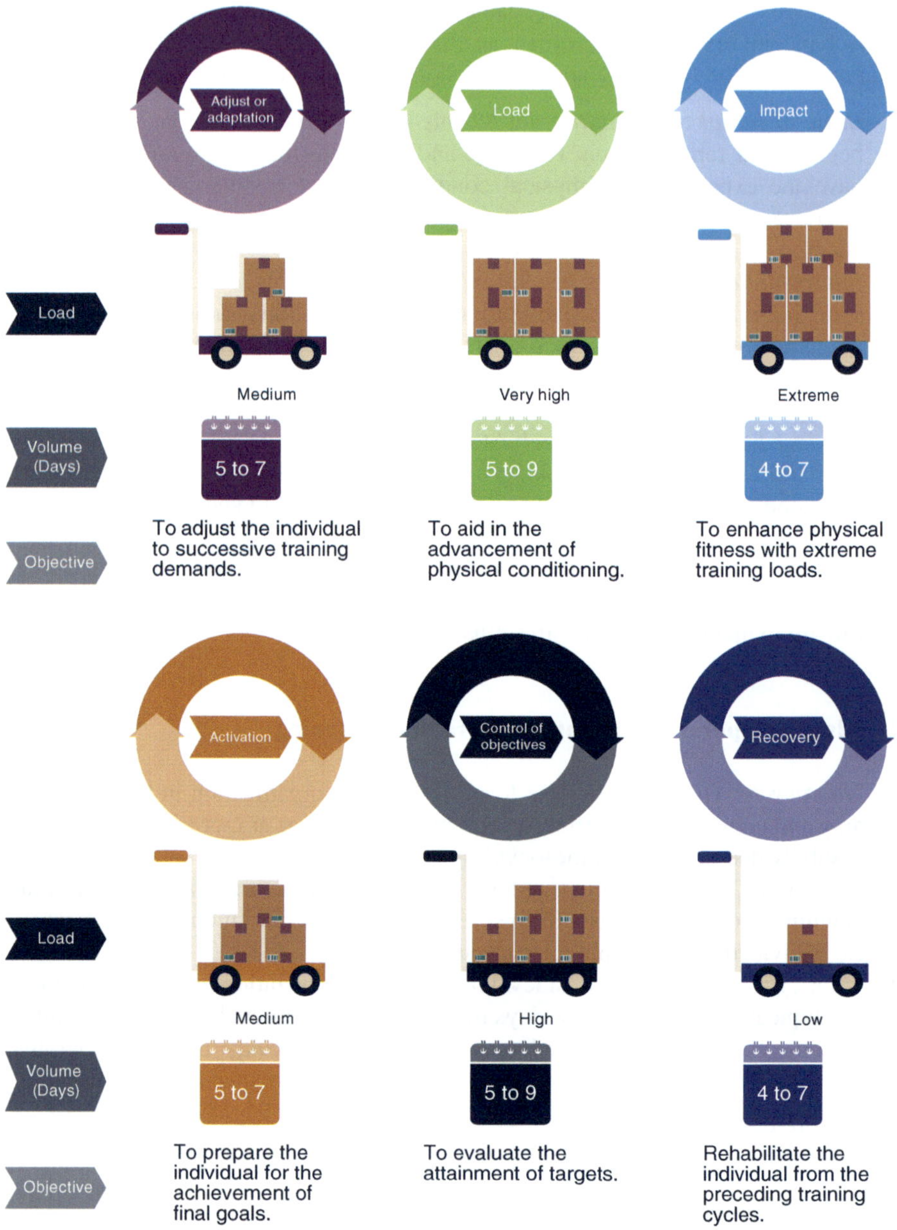

Fig. 8.2 Types of microcycles, modified by Vladimir Issurin [2]

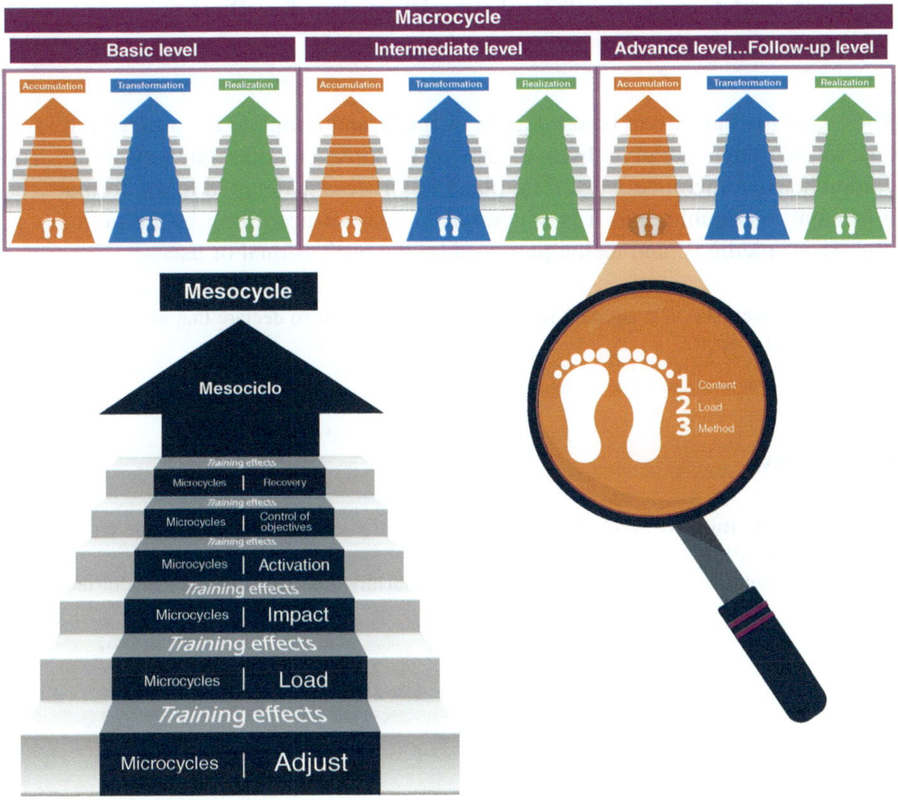

Fig. 8.3 Graphic representation of the planning structure

and recovery). During and after each microcycle, training effects (such as residual effects, acute effects, immediate effects, funneling effects, and cumulative effects) are obtained in order to evaluate the training process. Upon completion of each microcycle, the purpose of a larger unit, the mesocycle, is achieved, which may be an accumulation, transformation, or realization cycle. Then, a set of mesocycles (which varies depending on the patient's biopsychosocial factors and treatment goals) forms a level of training, which may be basic, intermediate, advanced, or follow-up. Finally, the macrocycle is the largest unit that encompasses all levels of training and achieves the proposed goals. It is important to clarify that each training unit (microcycle, mesocycle and macrocycle) requires basic planning, including the determination of training content, method, and load (hence the footprint symbol).

Format and Example of Training Planning for Parkinson's Patients

The Excel file below can be used as an example and template for prescribing exercise for neurodegenerative diseases such as Parkinson's and related disorders. The comprehensive therapeutic exercise planning process is detailed in the format. The document is editable, and it is suggested to adapt it according to the population, objectives, methods, and techniques used by the professional or user.

Competing Interests The author have no conflicts of interest to declare that are relevant to the content of this chapter.

References

1. Bompa TO, Buzzichelli C. Periodización del entrenamiento deportivo. 4th ed. España: Paidotribo; 2015.
2. Issurin V. Entrenamiento deportivo: Periodización en bloques. 5th ed. España: Paidotribo; 2020.

Glossary

Apathy Lack of interest or enthusiasm for daily activities and lack of motivation and excitement.

Articulatory Ability Refers to the ability of the muscles in the mouth and tongue to produce clear and precise sounds when speaking.

Chronic Fatigue Persistent and debilitating fatigue that is not relieved by rest, which can affect a person's ability to perform daily activities. It can have multiple causes, such as sleep disorders, infections, or autoimmune diseases.

Cognitive Executive Functions Refers to a set of mental skills that enable an individual to plan, organize, prioritize, initiate, sustain, monitor, and adjust behavior in line with established goals. These mental skills are important for learning, problem-solving, decision-making, and socially appropriate behavior.

Conditional Physical Abilities Physical skills that can be improved through practice and training. These abilities are directly related to the work and movement of the body (strength, speed, endurance, flexibility, etc.).

Coordination Physical Abilities Coordination abilities refer to an individual's ability to perform precise and efficient movements. In general terms, these abilities involve coordinating a set of movements to carry out a motor task properly. These abilities focus on the orderly practice of movements to achieve a specific goal and are based on perceptions and actions that help regulate and direct movement. The physical coordination skills are generally classified into orientation, adaptation, differentiation, reaction, coupling, balance, and rhythm.

Dementia A syndrome characterized by a progressive loss of cognitive function, including memory, reasoning, problem-solving, and the ability to perform daily activities.

Density Density in the context of training can be defined as the frequency with which stimuli are delivered to the individual in a given unit of time. It is expressed by numbers that indicate the ratio of exercise duration to recovery, such as 1:2. When exercise duration is greater, as in a 5:2 ratio, volume is prioritized, and the

C. A. A. Mejía, *Therapeutic Exercise for Parkinson's Disease and Related Disorders*, https://doi.org/10.1007/978-3-031-62119-2

work performed focuses generally on endurance. On the other hand, if recovery is greater, as in a 1:4 ratio, intensity is prioritized, and the focus generally is on speed, power, etc. Density is crucial in training planning because it affects the effectiveness of the load and prevents chronic fatigue. The appropriate density depends on factors such as the duration and intensity of the exercise, the level of fitness, the goal to be achieved, and the stage of training.

Diaphragmatic Breathing A type of breathing in which the diaphragm, a muscle located beneath the lungs, is used to inhale and exhale air more effectively.

Exercise Prescription The process of designing and planning a specific training program for an individual or group of individuals, considering their goals, current physical condition, physical limitations, and personal preferences. This process includes selecting appropriate exercises, designing a progression plan, and monitoring progress.

Exercise Planned and structured physical activity with the goal of improving health, physical fitness, or sports performance.

Frequency Frequency refers to how often a training session is performed in a given period of time, typically a week.

Glycolytic Metabolic Pathways These are the metabolic pathways used by the human body to produce energy through glycolysis, a process in which glucose is broken down to produce ATP, the primary source of cellular energy. These pathways are predominant during high-intensity and short-duration physical efforts (physical efforts lasting more than 6 s and up to a minute, in which the glycolytic metabolic pathway predominates in energy production), and do not necessarily involve the absence of oxygen. It is important to note that the term "anaerobic" is suggested to be avoided when referring to these pathways, as cellular oxygen presence is constant (Chamari and Padulo 2015).

Heart Rate (HR) Refers to the number of times the heart beats per minute. It is measured in beats per minute (bpm) and is a key indicator of cardiovascular system activity. Heart rate can vary depending on age, level of physical activity, health status, and other factors.

Hyposmia Partial loss of the sense of smell, which can occur for various reasons, such as illnesses, injuries, or exposure to toxic chemicals.

Intensity Intensity is defined as the level of stimulus an individual receives during exertion. In terms of physical training, intensity refers to the quality of the load (qualitative aspect) and is determined by various factors, including the execution speed, exercise complexity, and the duration of rests between sets and repetitions.

Intestinal Constipation Difficulty in evacuating the bowels, caused by hard or infrequent stools, which can lead to abdominal discomfort, pain, and other symptoms.

Kinesthetic Refers to the conscious perception of the position and movement of various parts of the body.

Lactate concentration in millimoles per liter ([Lact-] mmol L^{-1}) This measurement is used to quantify the amount of lactate present in a blood sample or other biological fluid. Lactate is a by-product of glycolytic metabolism, and its concentration in the blood may increase during intense exercise or in situations where oxygen delivery to tissues is lower than normal. Measurement of lactate concentration is important in evaluating exercise performance and monitoring the metabolic status of patients, as elevated levels may indicate muscle fatigue, lactic acidosis, or metabolic problems.

Load Control Refers to the proper management of the quantity, intensity, density, duration, and frequency of training to prevent overtraining and injuries.

Load Duration The period during which the training stimulus influences the body. It is closely related to the volume of the load.

Load When we talk about training load, we are referring to the amount of work or physical stimulus applied during a training session with the goal of producing a training effect that leads to adaptation in the body. This adaptation process can manifest itself as improved physical performance, increased strength, endurance, or cardiovascular capacity, among other things. It is important to note that training load should be adjusted on an individual basis as it depends on factors such as age, health status, previous training experience, and personal goals. In addition, exercise load should be progressive and increased gradually to avoid overtraining and injury. In summary, training load is a critical factor in designing an effective and safe exercise program.

Macropauses Longer breaks between exercise sets. These breaks are used to allow complete recovery between intense efforts and reduce the risk of injuries.

Maximum Heart Rate (MHR) Refers to the maximum number of ventricular contractions performed by the heart, reached in a maximal intensity effort with high muscular involvement until exhaustion. Maximum heart rate is the highest that a person can reach during intense exercise and depends on factors such as age, gender, ethnic origin, level of physical activity, and other biopsychosocial factors.

Means Refers to the resources and tools that can be used to conduct physical training through a method. These can include training equipment, sports facilities, mobile applications, etc.

Methods Refers to different approaches and strategies that can be used to plan training, types of active and passive therapy, among others.

Micropauses Short breaks taken during training to allow partial recovery and reduce fatigue between exercises or repetitions.

Multisystem Atrophies Refers to a group of neurodegenerative disorders that affect multiple systems of the body, including the brain, peripheral nervous system, autonomic system, and sensory and motor systems. These diseases are rare and typically progressive, meaning that symptoms worsen over time.

Muscle Electrostimulation The application of electrical currents through electrodes placed on the skin with the aim of inducing muscle contraction in a specific area of the body.

Muscle Hypotonia Refers to a decrease in muscle tone and may be related to various medical conditions, including neurological disorders, muscular diseases, and spinal cord injuries.

Neurodegenerative Refers to diseases that affect the nervous system and result in the progressive degeneration of nerve cells. These diseases can be inherited or acquired and can affect different areas of the brain and spinal cord, leading to a variety of neurological symptoms and disabilities.

Occupational Therapy Focuses on helping individuals perform activities of daily living (ADLs) more effectively, either after an injury, illness, or disability, or to improve emotional well-being and quality of life.

Orthostatic Hypotension A sudden drop in blood pressure that occurs when a person transitions from a seated or lying position to a standing position, which can lead to dizziness, weakness, fainting, and other symptoms.

Oxidative Mitochondrial Metabolic Pathways These are the metabolic pathways used by the human body to produce energy through the oxidation of nutrients in the presence of a higher amount of oxygen. These pathways are predominant during low to moderate intensity and long-duration physical efforts, allowing for sustained ATP production. It is important to note that the term "aerobic" is suggested to be avoided when referring to these pathways, as it can be confusing and does not necessarily imply low intensity. Efforts can be of high and low intensity sustained for a prolonged time, typically in exercises lasting longer than 1 min, with a predominance of the "oxidative mitochondrial phosphorylation" pathway (Chamari and Padulo 2015).

Pathological Stages The stages and/or level of progression of a disease or condition, which may vary depending on the type of disease and the individual.

Pathophysiology Refers to the study of abnormal physiological processes that occur in an organism because of a disease or injury. In the medical context, this term is used to describe how a disease affects the normal function of the body and how it develops.

Percentage of Anaerobic Threshold (%AT) The % AT or the activation threshold of glycolytic metabolic pathways is the exercise intensity point at which lactic acid production surpasses its elimination, resulting in a significant increase in blood lactate concentration. This change describes a shift from primarily utilizing the mitochondrial oxidative metabolic system (commonly referred to as aerobic) to the glycolytic system (known as anaerobic) for energy production. Various terms, such as maximum lactate steady state, Mader's aerobic-anaerobic threshold, Kindermann's anaerobic threshold, Keul and Stegmann's individual anaerobic threshold, Sjödin and Jacobs' blood lactate accumulation onset, and Orr's ventilatory threshold 2, are used to describe this phenomenon. The activation threshold of glycolytic metabolic pathways is typically reached at 80–95% of VO_2 max, which is theoretically equivalent to a blood lactate concentration of 4 mmol L^{-1} (lactate concentration in millimoles per liter), indicating high-intensity effort.

Percentage of Heart Rate Reserve (%HRR) Heart rate reserve is calculated by subtracting resting heart rate from maximum heart rate. This measure is used to adjust heart rate during physical exercise to maintain adequate and sustained effort, and to program training intensity. The term "heart rate reserve" is commonly used instead of "reserve beats" to avoid misunderstandings and standardize its use.

Percentage of Maximum Aerobic Velocity (% MAV) It is a term used in the field of sports performance, especially in endurance sports such as running, cycling, or skiing. MAV is the theoretical minimum speed required to achieve maximum oxygen consumption (VO_2 max). In other words, it is the speed at which the body operates at the maximum of its mitochondrial oxidative metabolic capacity (aerobic). MAV is like the starting point at which your body reaches its maximum capacity to absorb and efficiently use oxygen during exercise. When you reach MAV, you are in what is called the "beginning of the plateau" of VO_2 max. VO_2 max is the maximum amount of oxygen your body can use during intense exercise. The "plateau" is a part of the performance curve where VO_2 max peaks and remains stable for a while before declining. MAV marks the beginning of this plateau on the performance curve, which means that you are exercising at a high enough intensity to reach your maximum oxygen consumption, but you are not yet at the peak of that capacity. The typical unit of measurement for MAV is kilometers per hour (km/h) or meters per second (m/s), depending on user preference or the specific context of the exercise or activity.

Percentage of Maximum Heart Rate (%MHR) %MHR is the highest number of ventricular contractions that the heart can achieve during intense exercise until exhaustion, expressed as a percentage. This value depends on various factors, including age, gender, ethnic origin, level of physical activity, and other biopsychosocial factors. This indicator is crucial in training programs and exercise monitoring as it allows for personalized adaptation of training intensity. It determines exercise intensity in beats per minute (bpm), enabling assessment of a person's level within a specific intensity zone.

Percentage of Maximum Oxygen Consumption (% VO_2 max) Percentage of maximum oxygen consumption, or VO_2 max, is the maximum amount of oxygen a person can use during intense physical exercise. It is expressed in milliliters of oxygen per kilogram of body weight per minute (ml kg^{-1} min^{-1}) and is considered a crucial indicator for evaluating an individual's physiological status. VO_2 max is related to various central and peripheral aspects of the body, like lung function, cardiac output, blood volume, muscular capillarity, diffusion capacity, and mitochondrial activity. VO_2 max is heavily influenced by genetic factors and can be measured through several methods, including maximal and submaximal tests performed commonly on a treadmill or stationary bike. While maximal tests are accurate, they can be costly and pose health risks, especially in people with heart problems. Submaximal approaches and those unrelated to exercise are less accurate but more economical and less risky. Therefore, the use of submaximal tests in the clinical setting is suggested as a method for estimating VO_2 max. It is important to note that these tests may not provide the same level of accuracy as maximal tests, but they are a viable alternative in certain situations.

Phosphagen Metabolic Pathways A system of energy production that activates glycolytic metabolic pathways used by the human body for high-intensity and short-duration physical activities, i.e., explosive efforts lasting up to a maximum of 6 s. This system relies on the breakdown of creatine phosphate, a molecule stored in muscle cells, to produce ATP, the primary source of cellular energy.

Physical Activity Includes any type of movement generated by skeletal muscles that requires energy expenditure, such as walking, running, cycling, doing yoga, among other activities.

Physical Therapy A type of treatment that focuses on the movement and physical function of the body, using exercises and manual techniques to improve mobility, strength, and flexibility.

Psychosis A severe mental disorder characterized by a loss of contact with reality, hallucinations, delusions, and changes in personality.

REM Sleep Stages The phase of sleep in which vivid dreams occur, the brain is highly active, and muscles are relaxed. It is also known as paradoxical sleep.

Repetitions The action of performing a complete movement, exercise, or task.

Rowing Exercise An exercise that simulates the motion of rowing and can involve different muscle groups, including arms, shoulders, back, abdomen, and legs.

Sets A group of consecutive repetitions of an exercise.

Signs Objective findings observed by an outside person during a physical examination of a patient. These findings may include changes in vital signs, such as temperature, blood pressure, and heart rate, as well as changes in the patient's physical appearance, such as skin coloration or the presence of edema.

Sport Structured and competitive exercise in which rules are applied, and an organized framework is followed.

Swallowing Refers to the process of consuming food and liquids, which involves complex coordination of the muscles in the mouth, throat, and esophagus.

Symptoms Subjective manifestations experienced by a patient because of a medical condition or disease. Symptoms are an expression of what the patient feels and can vary depending on the underlying medical condition that causes them.

Treadmill A machine for running or walking in a fixed place, with a surface that simulates outdoor running.

Urinary Dysfunction Difficulties or problems with urination, such as urinary incontinence, urinary retention, or frequent and painful urination.

Virtual Reality Refers to the use of technology that allows the user to have an immersive and simulated experience in a virtual environment that can mimic or replicate real-life situations.

Volume The volume of training load refers to the total amount of work performed (quantitative aspect) during a training session and can be measured in various ways, such as the number of repetitions and sets completed, the weight lifted, or the distance covered.

Bibliography

1. Postuma RB, Berg D, Stern M, Poewe W, Olanow CW, Oertel W, et al. MDS clinical diagnostic criteria for Parkinson's disease. Mov Disord. 2015;30(12):1591–601.
2. Konczak J, Krawczewski K, Tuite P, Maschke M. The perception of passive motion in Parkinson's disease. J Neurol. 2007;254(5):655.
3. Maschke M, Gomez CM, Tuite PJ, Konczak J. Dysfunction of the basal ganglia, but not the cerebellum, impairs kinaesthesia. Brain. 2003;126(Pt 10):2312–22.
4. Putzki N, Stude P, Konczak J, Graf K, Diener H-C, Maschke M. Kinesthesia is impaired in focal dystonia. Mov Disord. 2006;21(6):754–60.
5. Mathiowetz V, Weber K, Kashman N, Volland G. Adult norms for the nine-hole peg test of finger dexterity. Occup Ther J Res. 1985;5(1):24–38.
6. Desmurget M, Grafton ST, Vindras P, Grea H, Turner RS. The basal ganglia network mediates the planning of movement amplitude. Eur J Neurosci. 2004;19(10):2871–80.
7. Kaji R, Urushihara R, Murase N, Shimazu H, Goto S. Abnormal sensory gating in basal ganglia disorders. J Neurol. 2005;252(Suppl. 4):IV13–IV6.
8. Wiener M, Turkeltaub P, Coslett HB. The image of time: a voxel-wise meta-analysis. NeuroImage. 2010;49(2):1728–40.
9. Grahn JA, Brett M. Rhythm perception in motor areas of the brain. J Cogn Neurosci. 2007;19(5):893–906.
10. Grahn JA, Rowe JB. Feeling the beat: premotor and striatal interactions in musicians and nonmusicians during beat perception. J Neurosci. 2009;29(23):7540–8.
11. Bienkiewicz MMN, Craig CM. Parkinson's is time on your side? Evidence for difficulties with sensorimotor synchronization. Front Neurol. 2015;6:249.
12. Nombela C, Hughes LE, Owen AM, Grahn JA. Into the groove: can rhythm influence Parkinson's disease? Neurosci Biobehav Rev. 2013;37(10):2564–70.
13. Thaut MH, et al. Rhythmic auditory stimulation in gait training for Parkinson's disease patients. Mov Disord. 1996;11:193–200. https://doi.org/10.1002/mds.870110213.
14. Thaut MH, McIntosh KW, McIntosh GC, Hoemberg V. Auditory rhythmicity enhances movement and speech motor control in patients with Parkinson's disease. Funct Neurol. 2001;16:163–72.
15. Jones D, et al. Everyday walking with Parkinson's disease: understanding personal challenges and strategies. Disabil Rehabil. 2008;30:1213–21. https://doi.org/10.1080/09638280701828955.
16. Selleck MA, Sataloff RT. The impact of the auditory system on phonation: a review. J Voice. 2014;28:688–93. https://doi.org/10.1016/j.jvoice.2014.03.018.

C. A. A. Mejía, *Therapeutic Exercise for Parkinson's Disease and Related Disorders*, https://doi.org/10.1007/978-3-031-62119-2

17. Rocha PA, Slade SC, Mcclelland J, Morris ME. Dance is more than therapy: qualitative analysis on therapeutic dancing classes for Parkinson's. Complement Ther Med. 2017;34:1–9.
18. Studer V, et al. Treadmill training with cues and feedback improves gait in people with more advanced Parkinson's disease. J Parkinsons Dis. 2017;7:729–39.
19. Amara AW, Memon AA. Effects of exercise on non-motor symptoms in Parkinson's disease. Clin Ther. 2018;40:8–15.
20. Uygur M, Bellumori M, Knight CA. Effects of a low-resistance, interval bicycling intervention in Parkinson's disease. Physiother Theory Pract. 2017;33:897–904.
21. Mak MK, Wong-Yu IS, Shen X, Chung CL. Long-term effects of exercise and physical therapy in people with Parkinson disease. Nat Rev Neurol. 2017;13:689–703.
22. Schootemeijer S, van der Kolk NM, Bloem BR, de Vries NM. Current perspectives on aerobic exercise in people with Parkinson's disease. Neurotherapeutics. 2020;17:1418–33.
23. Hackney M, Earhart GM. Effects of dance on movement control in Parkinson's disease: a comparison of Argentine tango and American ballroom. J Rehabil Med. 2009;41:475–81.
24. Ganesan M, Sathyaprabha TN, Gupta A, Pal PK. Effect of partial weight-supported treadmill gait training on balance in patients with Parkinson disease. PM R. 2014;6:22–33.
25. Cugusi L, et al. Effects of a Nordic Walking program on motor and non-motor symptoms, functional performance and body composition in patients with Parkinson's disease. NeuroRehabilitation. 2015;37:245–54.
26. Lee HJ, et al. Turo (QI Dance) program for Parkinson's disease patients: randomized, assessor blind, waiting-list control, partial crossover study. Explore. 2018;14:216–23.
27. Solla P, et al. Sardinian folk dance for individuals with Parkinson's disease: a randomized controlled pilot trial. J Alter Complement Med. 2019;25:305–16.
28. van der Kolk NM. Effectiveness of home-based and remotely supervised aerobic exercise in Parkinson's disease: a double-blind, randomised controlled trial. Lancet Neurol. 2019;18:998–1008.
29. Sage MD, Almeida QJ. Symptom and gait changes after sensory attention focused exercise vs aerobic training in Parkinson's disease. Mov Disord. 2009;24:1132–8.
30. Li ZL, et al. Comparison of Wuqinxi Qigong with stretching on single- and dual-task gait, motor symptoms and quality of life in Parkinson's disease: a preliminary randomized control study. Int J Environ Res Public Health. 2022;19:8042.
31. Sacheli MA, et al. Exercise increases caudate dopamine release and ventral striatal activation in Parkinson's disease. Mov Disord. 2019;34:1891–900.
32. Nadeau A, Pourcher E, Corbeil P. Effects of 24 wk of treadmill training on gait performance in Parkinson's disease. Med Sci Sports Exerc. 2014;46:645–55.
33. Schenkman M, et al. Effect of high-intensity treadmill exercise on motor symptoms in patients with de novo Parkinson disease: a phase 2 randomized clinical trial. JAMA Neurol. 2017;75:219–26.
34. Altmann LJ, et al. Aerobic exercise improves mood, cognition, and language function in Parkinson's disease: results of a controlled study. J Int Neuropsychol Soc. 2016;22:878–89.
35. Canning CG, Allen NE, Dean CM, Goh L, Fung VS. Home-based treadmill training for individuals with Parkinson's disease: a randomized controlled pilot trial. Clin Rehabil. 2012;26:817–26.
36. Hashimoto H, Takabatake S, Miyaguchi H, Nakanishi H, Naitou Y. Effects of dance on motor functions, cognitive functions, and mental symptoms of Parkinson's disease: a quasi-randomized pilot trial. Complement Ther Med. 2015;23:210–9.
37. Wan ZR, et al. Effects of health qigong exercises on physical function on patients with Parkinson's disease. J Multidiscip Health. 2021;14:941–50.
38. Arfa-Fatollahkhani P, et al. Effects of treadmill training on the balance, functional capacity and quality of life in Parkinson's disease: a randomized clinical trial. J Complement Integr Med. 2019;17:1154–8.

39. Cakit BD, Saracoglu M, Genc H, Erdem HR, Inan L. The effects of incremental speed-dependent treadmill training on postural instability and fear of falling in Parkinson's disease. Clin Rehabil. 2007;21:698–705.
40. Tollár J, Nagy F, Hortobágyi T. Vastly different exercise programs similarly improve Parkinsonian symptoms: a randomized clinical trial. Gerontology. 2019;65:120–7.
41. Protas EJ, et al. Gait and step training to reduce falls in Parkinson's disease. NeuroRehabilitation. 2005;20:183–90.
42. Zhao JG, Zeng XT, Wang J, Liu L. Association between calcium or vitamin D supplementation and fracture incidence in community-dwelling older adults. JAMA. 2017;318:2466–82.
43. Reuter I, et al. Effects of a flexibility and relaxation programme, walking, and Nordic Walking on Parkinson's disease. J Aging Res. 2011;2011:232473.
44. Karlsen KH, Larsen JP, Tandberg E, Maeland JG. Influence of clinical and demographic variables on quality of life in patients with Parkinson's disease. J Neurol Neurosurg Psychiatr. 1999;66:431–5.
45. Barnish J, Atkinson RA, Barran SM, Barnish MS. Potential benefit of singing for people with Parkinson's disease: a systematic review. J Parkinsons Dis. 2016;6:473–84. https://doi.org/10.3233/JPD-160837.
46. Barnish MS, Horton SMC, Butterfint ZR, Clark AB, Atkinson RA, Deane KHO. Speech and communication in Parkinson's disease: a cross-sectional exploratory study in the UK. BMJ Open. 2017;7:e014642.
47. McAuliffe MJ, Baylor CR, Yorkston KM. Variable associated with communicative participation in Parkinson's disease and its relationship to measures of health-related quality of life. Int J Speech Lang Pathol. 2017;19:407–17.
48. Chaiklin H. Marian Chace: her papers. Columbia, MD: American Dance Therapy Association; 1975.
49. Westbrook BK, McKibben H. Dance/movement therapy with groups of outpatients with Parkinson's disease. Am J Dance Ther. 1989;11(1):27–38.
50. Hackney ME, Earhart GM. Effects of dance on gait and balance in Parkinson's disease: a comparison of partnered and nonpartnered dance movement. Neurorehabil Neural Repair. 2010;24(4):384–92.
51. Hackney ME, Kantorovich S, Levin R, Earhart GM. Effects of tango on functional mobility in Parkinson's disease: a preliminary study. J Neurol Phys Ther. 2007;31:173–9.
52. Marchant D, Sylvester JL, Earhart GM. Effects of a short duration, high dose contact improvisation dance workshop on Parkinson's disease: a pilot study. Complementary Ther Med. 2010;18(5):184–90.
53. Duncan RP, Earhart GM. Randomized controlled trial of community-based dancing to modify disease progression in Parkinson disease. Neurorehabil Neural Repair. 2012;26(2):132–43.
54. Hackney ME, Earhart GM. Short duration, intensive tango dancing for Parkinson disease: an uncontrolled pilot study. Complement Ther Med. 2009;17(4):203–7.
55. Batson G. Feasibility of an intensive trial of modern dance for adults with Parkinson disease. Complementary Health Pract Rev. 2010;15(2):65–83.
56. Hackney ME, Kantorovich S, Earhart GM. A study of the effects of argentine tango as a form of partnered dance for those with Parkinson disease and the healthy elderly. Am J Dance Ther. 2007;29(2):109–27.
57. Heiberger L, Maurer C, Amtage F, Mendez-Balbuena I, Schulte-Mönting J, Hepp-Reymond M-C, et al. Impact of a weekly dance class on the functional mobility and on the quality of life of individuals with Parkinson's disease. Front Aging Neurosci. 2011;3(14):1–15.
58. Volpe D, Signorini M, Marchetto A, Lynch T, Morris ME. A comparison of Irish set dancing and exercises for people with Parkinson's disease: a phase II feasibility study. BMC Geriatr. 2013;13:54.

59. Jankovic J. Gait disorders. Neurol Clin. 2015;33(1):249–68.
60. de Dreu MJ, van der Wilk AS, Poppe E, Kwakkel G, Wegen EE. Rehabilitation, exercise therapy and music in patients with Parkinson's disease: a meta-analysis of the effects of music-based movement therapy on walking ability, balance and quality of life. Parkinsonism Relat Disord. 2012;18(Suppl. 1):S114–9.
61. Braunlich K, Seger CA, Jentink KG, Buard I, Kluger BM, Thaut MH. Rhythmic auditory cues shape neural network recruitment in Parkinson's disease during repetitive motor behavior. Eur J Neurosci. 2019;49(6):849–58.
62. Chen JL, Penhune VB, Zatorre RJ. Listening to musical rhythms recruits motor regions of the brain. Cereb Cortex. 2008;18(12):2844–54.
63. Koshimori Y, Thaut MH. Future perspectives on neural mechanisms underlying rhythm and music-based neurorehabilitation in Parkinson's disease. Ageing Res Rev. 2018 Nov;47:133–9.
64. Handojoseno AA, Gilat M, Ly QT, Chamtie H, Shine JM, Nguyen TN, et al. An EEG study of turning freeze in Parkinson's disease patients: the alteration of brain dynamic on the motor and visual cortex. In: Engineering in medicine and biology society (EMBC) 37th annual international conference of the IEEE. IEEE; 2015. p. 6618–21.
65. Ly QT, Handojoseno AA, Gilat M, Nguyen N, Chai R, Tran Y, et al. Detection of gait initiation failure in Parkinson's disease patients using EEG signals. In: Engineering in medicine and biology society (EMBC), 2016 IEEE 38th annual international conference of the IEEE; 2016. p. 1599–602.
66. Pelzer EA, Hintzen A, Goldau M, von Cramon DY, Timmermann L, Tittgemeyer M. Cerebellar networks with basal ganglia: feasibility for tracking cerebello-pallidal and subthalamo-cerebellar projections in the human brain. Eur J Neurosci. 2013;38:3106–14.
67. Petter EA, Lusk NA, Hesslow G, Meck WH. Interactive roles of the cerebellum and striatum in sub-second and supra-second timing: support for an initiation, continuation, adjustment, and termination (ICAT) model of temporal processing. Neurosci Biobehav Rev. 2016;71:739–55.
68. Shine JM, Matar E, Ward PB, Frank MJ, Moustafa AA, Pearson M, Naismith SL, Lewis SJ. Freezing of gait in Parkinson's disease is associated with functional decoupling between the cognitive control network and the basal ganglia. Brain. 2013;136(Pt 12):3671–81.
69. Szewczyk-Krolikowski K, Menke RA, Rolinski M, Duff E, Salimi-Khorshidi G, Filippini N, Zamboni G, Hu MT, Mackay CE. Functional connectivity in the basal ganglia network differentiates PD patients from controls. Neurology. 2014;83(3):208–14.
70. McIntosh GC, Brown SH, Rice RR, Thaut MH. Rhythmic auditory-motor facilitation of gait patterns in patients with Parkinson's disease. J Neurol Neurosurg Psychiatry. 1997;62:22–6.
71. Miller RA, Thaut MH, McIntosh GC, Rice RR. Components of EMG symmetry and variability in parkinsonian and healthy elderly gait. Electroencephalogr Clin Neurophysiol. 1996a;101(1):1–7.
72. Nieuwboer A, Kwakkel G, Rochester L, Jones D, van Wegen E, Willems AM, Chavret F, Hetherington V, Baker K, Lim I. Cueing training in the home improves gait-related mobility in Parkinson's disease: the RESCUE trial. J Neurol Neurosurg Psychiatry. 2007;78(2):134–40. Erratum in: J Neurol Neurosurg Psychiatry. 2010;81(12):1414. J Neurol Neurosurg Psychiatry. 2010;81(1):126
73. Rocha PA, Porfírio GM, Ferraz HB, Trevisani VF. Effects of external cues on gait parameters of Parkinson's disease patients: a systematic review. Clin Neurol Neurosurg. 2014;124:127–34.
74. Thaut MH, McIntosh GC, Hoemberg V. Neurobiological foundations of neurologic music therapy: rhythmic entrainment and the motor system. Front Psychol. 2014a;5:1185.
75. Thaut MH, Trimarchi PD, Parsons LM. Human brain basis of musical rhythm perception: common and distinct neural substrates for meter, tempo, and pattern. Brain Sci. 2014b;4(2):428–52.
76. Formaggio E, Storti SF, Boscolo Galazzo I, Gandolfi M, Geroin C, Smania N, Spezia L, Waldner A, Fiaschi A, Manganotti P. Modulation of event-related desynchronization in robot-assisted hand performance: brain oscillatory changes in active, passive and imagined movements. J Neuroeng Rehabil. 2013;10:24.

77. Manganotti P, Gerloff C, Toro C, Katsuta H, Sadato N, Zhuang Leocani L, Hallett M. Task-related coherence and task-related spectral power changes during sequential finger movements. Electroencephalogr Clin Neurophysiol. 1998;109(1):50–62.
78. Calabrò RS, Naro A, Russo M, Bramanti P, Carioti L, Balletta T, Buda A, Manuli A, Filoni S, Bramanti A. Shaping neuroplasticity by using powered exoskeletons in patients with stroke: a randomized clinical trial. J Neuroeng Rehabil. 2018;15(1):35.
79. Calabrò RS, Naro A, Russo M, Leo A, De Luca R, Balletta T, Buda A, La Rosa G, Bramanti A, Bramanti P. The role of virtual reality in improving motor performance as revealed by EEG: a randomized clinical trial. J Neuroeng Rehabil. 2017;14(1):53.
80. Jenkinson N, Brown P. New insights into the relationship between dopamine, beta oscillations and motor function. Trends Neurosci. 2011;34:611–8.
81. Koshimori Y, Strafella AP, Valli M, et al. Motor synchronization to rhythmic auditory stimulation (RAS) attenuates dopaminergic responses in ventral striatum in young healthy adults: [11C]-(+)-PHNO PET study. Front Neurosci. 2019;13:106.
82. Little S, Brown P. The functional role of beta oscillations in Parkinson's disease. Parkinsonism Relat Disord. 2014;20(Suppl. 1):S44–8.
83. Zigmond MJ, Cameron JL, Hoffer BJ, et al. Neurorestoration by physical exercise: moving forward. Parkinsonism Relat Disord. 2012;18(S1):S147–50. https://doi.org/10.1016/S1353-8020(11)70046-3.
84. Becker BE. Aquatic therapy: scientific foundations and clinical rehabilitation applications. PM R. 2009;1:859–72. https://doi.org/10.1016/j.pmrj.2009.05.017.
85. Hall J, Swinkels A, Briddon J, et al. Does aquatic exercise relieve pain in adults with neurologic or musculoskeletal disease? A systematic review and meta-analysis of randomized controlled trials. Arch Phys Med Rehabil. 2008;89:873–83. https://doi.org/10.1016/j.apmr.2007.09.054.
86. Kamioka H, Tsutani K, Okuizumi H, et al. Effectiveness of aquatic exercise and balneotherapy: a summary of systematic reviews based on randomized controlled trials of water immersion therapies. J Clin Epidemiol. 2010;20:2–12.
87. Villalta EM, Peiris CL. Early aquatic physical therapy improves function and does not increase risk of wound-related adverse events for adults after orthopedic surgery: a systematic review and meta-analysis. Arch Phys Med Rehabil. 2013;94:138–48. https://doi.org/10.1016/j.apmr.2012.07.020.
88. Jung T, Kawasaki M, Jara M, et al. The effects of aquatic exercise on balance outcomes in individuals with Parkinson's disease. In: International Symposium on Adapted Physical Activity (ISAPA), Paris, 2011; 2011. p. 129.
89. Kawasaki M. The effect of aquatic exercise on balance outcomes in individuals with Parkinson disease. Med Sci Sport Exerc. 2009;41:102.
90. Vivas J, Arias P, Cudeiro J. Aquatic therapy versus conventional land-based therapy for Parkinson's disease: an open-label pilot study. Arch Phys Med Rehabil. 2011;92:1202–10. https://doi.org/10.1016/j.apmr.2011.03.017.
91. Ayán C, Cancela J. Effects of aquatic exercise on persons with Parkinson's disease: a preliminary study. Sci Sport. 2012;27:300–4. https://doi.org/10.1016/j.scispo.2011.12.006.
92. Ayán C, Cancela J. Feasibility of 2 different water-based exercise training programs in patients with Parkinson's disease: a pilot study. Arch Phys Med Rehabil. 2012;93:1709–14. https://doi.org/10.1016/j.apmr.2012.03.029.
93. Crizzle A, Newhouse J. Water exercise for individuals with Parkinson's disease: a pilot study. ATJ. 2007;9:22–5.
94. Kargarfard M, Chitsaz A, Azizi S. Effects of an 8-week aquatic exercise training on balance in patients with Parkinson's disease. J Isfahan Med Sch. 2012;30:1.
95. Sage M, Johnston R, Almeida Q. Comparison of exercise strategies for motor symptom improvement in Parkinson's disease. Neurodegen Dis Manag. 2011;1:387–95. https://doi.org/10.2217/nmt.11.49.

96. Therrien J, Fiegle L, Chong R, et al (2008) Effect of 8-week aquatic exercise training on postural control and quality of life in Parkinson's disease. Student Research Project Georgia Health Science University. http://www.georgiahealth.edu/alliedhealth/pt/research.html. Accessed 20 May 2013.
97. Goodwin VA, Richards SH, Taylor RS, et al. The effectiveness of exercise interventions for people with Parkinson's disease: a systematic review and meta-analysis. Mov Disord. 2008;15:631–40. https://doi.org/10.1002/mds.21922.
98. Tomlinson CL, Patel S, Meek C, Herd CP, Clarke CE, Stowe R, et al. Physiotherapy intervention in Parkinson's disease: systematic review and meta-analysis. BMJ. 2012;345:e5004.
99. Wróblewska A, Gajos A, Smyczyńska U, Bogucki A. The therapeutic effect of nordic walking on freezing of gait in Parkinson's disease: a pilot study. Parkinsons Dis. 2019:3846279.
100. Public Health Agency of Canada, Mapping connections: an understanding of neurological conditions in Canada. 2014:1–98. http://www.phac-aspc.gc.ca/publicat/cd-mc/mc-ec/index-eng.php. Accessed 26 Aug 2016.
101. Parkinson Canada, Exercises by Parkinson Society of Canada. 2012:1–12. https://www.parkinsons.va.gov/NorthWest/Documents/Pt_ed_handouts/Exercise_for_PD_1-20-12.pdf. Accessed 24 June 2019.
102. Li JX, Xu DQ, Hong Y. Changes in muscle strength, endurance, and reaction of the lower extremities with Tai Chi intervention. J Biomech. 2009;42:967–71. https://doi.org/10.1016/j.jbiomech.2009.03.001.
103. Law N-Y, Li JX. The temporospatial and kinematic characteristics of typical Tai Chi movements: repulse monkey and wave-hand in cloud. Res Sport Med. 2014;22:111–23. https://doi.org/10.1080/15438627.2014.881819.
104. Li JX, Law N-Y. Kinetics of the lower limb during two typical Tai Chi movements in the elderly. Res Sports Med. 2018;26:112–23. https://doi.org/10.1080/15438627.2017.1393753.
105. Law N-Y, Li JX. Biomechanics analysis of seven Tai Chi movements. Sport Med Heal Sci. 2022;20:1–68. https://doi.org/10.1016/j.smhs.2022.06.002.
106. Li F, Harmer P, Fitzgerald K, Eckstrom E, Stock R, Galver J, Maddalozzo G, Batya SS. Tai chi and postural stability in patients with Parkinson's disease. N Engl J Med. 2012;366:511–9. https://doi.org/10.1056/NEJMoa1107911.
107. Jankovic J. Parkinson's disease: clinical features and diagnosis. J Neurol Neurosurg Psychiatry. 2008;79(4):368–76.
108. Sherrington C, Whitney JC, Lord SR, Herbert RD, Cumming RG, Close JC. Effective exercise for the prevention of falls: a systematic review and meta-analysis. J Am Geriatr Soc. 2008;56:2234–43.
109. Gao Q, Leung A, Yang Y, Wei Q, Guan M, Jia C, He C. Effects of Tai Chi on balance and fall prevention in Parkinson's disease: a randomized controlled trial. Clin Rehabil. 2014;28:748–53. https://doi.org/10.1177/0269215514521044.
110. Martin JP. The basal ganglia and posture. Philadelphia: Lippincott; 1967.
111. Mille M-L, Creath RA, Prettyman MG, Hilliard MJ, Martinez KM, MacKinnon CD, Rogers MW. Posture and locomotion coupling: a target for rehabilitation interventions in persons with Parkinson's disease. Parkinson's Dis. 2012;(1):754186.
112. Rogers MW, Hilliard MJ, Martinez KM, Zhang Y, Simuni T, Mille ML. Perturbations of ground support alter posture and locomotion coupling during step initiation in Parkinson's disease. Exp Brain Res. 2011;208(4):557–67. https://doi.org/10.1007/s00221-010-2504-z.
113. Mille ML, Hilliard MJ, Martinez KM, Simuni T, Zhang Y, Rogers MW. Short-term effects of posture-assisted step training on rapid step initiation in Parkinson's disease. J Neurol Phys Ther. 2009;33(2):88–95.
114. Park JH, Stelmach GE. Force development during target-directed isometric force production in Parkinson's disease. Neurosci Lett. 2007;412(2):173–8. https://doi.org/10.1016/j.neulet.2006.11.009.

115. Mille ML, Johnson Hilliard M, Martinez KM, Simuni T, Rogers MW. Acute effects of a lateral postural assist on voluntary step initiation in patients with Parkinson's disease. Mov Disord. 2007;22(1):20–7. https://doi.org/10.1002/mds.21139.
116. Sturkenboom IHWM, Thijssen MCE, Gons-van Elsacker JJ, Maasdam A, Schulten M, Vijver-Visser D, Steultjens EJM, Bloem BR, Munneke M. Ergotherapie bij de ziekte van Parkinson, een richtlijn van Ergotherapie Nederland. Utrecht/Den Haag: Ergotherapie Nederland/Uitgeverij Lemma; 2008.
117. Sturkenboom IHWM, Thijssen MCE, Gons-van Elsacker JJ, Maasdam A, Schulten M, Vijver-Visser D, Steultjens EJM, Bloem BR, Munneke M. Guidelines for occupational therapy in Parkinson's disease rehabilitation. Nijmegen/Miami: ParkinsonNet/NPF; 2012. [online pdf http://www.parkinson.org/Search-Pages/Search.aspx?pKeywords=guidelines]
118. Sangarapillai K, Norman BM, Almeida QJ. Analyzing the effects of PDSAFEx™ on the motor symptoms of Parkinson's disease: a retrospective study. Neuro Rehabil. 2020;46:589–93.
119. Keogh JWL, O'Reilly S, O'Brien E, Morrison S, Kavanagh JJ. Can resistance training improve upper limb postural tremor, force steadiness and dexterity in older adults? A systematic review. Sports Med. 2019;49:1199–216.
120. Kadkhodaie M, et al. Effect of eccentric-based rehabilitation on hand tremor intensity in Parkinson disease. Neurol Sci. 2020;41:637–43.
121. Landers MR, Navalta JW, Murtishaw AS, Kinney JW, Pirio Richardson S. A high-intensity exercise boot camp for persons with Parkinson disease: a phase II, pragmatic, randomized clinical trial of feasibility, safety, signal of efficacy, and disease mechanisms. J Neurol Phys Ther. 2019;43:12–25.
122. Frazzitta G, et al. Intensive rehabilitation treatment in early Parkinson's disease: a randomized pilot study with a 2-year follow-up. Neurorehabil Neural Repair. 2015;29:123–31.
123. Chen K, et al. Effect of exercise on quality of life in Parkinson's disease: a systematic review and meta-analysis. Parkinsons Dis. 2020;2020:3257623.
124. Carapellotti AM, Stevenson R, Doumas M. The efficacy of dance for improving motor impairments, non-motor symptoms, and quality of life in Parkinson's disease: a systematic review and meta-analysis. PLoS One. 2020;15:e0236820.
125. Radder DLM, et al. Physiotherapy in Parkinson's disease: a meta-analysis of present treatment modalities. Neurorehabil Neural Repair. 2020;34:871–80.
126. Song R, et al. The impact of Tai Chi and Qigong mind-body exercises on motor and non-motor function and quality of life in Parkinson's disease: a systematic review and meta-analysis. Parkinsonism Relat Disord. 2017;41:3–13.
127. Deuel LM, Seeberger LC. Complementary therapies in Parkinson disease: a review of acupuncture, Tai Chi, Qi Gong, Yoga, and Cannabis. Neurotherapeutics. 2020;17:1434–55.
128. Ni M, Mooney K, Signorile JF. Controlled pilot study of the effects of power yoga in Parkinson's disease. Complement Ther Med. 2016;25:126–31.
129. Hauser RA, Auinger P. Determination of minimal clinically important change in early and advanced Parkinson's disease. Mov Disord. 2011;26:813–8.
130. Tomlinson CL, et al. Physiotherapy for Parkinson's disease: a comparison of techniques. Cochrane Database Syst Rev. 2014;(6):Cd002815.
131. Ghai S, Ghai I, Effenberg AO. Effect of rhythmic auditory cueing on aging gait: a systematic review and meta-analysis. Aging Dis. 2017:131–200. https://doi.org/10.14336/ad.2017.1031.
132. Spaulding SJ, et al. Cueing and gait improvement among people with Parkinson's disease: a meta-analysis. Arch Phys Med Rehabil. 2013;94:562–70. https://doi.org/10.1016/j.apmr.2012.10.026.
133. Thaut M, McIntosh GC, Hoemberg V. Neurobiological foundations of neurologic music therapy: rhythmic entrainment and the motor system. Front Psychol. 2015;5:1185.
134. Ghai S, Ghai I, Effenberg AO. Effect of rhythmic auditory cueing on gait in Cerebral palsy: a systematic review and metaanalysis. Neuropsychiatr Dis Treat. 2017:1–17. Accepted, In Press

135. Lim I, van Wegen E, de Goede C, Deutekom M, Nieuwboer A, Willems A, Jones D, Rochester L, Kwakkel G. Effects of external rhythmical cueing on gait in patients with Parkinson's disease: a systematic review. Clin Rehabil. 2005;19(7):695–713.
136. Cameron MH, Wagner JM. Gait abnormalities in multiple sclerosis: pathogenesis, evaluation, and advances in treatment. Curr Neurol Neurosci Rep. 2011;11:507–15.
137. Masters RSW, Maxwell J. The theory of reinvestment. Int Rev Sport Exer Psychol. 2008;1:160–83.
138. Ghai S, Driller M, Masters R. The influence of below-knee compression garments on knee-joint proprioception. Gait Posture. 2016. In Press; https://doi.org/10.1016/j.gaitpost.2016.08.008.
139. Masters RSW. Knowledge, knerves and know-how: the role of explicit versus implicit knowledge in the breakdown of a complex motor skill under pressure. Brit J Psychol. 1992;83:343–58.
140. Ghai S. Proprioception and performance: the role of below-knee compression garments and secondary tasks (master's dissertation). University of Waikato; 2016.
141. Kim SJ, et al. Changes in gait patterns with rhythmic auditory stimulation in adults with cerebral palsy. Neuro Rehabil. 2011;29:233–41.
142. Effenberg AO, Fehse U, Schmitz G, Krueger B, Mechling H. Movement sonification: effects on motor learning beyond rhythmic adjustments. Front Neurosci. 2016;10:219.
143. Thaut MH, Miltner R, Lange HW, Hurt CP, Hoemberg V. Velocity modulation and rhythmic synchronization of gait in Huntington's disease. Mov Disord. 1999b;14(5):808–19.
144. Baram Y, Miller A. Auditory feedback control for improvement of gait in patients with multiple sclerosis. J Neurol Sci. 2007;254:90–4.
145. Shannon K. The effect of rhythmic auditory stimulation on the gait parameters of patients with incomplete spinal cord injury: an exploratory pilot study. Int J Rehabil Res. 2008;31:155–7.
146. Liberati, A. et al. The PRISMA statement for reporting systematic reviews and meta-analyses of studies that evaluate health care interventions: explanation and elaboration. Ann Intern Med 2009;151:W-65–W-94.
147. Borenstein M, Hedges LV, Higgins J, Rothstein HR. A basic introduction to fixed-effect and random-effects models for meta-analysis. Res Synthesis Met. 2010;1:97–111.
148. Ito N, Hayshi A, Lin W, Ohkoshi N, Watanabe M, Shoji S. Music therapy in Parkinson's disease: improvement of parkinsonian gait and depression with rhythmic auditory stimulation. In: Nakada T, editor. Integrated human brain science: theory, method application (music). New York: Elsevier Science; 2000. p. 435–43.
149. Willems AM, et al. The use of rhythmic auditory cues to influence gait in patients with Parkinson's disease, the differential effect for freezers and non-freezers, an explorative study. Disabil Rehabil. 2006;28:721–8. https://doi.org/10.1080/09638280500386569.
150. Rochester L, et al. The effect of external rhythmic cues (auditory and visual) on walking during a functional task in homes of people with Parkinson's disease. Arch Phys Med Rehabil. 2005;86:999–1006. https://doi.org/10.1016/j.apmr.2004.10.040.
151. Lazzara G, Lazarus CL, Logemann JA. Impact of thermal stimulation on the triggering of the swallowing reflex. Dysphagia. 1986;1:73–7.
152. Rosenbek JC, Robbins J, Willford WO, Kirk G, Schiltz A, Sowell T, et al. Comparing treatment intensities of tactile-thermal application. Dysphagia. 1998;13:1–9.
153. Hamdy S, Jilani S, Price V, Parker C, Hall N, Power M. Modulation of human swallowing behaviour by thermal and chemical stimulation in health and after brain injury. Neurogastroenterol Motil. 2003;15:69–77.
154. Power M, Fraser C, Hobson A, Rothwell JC, Mistry S, Nicholson DA, et al. Changes in pharyngeal corticobulbar excitability and swallowing behavior after oral stimulation. Am J Physiol Gastrointest Liver Physiol. 2004;286:G45–50.
155. Braak H, Del Tredici K, Rub U, De Vos RA, Cansen Steur EN, Braak E. Staging of brain pathology related to sporadic Parkinson's disease. Neurobiol Aging. 2003;24:197–211.
156. Rosenbek JC, Robbins JA, Roecker EB, Coyle JL. Penetration-aspiration scale. Dysphagia. 1996;11:93–8.

157. Eisenhuber E, Schima W, Schober E, Pokieser P, Stadler A, Scharitzer M, et al. Videofluoroscopic assessment of patients with dysphagia: pharyngeal retention is a predictive factor for aspiration. AJR Am J Roentgenol. 2002;178:393–8.
158. de Vos RAI, Jansen Steur ENH, Yilmazer D, Braak H, Braak E. Pathological and clinical features of Parkinson's disease with and without dementia. In: Perry RH, McKeith IG, Perry EK, editors. Dementia with Lewy bodies. New York: Cambridge University Press; 1996. p. 255–67.
159. Jellinger K. Pathology of Parkinson's disease. Changes other than the nigrostriatal pathway. Mol Chem Neuropathol. 1991;14:153–97.
160. Nilsson H, Ekberg O, Olsson R, Hindfelt B. Quantitative assessment of oral and pharyngeal function in Parkinson's disease. Dysphagia. 1996;11:144–50.
161. Logemann JA. Evaluation and treatment of swallowing disorders. 2nd ed. Austin: Pro-Ed; 1998.
162. Leopold NA, Kagel MC. Laryngeal deglutition movement in Parkinson's disease. Neurology. 1997;48:373–6.
163. Nagaya M, Kachi T, Yamada T, Igata I. Videofluorographic study of swallowing in Parkinson's disease. Dysphagia. 1998;13:95–100.
164. Woodford HJ, Walker RW. Emergency hospital admissions in idiopathic Parkinson's disease. Mov Disord. 2005;20:1104–8.
165. Hunter P, Crameri J, Austin S, Woodward M, Hughes A. Response of parkinsonian swallowing dysfunction to dopaminergic stimulation. J Neurol Neurosurg Psychiatry. 1997;63:579–83.
166. Fonda D, Schwartz J, Clinnick S. Parkinsonian medication one hour before meals improves symptomatic swallowing: a case study. Dysphagia. 1995;10:165–6.
167. Pitts T, Bolser D, Rosenbek J, Troche M, Sapienza C. Voluntary cough production and swallow dysfunction in Parkinson's disease. Dysphagia. 2008;23:221–340.
168. Garcia-Agundez A, Folkerts A-K, Konrad R, Caseman P, Göbel S, Kalbe E. PDDanceCity: an exergame for patients with idiopathic Parkinson's disease and cognitive impairment. In: Mensch und Computer 2017-Tagungsband; 2017.
169. Barry G, Galna B, Rochester L. The role of exergaming in Parkinson's disease rehabilitation: a systematic review of the evidence. J Neuroeng Rehabil. 2014;11(1):33.
170. Allen NE, et al. An interactive videogame for arm and hand exercise in people with Parkinson's disease: a randomized controlled trial. Parkinsonism Relat Disord. 2017;
171. Liao Y-Y, Yang Y-R, Cheng S-J, Wu Y-R, Fuh J-L, Wang R-Y. Virtual reality–based training to improve obstacle-crossing performance and dynamic balance in patients with Parkinson's disease. Neurorehabil Neural Repair. 2015;29(7):658–67.
172. Shih M-C, Wang R-Y, Cheng S-J, Yang Y-R. Effects of a balance-based exergaming intervention using the Kinect sensor on posture stability in individuals with Parkinson's disease: a single-blinded randomized controlled trial. J Neuroeng Rehabil. 2016;13(1):78.
173. Ribas CG, da Silva LA, Corrêa MR, Teive HG, Valderramas S. Effectiveness of exergaming in improving functional balance, fatigue and quality of life in Parkinson's disease: a pilot randomized controlled trial. Parkinsonism Relat Disord. 2017;
174. Zimmermann R, et al. Cognitive training in Parkinson disease Cognition-specific vs nonspecific computer training. Neurology. 2014;82(14):1219–26.
175. Song J, et al. Home-based step training using videogame technology in people with Parkinson's disease: a single-blinded randomised controlled trial. Clin Rehabil. 2017:0269215517721593.
176. Ferraz DD, Trippo KV, Duarte GP, Neto MG, Santos KOB, Oliveira FJ. The effects of functional training, bicycle exercise and exergaming on walking capacity of elderly with Parkinson's disease: a pilot randomized controlled single-blinded trial. Arch Phys Med Rehabil. 2018;
177. Tollár J, Nagy F, Hortobágyi T. Vastly different exercise programs similarly improve parkinsonian symptoms: a randomized clinical trial. Gerontology. 2018:1–8.

178. Pompeu JE, et al. Effect of Nintendo Wii™-based motor and cognitive training on activities of daily living in patients with Parkinson's disease: a randomised clinical trial. Physiotherapy. 2012;98(3):196–204.
179. Giuffrida JP, Riley DE, Maddux BN, Heldman DA. Clinically deployable Kinesia™ technology for automated tremor assessment. Mov Disord. 2009;24(5):723–30.
180. Craig P, Dieppe P, MacIntyre S, Michie S, Nazareth I, Petticrew M, Medical Research Council. Developing and evaluating complex interventions: new guidance. London: MRC; 2008.
181. Ramig LO, Countryman S, Thompson LL, Horii Y. Comparison of two forms of intensive speech treatment for Parkinson disease. J Speech Hear Res. 1995;38:1232–51.
182. Ramig LO. Intensive voice treatment (LSVT®) for patients with Parkinson's disease: a 2 year follow up. J Neurol Neurosurg Psychiatry. 2001;71:493–8. https://doi.org/10.1136/jnnp.71.4.493.
183. Berganzo K, Tijero B, González-Eizaguirre A, et al. Motor and non-motor symptoms of Parkinson's disease and their impact on quality of life and on different clinical subgroups. Síntomas no motores y motores en la enfermedad de Parkinson y su relación con la calidad de vida y los distintos subgrupos clínicos. Neurologia. 2016;31:585–91. https://doi.org/10.1016/j.nrl.2014.10.010.
184. Pereira APS, Marinho V, Gupta D, Magalhães F, Ayres C, Teixeira S. Music therapy and dance as gait rehabilitation in patients with Parkinson disease: a review of evidence. J Geriatr Psychiatr Neurol. 2019;32:49–56.
185. Fan B, Jabeen R, Bo B, et al. What and how can physical activity prevention function on Parkinson's disease? Oxidative Med Cell Longev. 2020;2020:4293071. https://doi.org/10.1155/2020/4293071.
186. Shanahan J, Morris ME, Bhriain ON, et al. Dance for people with Parkinson disease: what is the evidence telling us? Arch Phys Med Rehabil. 2015;96:141–53. https://doi.org/10.1016/j.apmr.2014.08.017.
187. Delabary MDS, Komeroski IG, Monteiro EP, Costa RR, Haas AN. Effects of dance practice on functional mobility, motor symptoms and quality of life in people with Parkinson's disease: a systematic review with meta-analysis. Aging Clin Exp Res. 2018;30:727–35.
188. Visser M, Leentjens AF, Marinus J, et al. Reliability and validity of the Beck depression inventory in patients with Parkinson's disease. Mov Disord. 2006;21:668–72. https://doi.org/10.1002/mds.20792.
189. Lee NY, Lee DK, Song HS. Effect of virtual reality dance exercise on the balance, activities of daily living, and depressive disorder status of Parkinson's disease patients. J Phys Ther Sci. 2015;27:145–7. https://doi.org/10.1589/jpts.27.145.
190. Michels K, Dubaz O, Hornthal E, Bega D. "Dance therapy" as a psychotherapeutic movement intervention in Parkinson's disease. Complement Ther Med. 2018;40:248–52.
191. Romenets SR, Anang J, Fereshtehnejad SM, Pelletier A, Postuma R. Tango for treatment of motor and non-motor manifestations in Parkinson's disease: a randomized control study. Complement Ther Med. 2015;23:175–84.
192. Seppi K, Ray Chaudhuri K, Coelho M, et al. Update on treatments for nonmotor symptoms of Parkinson's disease-an evidence-based medicine review. Mov Disord. 2019;34:180–98. https://doi.org/10.1002/mds.27602. (Erratum in: Mov Disord (2019) 34:765)
193. Rivera-Martinez S, Wells MR, Capobianco JD. A retrospective study of cranial strain patterns in patients with idiopathic Parkinson's disease. J Am Osteopath Assoc. 2002;102:417–22.
194. Boehm KM, Lawner BJ, McFee RB. Study raises important issues about the potential benefit of osteopathy in the cranial field to patients with Parkinson's disease. J Am Osteopath Assoc. 2003;103:354–5.
195. Dennison PE, Dennison G. Brain-gym—das Handbuch. Kirchzarten: VAK Verlag; 2013.
196. Sulzer P, Becker S, Maetzler W, Kalbe E, vanNueten L, Timmers M, Machetanz G, Streffer J, Salvadore G, Scholz E, Tkaczynska Z, Brockmann K, Berg D, Liepelt-Scarfone I. Validation of a novel Montreal Cognitive Assessment scoring algorithm in non-demented Parkinson's disease patients. J Neurol. 2018;265:1976–84.

197. Müller T, Schäfer S, Kuhn W, Przuntek H. Correlation between tapping and inserting of pegs in Parkinson's disease. Can J Neurol Sci. 2000;27:311–5.
198. Tait JL, Duckham RL, Milte CM, Main LC, Daly RM. Influence of sequential vs. simultaneous dual-task exercise training on cognitive function in older adults. Front Aging Neurosci. 2017; https://doi.org/10.3389/fnagi.2017.00368/full.
199. Feng Y-S, Yang S-D, Tan Z-X, Wang M-M, Xing Y, Dong F, et al. The benefits and mechanisms of exercise training for Parkinson's disease. Life Sci. 2020;245:117345.
200. Fritz NE, Cheek FM, Nichols-Larsen DS. Motor-cognitive dual-task training in persons with neurologic disorders: a systematic review. J Neurol Phys Ther. 2015;39(3):142–53.
201. Theill N, Schumacher V, Adelsberger R, Martin M, Jäncke L. Effects of simultaneously performed cognitive and physical training in older adults. BMC Neurosci. 2013; https://doi.org/10.1186/1471-2202-14-103.
202. Corregidor-Sánchez AI, Segura-Fragoso A, Rodríguez-Hernández M, Criado-Alvarez JJ, González-Gonzalez J, Polonio-López B. Can exergames contribute to improving walking capacity in older adults? A systematic review and meta-analysis. Maturitas. 2020;1(132):40–8.
203. da Silva FC, da IopR R, de Oliveira LC, Boll AM, de Alvarenga JGS, Gutierres Filho PJB, et al. Effects of physical exercise programs on cognitive function in Parkinson's disease patients: a systematic review of randomized controlled trials of the last 10 years. PLoS One. 2018; https://doi.org/10.1371/journal.pone.0193113.
204. Argent R, Daly A, Caulfield B. Patient involvement with home-based exercise programs: can connected health interventions influence adherence? JMIR Mhealth Uhealth. 2018;6(3):e47.
205. Mazza M, Kammler-Sücker K, Leménager T, Kiefer F, Lenz B. Virtual reality: a powerful technology to provide novel insight into treatment mechanisms of addiction. Transl Psychiatry 2021;11(1):1–11.
206. Schultheis MT, Rizzo AA. The application of virtual reality technology in rehabilitation. Rehabil Psychol. 2001;46(3):296.
207. Raffegeau TE, Krehbiel LM, Kang N, Thijs FJ, Altmann LJ, Cauraugh JH, Hass CJ. A meta-analysis: Parkinson's disease and dual-task walking. Parkinsonism Relat Disord. 2019;62:28–35.
208. Heinzel S, Maechtel M, Hasmann SE, Hobert MA, Heger T, Berg D, Maetzler W. Motor dual-tasking deficits predict falls in Parkinson's disease: a prospective study. Parkinsonism Relat Disord. 2016;26:73–7.
209. Johansson H, Ekman U, Rennie L, Peterson DS, Leavy B, Franzén E. Dual-task effects during a motor-cognitive task in Parkinson's disease: patterns of prioritization and the influence of cognitive status. Neurorehabil Neural Repair. 2021;35(4):356–66.
210. Strouwen C, Molenaar EA, Münks L, Keus SH, Zijlmans JC, Vandenberghe W, Bloem BR, Nieuwboer A. Training dual tasks together or apart in Parkinson's disease: results from the DUALITY trial. Mov Disord. 2017;32(8):1201–10.
211. Valenzuela CSM, Moscardó LD, López-Pascual J, Serra-Añó P, Tomás JM. Effects of dual-task group training on gait, cognitive executive function, and quality of life in people with Parkinson disease: results of randomized controlled DUALGAIT trial. Arch Phys Med Rehabil. 2020;101(11):1849–56.
212. Wu J, Zhang H, Chen Z, Fu R, Yang H, Zeng H, Ren Z. Benefits of virtual reality balance training for patients with Parkinson disease: systematic review, meta-analysis, and meta-regression of a randomized controlled trial. JMIR Serious Games. 2022;10(1):e30882.
213. Dockx K, Bekkers EM, Van den Bergh V, Ginis P, Rochester L, Hausdorff JM, Mirelman A, Nieuwboer A. Virtual reality for rehabilitation in Parkinson's disease. Cochrane Database Syst Rev. 2016;12(12):CD010760.
214. Jung SH, Hasegawa N, Mancini M, King LA, Carlson-Kuhta P, Smulders K, Peterson DS, Barlow N, Harker G, Morris R. Effects of the agility boot camp with cognitive challenge (ABC-C) exercise program for Parkinson's disease. NPJ Parkinson's Dis. 2020;6(1):1–8.

215. King L, Salarian A, Mancini M, Priest K, Nutt J, Serdar A, Wilhelm J, Schlimgen J, Smith M, Horak F. Exploring outcome measures for exercise intervention in people with Parkinson's disease. Parkinson's Dis. 2013;(1):572134.
216. Triegaardt J, Han TS, Sada C, Sharma S, Sharma P. The role of virtual reality on outcomes in rehabilitation of Parkinson's disease: meta-analysis and systematic review in 1031 participants. Neurol Sci. 2020;41(3):529–36.
217. Chen Y, Gao Q, He C-Q, Bian R. Effect of virtual reality on balance in individuals with Parkinson disease: a systematic review and meta-analysis of randomized controlled trials. Phys Ther. 2020;100(6):933–45.
218. Silsupadol P, Lugade V, Shumway-Cook A, van Donkelaar P, Chou L-S, Mayr U, Woollacott MH. Training-related changes in dual-task walking performance of elderly persons with balance impairment: a double-blind, randomized controlled trial. Gait Posture. 2009;29(4):634–9.
219. Pedroso RV, Coelho FG, Santos-Galduróz RF, Costa JL, Gobbi S, Stella F. Balance, executive functions and falls in elderly with Alzheimer's disease (AD): a longitudinal study. Arch Gerontol Geriatr. 2012;54(2):348–51.
220. Hiyamizu M, Morioka S, Shomoto K, Shimada T. Effects of dual task balance training on dual task performance in elderly people: a randomized controlled trial. Clin Rehabil. 2012;26:58–67.
221. Fernandes Â, Rocha N, Santos R, Tavares JMR. Effects of dual-task training on balance and executive functions in Parkinson's disease: a pilot study. Somatosens Mot Res. 2015;32(2):122–7.
222. Li Z, Chen J, Cheng J, Huang S, Hu Y, Wu Y, et al. Acupuncture Modulates the cerebello-thalamo-cortical circuit and cognitive brain regions in patients of Parkinson's disease with tremor. Front Aging Neurosci. 2018;10:206.
223. Toosizadeh N, Lei H, Schwenk M, Sherman SJ, Sternberg E, Mohler J, et al. Does integrative medicine enhance balance in aging adults? Proof of concept for the benefit of electroacupuncture therapy in Parkinson's disease. Gerontology. 2015;61(1):3–14.
224. Aroxa FH, Gondim IT, Santos EL, Coriolano MD, Asano AG, Asano NM. Acupuncture as adjuvant therapy for sleep disorders in Parkinson's disease. J Acupunct Meridian Stud. 2017;10(1):33–8.
225. Vergara-Diaz G, Osypiuk K, Hausdorff JM, Bonato P, Gow BJ, Miranda JG, et al. Tai Chi for reducing dual-task gait variability, a potential mediator of fall risk in Parkinson's disease: a pilot randomized controlled trial. Glob Adv Health Med. 2018;7:2164956118775385.
226. Zhang TY, Hu Y, Nie ZY, Jin RX, Chen F, Guan Q, et al. Effects of Tai Chi and Multimodal exercise training on movement and balance function in mild to moderate idiopathic Parkinson disease. Am J Phys Med Rehabil. 2015;94(10 Suppl. 1):921–9.
227. Kurt EE, Buyukturan B, Buyukturan O, Erdem HR, Tuncay F. Effects of Ai Chi on balance, quality of life, functional mobility, and motor impairment in patients with Parkinson's disease. Disabil Rehabil. 2018;40(7):791–7.
228. Schmitz-Hubsch T, Pyfer D, Kielwein K, Fimmers R, Klockgether T, Wullner U. Qigong exercise for the symptoms of Parkinson's disease: a randomized, controlled pilot study. Mov Disord. 2006;21(4):543–8.
229. Lee HJ, Kim SY, Chae Y, Kim MY, Yin C, Jung WS, et al. Turo (Qi Dance) Program for Parkinson's disease patients: randomized, assessor blind, waiting-list control, partial cross-over study. Explore (NY). 2018;14(3):216–23.
230. Liu XL, Chen S, Wang Y. Effects of health Qigong exercises on relieving symptoms of Parkinson's disease. Evid Based Complement Alternat Med. 2016;2016:5935782.
231. Xiao CM, Zhuang YC. Effect of health Baduanjin Qigong for mild to moderate Parkinson's disease. Geriatr Gerontol Int. 2016;16(8):911–9.
232. Xiao C, Zhuang Y, Kang Y. Effect of health Qigong Baduanjin on fall prevention in individuals with Parkinson's disease. J Am Geriatr Soc. 2016;64(11):e227–e8.

233. Ni M, Signorile JF, Mooney K, Balachandran A, Potiaumpai M, Luca C, et al. Comparative effect of power training and high-speed yoga on motor function in older patients with Parkinson disease. Arch Phys Med Rehabil. 2016;97(3):345–54 e15.
234. Bega D, Stein J. Yoga versus resistance training in mild to moderate severity Parkinson's disease: a 12-week pilot study. J Yoga Phys Ther. 2016;06(01)
235. Kwok JYY, Kwan JCY, Auyeung M, Mok VCT, Lau CKY, Choi KC, et al. Effects of mindfulness yoga vs stretching and resistance training exercises on anxiety and depression for people with Parkinson disease: a randomized clinical trial. JAMA Neurol. 2019;76(7):755–63.
236. Venderova K, Ruzicka E, Vorisek V, Visnovsky P. Survey on cannabis use in Parkinson's disease: subjective improvement of motor symptoms. Mov Disord. 2004;19(9):1102–6.
237. Balash Y, Bar-Lev Schleider L, Korczyn AD, Shabtai H, Knaani J, Rosenberg A, et al. Medical cannabis in Parkinson disease: real-life patients' experience. Clin Neuropharmacol. 2017;40(6):268–72.
238. Shohet A, Khlebtovsky A, Roizen N, Roditi Y, Djaldetti R. Effect of medical cannabis on thermal quantitative measurements of pain in patients with Parkinson's disease. Eur J Pain. 2017;21(3):486–93.
239. Leehey MA, Liu Y, Hart F, Epstein C, Cook M, Sillau S, et al. Safety and tolerability of cannabidiol in Parkinson disease: an open label, dose-escalation study. Cannabis Cannabinoid Res. 2020;
240. Hinnell C, Hurt CS, Landau S, Brown RG, Samuel M, Group P-PS. Nonmotor versus motor symptoms: how much do they matter to health status in Parkinson's disease? Mov Disord. 2012;27(2):236–41.
241. Santos-Garcia D, de la Fuente-Fernandez R. Impact of non-motor symptoms on health-related and perceived quality of life in Parkinson's disease. J Neurol Sci. 2013;332(1–2):136–40.
242. Wang Y, Xie CL, Wang WW, Lu L, Fu DL, Wang XT, et al. Epidemiology of complementary and alternative medicine use in patients with Parkinson's disease. J Clin Neurosci. 2013;20(8):1062–7.
243. Suchowersky O, Gronseth G, Perlmutter J, Reich S, Zesiewicz T, Weiner WJ. Practice parameter: neuroprotective strategies and alternative therapies for Parkinson disease (an evidence-based review). Neurology. 2006;66:976–82.
244. Li F, Harmer P. Economic evaluation of a Tai Ji Quan intervention to reduce falls in people with Parkinson disease, Oregon, 2008–2011. Prev Chronic Dis. 2015;12:E120.
245. Jiang T, Li G, Xu J, Gao S, Chen X. The challenge of the pathogenesis of Parkinson's disease: Is autoimmunity the culprit? Front Immunol. 2018;9:2047.
246. Hatano T, Saiki S, Okuzumi A, Mohney RP, Hattori N. Identification of novel biomarkers for Parkinson's disease by metabolomic technologies. J Neurol Neurosurg Psychiatry. 2016;87:295–301.
247. Pedersen M, Zalesky A, Omidvarnia A, Jackson GD. Multilayer network switching rate predicts brain performance. Proc Natl Acad Sci U S A. 2018;115:13376–81.
248. Su J, Huang P, Qin M, Lu Q, Sang X, Cai Y, et al. Reduction of HIP2 expression causes motor function impairment and increased vulnerability to dopaminergic degeneration in Parkinson's disease models. Cell Death Dis. 2018;9:1020.
249. Peterka M, Odorfer T, Schwab M, Volkmann J, Zeller D. Daniel LSVT-BIG therapy in Parkinson's disease: physiological evidence for proprioceptive recalibration. BMC Neurol. 2020; https://doi.org/10.1186/s12883-020-01858-2.
250. Pu L, Qureshi NK, Ly J, Zhang B, Cong F, Tang WC, Liang Z. Therapeutic benefits of music-based synchronous finger tapping in Parkinson's disease—an fNIRS study protocol for randomized controlled trial in Dalian, China. Trials. 2020; https://doi.org/10.1186/s13063-020-04770-9.
251. Harrison EC, Horin AP, Earhart GM. Internal cueing improves gait more than external cueing in healthy adults and people with Parkinson disease. Sci Rep. 2018; https://doi.org/10.1038/s41598-018-33942-6.

252. Zhen K, Zhang S, Tao X, Li G, Lv Y, Yu L. A systematic review and meta-analysis on effects of aerobic exercise in people with Parkinson's disease. NPJ Parkinson's Dis. 2022; https://doi.org/10.1038/s41531-022-00418-4.
253. Barnish MS, Barran SM. A systematic review of active group-based dance, singing, music therapy and theatrical interventions for quality of life, functional communication, speech, motor function and cognitive status in people with Parkinson's disease. BMC Neurol. 2020; https://doi.org/10.1186/s12883-020-01938-3.
254. Mandelbaum R, Lo AC. Examining dance as an intervention in Parkinson's disease: a systematic review. Am J Dance Ther. 2014; https://doi.org/10.1007/s10465-014-9181-6.
255. Calabrò RS, Naro A, Filoni S, Pullia M, Billeri L, Tomasello P, Portaro S, Di Lorenzo G, Tomaino C, Bramanti P. Placido walking to your right music: a randomized controlled trial on the novel use of treadmill plus music in Parkinson's disease. J Neuroeng Rehabil. 2019;16:1–4. https://doi.org/10.1186/s12984-019-0533-9.
256. Ayán Pérez C, Cancela JM. Effectiveness of water-based exercise in people living with Parkinson's disease: a systematic review. Eur Rev Aging Phys Act. 2013; https://doi.org/10.1007/s11556-013-0135-7.
257. Gilat M, Ginis P, Zoetewei D, De Vleeschhauwer J, Hulzinga F, D'Cruz N, Nieuwboer A. A systematic review on exercise and training-based interventions for freezing of gait in Parkinson's disease. NPJ Parkinson's Dis. 2021; https://doi.org/10.1038/s41531-021-00224-4.
258. Law NY, Li JX, Zhu Q, Nantel J. Effects of a biomechanical-based Tai Chi program on gait and posture in people with Parkinson's disease: study protocol for a randomized controlled trial. Trials. 2023; https://doi.org/10.1186/s13063-023-07146-x.
259. Yang Y, Hao YL, Tian WJ, Gong L, Zhang K, Shi QG, Sun DF, Li CL, Zhao ZL. The effectiveness of Tai Chi for patients with Parkinson's disease: study protocol for a randomized controlled trial. Trials. 2015; https://doi.org/10.1186/s13063-015-0639-8.
260. Creath RA, Prettyman M, Shulman L, Hilliard M, Martinez K, CD MK, Mille ML, Simuni T, Zhang J, Rogers MW, Mark W. Self-triggered assistive stimulus training improves step initiation in persons with Parkinson's disease. J Neuroeng Rehabil. 2013; https://doi.org/10.1186/1743-0003-10-11.
261. Sturkenboom IH, Graff MJ, Borm GF, Adang EM, Nijhuis-van der Sanden MW, Bloem BR, Munneke M. Effectiveness of occupational therapy in Parkinson's disease: study protocol for a randomized controlled trial. Trials. 2013; https://doi.org/10.1186/1745-6215-14-34.
262. Langer A, Hasenauer S, Gassner L, Pokan R, Dabnichki P, Wizany L, Gruber J, Roth D, Zimmel S, Treven M, Schmoeger M. A randomised controlled trial on effectiveness and feasibility of sport climbing in Parkinson's disease. NPJ Parkinson's Dis. 2021; https://doi.org/10.1038/s41531-021-00193-8.
263. Ghai S, Ghai I, Schmitz G, Effenberg AO. Effect of rhythmic auditory cueing on parkinsonian gait: a systematic review and meta-analysis. Sci Rep. 2018; https://doi.org/10.1038/s41598-017-16232-5.
264. Ledger S, Galvin R, Lynch D, Stokes EK. A randomised controlled trial evaluating the effect of an individual auditory cueing device on freezing and gait speed in people with Parkinson's disease. BMC Neurol. 2008; https://doi.org/10.1186/1471-2377-8-46.
265. Regan J, Walshe M, Tobin WO. Immediate effects of thermal–tactile stimulation on timing of swallow in idiopathic Parkinson's disease. Dysphagia. 2009; https://doi.org/10.1007/s00455-009-9244-x.
266. Garcia-Agundez A, Folkerts AK, Konrad R, Caserman P, Tregel T, Goosses M, Göbel S, Kalbe E. Recent advances in rehabilitation for Parkinson's Disease with exergames: a systematic review. J Neuroeng Rehabil. 2019; https://doi.org/10.1186/s12984-019-0492-1.
267. Sackley CM, Smith CH, Rick C, Brady MC, Ives N, Patel R, Roberts H, Dowling F, Jowett S, Wheatley K, Patel S. Lee Silverman voice treatment versus standard NHS speech and language therapy versus control in Parkinson's disease (PD COMM pilot): study protocol for a randomized controlled trial. Trials. 2014; https://doi.org/10.1186/1745-6215-15-213.

268. Wang LL, Sun CJ, Wang Y, Zhan TT, Yuan J, Niu CY, Yang J, Huang S, Cheng L. Effects of dance therapy on non-motor symptoms in patients with Parkinson's disease: a systematic review and meta-analysis. Aging Clin Exp Res. 2022; https://doi.org/10.1007/s40520-021-02030-7.
269. Kuhn W, Neufeld T, Müller T. Kinesiology training in patients with Parkinson's disease: results of a pilot study. J Neural Transm. 2020; https://doi.org/10.1007/s00702-019-02123-8.
270. Jäggi S, Wachter A, Adcock M, de Bruin ED, Möller JC, Marks D, Schweinfurther R, Giannouli E. Feasibility and effects of cognitive–motor exergames on fall risk factors in typical and atypical Parkinson's inpatients: a randomized controlled pilot study. Eur J Med Res. 2023; https://doi.org/10.1186/s40001-022-00963-x.
271. Yun SJ, Hyun SE, Oh BM, Seo HG. Fully immersive virtual reality exergames with dual-task components for patients with Parkinson's disease: a feasibility study. J Neuroeng Rehabil. 2023; https://doi.org/10.1186/s12984-023-01215-7.
272. Deuel Lisa M, Seeberger Lauren C. Complementary therapies in Parkinson disease: a review of acupuncture, Tai Chi, Qi Gong, Yoga, and cannabis. Neurotherapeutics. 2020; https://doi.org/10.1007/s13311-020-00900-y.
273. Li G, Huang P, Cui SS, Tan YY, He YC, Shen X, Jiang QY, Huang P, He GY, Li BY, Li YX. Mechanisms of motor symptom improvement by long-term Tai Chi training in Parkinson's disease patients. Translational. Neurodegeneration. 2022; https://doi.org/10.1186/s40035-022-00280-7.

Index

C. A. A. Mejía, *Therapeutic Exercise for Parkinson's Disease and Related Disorders*, https://doi.org/10.1007/978-3-031-62119-2

GPSR Compliance

The European Union's (EU) General Product Safety Regulation (GPSR) is a set of rules that requires consumer products to be safe and our obligations to ensure this.

If you have any concerns about our products, you can contact us on ProductSafety@springernature.com

In case Publisher is established outside the EU, the EU authorized representative is:

Springer Nature Customer Service Center GmbH
Europaplatz 3
69115 Heidelberg, Germany

Batch number: 10732090

Printed by Printforce, the Netherlands